Positive Psychiatry

A Clinical Handbook

Positive Psychiatry

A Clinical Handbook

Edited by

Dilip V. Jeste, M.D.

Senior Associate Dean for Healthy Aging and Senior Care,
Estelle and Edgar Levi Chair in Aging, Director, Sam and
Rose Stein Institute for Research on Aging, and
Distinguished Professor of Psychiatry and Neurosciences,
University of California, San Diego, La Jolla, California

Barton W. Palmer, Ph.D.

Professor, Department of Psychiatry,
University of California, San Diego, La Jolla, California

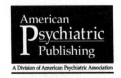

American Psychiatric Publishing
A Division of American Psychiatric Association

Washington, DC
London, England

Copyright © 2015 American Psychiatric Association
ALL RIGHTS RESERVED

Manufactured in the United States of America on acid-free paper
19   18   17   16   15   5   4   3   2   1
First Edition

Typeset in Minion and Gill Sans

American Psychiatric Publishing
A Division of American Psychiatric Association
1000 Wilson Boulevard
Arlington, VA 22209-3901
www.appi.org

Library of Congress Cataloging-in-Publication Data
Positive psychiatry : a clinical handbook / edited by Dilip V. Jeste and Barton W. Palmer. — First edition.
    p. ; cm.
  Includes bibliographical references and index.
  ISBN 978-1-58562-495-9 (pbk. : alk. paper)
  I. Jeste, Dilip V., editor. II. Palmer, Barton W. (Barton Wayne), editor.
III. American Psychiatric Publishing, publisher.
  [DNLM: 1. Psychotherapy—methods. 2. Happiness. 3. Personal Satisfaction. 4. Psychiatry—methods. 5. Resilience, Psychological. WM 420]
  RC480.5
  616.89'14—dc23

2015002631

British Library Cataloguing in Publication Data
A CIP record is available from the British Library.

We dedicate this book to our families for tolerating the long hours we worked on this book and for personifying resilience and wisdom.

—Dilip and Barton

Contents

Part I

Positive Psychosocial Factors

Part II
Positive Outcomes

Part III
Interventions in Positive Psychiatry

Part IV

Special Topics in Positive Psychiatry

Contributors

Per Bech, M.D., D.M.Sc.
Professor of Psychiatry, Psychiatric Research Unit, Mental Health Centre North Zealand, University of Copenhagen, Copenhagen, Denmark

Carl C. Bell, M.D., DLFAPA, FACPsych
Staff Psychiatrist, Jackson Park Hospital Family Medicine Clinic; Professor, Department of Psychiatry and School of Public Health, University of Illinois at Chicago, Chicago, Illinois

Dan G. Blazer, M.D., M.P.H., Ph.D.
J.P. Gibbons Professor of Psychiatry and Behavioral Sciences Emeritus, Duke University Medical Center, Durham, North Carolina

Samantha Boardman, M.D.
Clinical Instructor in Psychiatry and Public Health and Assistant Attending Psychiatrist, Weill Cornell Medical College, New York, New York

Anne M. Day, Ph.D.
Postdoctoral Research Fellow, Center for Alcohol and Addiction Studies, Brown University, Providence, Rhode Island

Colin A. Depp, Ph.D.
Associate Professor, Department of Psychiatry, University of California, San Diego, La Jolla, California

P. Murali Doraiswamy, M.D.
Professor of Psychiatry and Behavioral Sciences, Duke University School of Medicine, Durham, North Carolina

Lisa T. Eyler, Ph.D.
Associate Professor, Department of Psychiatry, University of California, San Diego, La Jolla, California; Clinical Research Psychologist, Mental Illness Research, Education and Clinical Center, VA San Diego, San Diego, California

Maja K. Gawronska, M.A.
Program Manager, Department of Psychiatry, University of California, San Diego, La Jolla, California

Alexandrea L. Harmell, M.S.
Doctoral Student, San Diego State University/University of California, San Diego Joint Doctoral Program in Clinical Psychology, La Jolla, California

Leslie R.M. Hausmann, Ph.D.
Core Faculty, Center for Health Equity Research and Promotion (CHERP), VA Pittsburgh Healthcare System; Assistant Professor of Medicine, School of Medicine, University of Pittsburgh, Pittsburgh, Pennsylvania

Dilip V. Jeste, M.D.
Senior Associate Dean for Healthy Aging and Senior Care, Estelle and Edgar Levi Chair in Aging, Director, Sam and Rose Stein Institute for Research on Aging, and Distinguished Professor of Psychiatry and Neurosciences, University of California, San Diego, La Jolla, California

Christopher W. Kahler, Ph.D.
Professor and Chair, Department of Behavioral and Social Sciences, Brown University, Providence, Rhode Island

Robert M. Kaplan, Ph.D.
Chief Science Officer, Agency for Healthcare Research and Quality, U.S. Department of Health and Human Services, Rockville, Maryland

Todd B. Kashdan, Ph.D.
Professor, Department of Psychology, and Senior Scientist, Center for Consciousness and Transformation, George Mason University, Fairfax, Virginia

Warren A. Kinghorn, M.D., Th.D.
Assistant Professor of Psychiatry and Pastoral and Moral Theology, Duke University Medical Center and Duke Divinity School, Durham, North Carolina

Evan M. Kleiman, Ph.D.
College Fellow, Department of Psychology, Harvard University, Cambridge, Massachusetts

Helen Lavretsky, M.D., M.S.
Professor of Psychiatry, University of California, Los Angeles; Director, Late-Life Mood, Stress, and Wellness Research Program, Semel Institute for Neuroscience and Human Behavior, Geffen School of Medicine at University of California, Los Angeles, California

Julie A. Lord, M.D.
Private Practice of Psychiatry

María J. Marquine, Ph.D.
Postdoctoral Fellow, University of California, San Diego, La Jolla, California

A'verria Sirkin Martin, Ph.D.
Postdoctoral Research Fellow, Department of Psychiatry, University of California, San Diego, La Jolla, California

Brent T. Mausbach, Ph.D.
Associate Professor in Residence, Department of Psychiatry, University of California, San Diego, La Jolla, California

Piper S. Meyer, Ph.D.
Director, Minnesota Center for Mental Health, University of Minnesota, St. Paul, Minnesota

Paul J. Mills, Ph.D.
Professor-in-Residence, Department of Psychiatry, University of California, San Diego, La Jolla, California

Raeanne C. Moore, Ph.D.
Postdoctoral Fellow, Department of Psychiatry, University of California, San Diego, La Jolla, California

Ruth M. O'Hara, Ph.D.
Associate Professor (Research) of Psychiatry and Behavioral Sciences, Stanford University School of Medicine, Stanford, California

Barton W. Palmer, Ph.D.
Professor, Department of Psychiatry, University of California, San Diego, La Jolla, California

Acacia C. Parks, Ph.D.
Assistant Professor of Psychology, Hiram College, Hiram, Ohio; Associate Editor, *Journal of Positive Psychology*

David C. Rettew, M.D.
Associate Professor of Psychiatry and Pediatrics, Training Director, Child and Adolescent Psychiatry Fellowship, and Director, Pediatric Psychiatry Clinic, University of Vermont College of Medicine, Burlington, Vermont

Christine Rufener, Ph.D.
Assistant Professor, Department of Psychiatry, University of California, San Diego; Staff Psychologist, VA San Diego Healthcare System, San Diego, California

Elyn R. Saks, J.D., Ph.D.
Orrin B. Evans Professor of Law, Psychology, and Psychiatry and the Behavioral Sciences, University of Southern California, Los Angeles, California

Martin E. P. Seligman, Ph.D.
Zellerbach Family Professor of Psychology and Director of the Positive Psychology Center, University of Pennsylvania, Philadelphia, Pennsylvania

Daniel D. Sewell, M.D.
Clinical Professor of Psychiatry, University of California, San Diego, La Jolla, California

Ajai R. Singh, M.D.
Editor, *Mens Sana Monographs*, Mumbai, India

Wendy B. Smith, M.A., Ph.D., BCB
Senior Scientific Advisor for Research Development and Outreach, Office of Behavioral and Social Sciences Research, Office of the Director, National Institutes of Health, Bethesda, Maryland

Nichea S. Spillane, Ph.D.
Assistant Professor (Research), Center for Alcohol and Addiction Studies, Brown University, Providence, Rhode Island

Richard F. Summers, M.D.
Clinical Professor of Psychiatry and Co-Director of Residency Training, Department of Psychiatry, Perelman School of Medicine, University of Pennsylvania, Philadelphia, Pennsylvania

George E. Vaillant, M.D.
Professor, Department of Psychiatry, Massachusetts General Hospital, Harvard Medical School, Boston, Massachusetts

Taya C. Varteresian, D.O., M.S.
Psychiatrist, LA County Department of Mental Health; Health Science Assistant Clinical Professor, University of California, Irvine, Irvine, California

Katherine Wachmann, Ph.D.
Postdoctoral Fellow, Ludwig Boltzmann Gesellschaft, Vienna, Austria

Zvinka Z. Zlatar, Ph.D.
Postdoctoral Fellow, University of California, San Diego, La Jolla, California

Disclosure of Competing Interests

The following contributors to this book have indicated a financial interest in or other affiliation with a commercial supporter, a manufacturer of a commercial product, a provider of a commercial service, a nongovernmental organization, and /or a government agency, as listed below:

P. Murali Doraiswamy, M.D.—*Grants* (to institution): Alzheimer Drug Discovery Foundation, Avid/Lilly, Department of Defense, Elan, Forum Pharma, Janssen, National Institutes of Health, Neuronetrix, Northern California Research Institute, Novartis, Pfizer/Medivation, University of California, San Diego; *Consultancy:* Abbvie, Accera, Anthrotonix, AstraZeneca, Avid/Lilly, Baxter, Cognoptix, Danone, EnVivo, Genomind, Lundbeck/Takeda, Muses Lab, Neurocog Trials, Piramal, Sonexa, Targacept, TauRx, University of Copenhagen; *Lectures, including service on speakers' bureaus:* Alzheimer's Association, Lundbeck; *Royalties:* St. Martin's Press; *Development of educational presentations:* Postgraduate Press; *Stock/stock options:* Clarimedix, Adverse Events Inc., Maxwell Health, Muses Lab; *Travel/accommodations/meeting expenses unrelated to activities listed above:* Biogen, X-prize.

Helen Lavretsky, M.D., M.S.—*Research grants:* Alzheimer's Research and Prevention Foundation, Forest Research Institute, National Institute of Mental Health/National Institutes of Health.

David C. Rettew, M.D.—*Royalties: Psychology Today,* WW Norton.

Daniel D. Sewell, M.D.—The author is a paid consultant for ActivCore Inc., a corporation that provides residential care to individuals living with dementia.

Richard F. Summers, M.D.—*Royalties:* Guilford Press.

The following contributors to this book have indicated no competing interests to disclose during the year preceding manuscript submission:

Per Bech, M.D., D.M.Sc.
Dan G. Blazer, M.D., M.P.H., Ph.D.
Samantha Boardman, M.D.
Anne M. Day, Ph.D.
Colin A. Depp, Ph.D.
Lisa T. Eyler, Ph.D.
Maja K. Gawronska, M.A.
Alexandrea L. Harmell, M.S.
Leslie R. M. Hausmann, Ph.D.
Dilip V. Jeste, M.D.
Christopher W. Kahler, Ph.D.
Robert M. Kaplan, Ph.D.
Todd B. Kashdan, Ph.D.
Warren A. Kinghorn, M.D., Th.D.
Evan M. Kleiman, Ph.D.
María J. Marquine, Ph.D.
A'verria Sirkin Martin, Ph.D.
Brent T. Mausbach, Ph.D.
Piper S. Meyer, Ph.D.
Paul J. Mills, Ph.D.
Raeanne C. Moore, Ph.D.
Ruth M. O'Hara, Ph.D.
Barton W. Palmer, Ph.D.
Acacia C. Parks, Ph.D.
Christine Rufener, Ph.D.
Elyn R. Saks, J.D., Ph.D.
Martin E. P. Seligman, Ph.D.
Ajai R. Singh, M.D.
Wendy B. Smith, M.A., Ph.D., BCB
Nichea S. Spillane, Ph.D.
George E. Vaillant, M.D.
Katherine Wachmann, Ph.D.
Zvinka Z. Zlatar, Ph.D.

Foreword

MARTIN E. P. SELIGMAN, PH.D.

"I just want to be happy, doctor" were the opening words I heard not infrequently on first meeting a patient. "You mean you don't want to be depressed," I would reply. This was a case of "Doctor, I hope you can cure what I have." "Mister, I hope you have what I can cure."

My background was in treating depression. I had taken 2 years of psychiatric residency at the Hospital of the University of Pennsylvania under Albert Stunkard and Aaron Beck in 1970 and 1971. I followed the considerable progress that was being made in the diagnosis and treatment of depression, so when a new patient asked me about being "happy," I did know something about how to treat depression, but I knew nothing about how to help make people happy. In fact, I thought that happiness and depression were exact opposites. I believed that if I got rid of my patient's dysphorias and minimized his or her sadness, anxiety, and anger, then I would have a happy patient. This is what Freud and Schopenhauer told us. In their views, the best that we can ever hope for in life, the best that we can ever hope for in therapy, is to hold suffering and misery as close to zero as possible. I have come to believe this view is empirically false, morally insidious, and a therapeutic dead end.

When you lie in bed at night, you are, for the most part, not thinking about how to go from –8 to –2 in your life, you are thinking about how to go from +3 to +9. The same is true of most of our patients. However, therapy is almost entirely about minimizing misery and suffering and not about building well-being. We somehow make the glib assumption that if misery is minimized, our patients will know how to find their way to well-being. However, research in positive psychology over the last 15 years has shown that the skills for having more positive emotions, for having more engagement at work and with the people we love, for having better relationships, for finding meaning and purpose in our existence, and for achievement and mastery are entirely different from the skills for fighting sadness, anxiety, and anger. These skills do not magically appear simply because misery abates; they must be built (Seligman 2011).

These thoughts were on my mind when I found myself elected president of the American Psychological Association in 1998. My main presidential initiative was the founding of positive psychology (Seligman and Csikszentmihalyi 2000). Clinical psychology, like psychiatry, has traditionally been about the relief of suffering. One gaping hole in psychological knowledge resulted: psychology knew little about what made life worth living or about what nonsuffering people pursue when they are not oppressed. I suggested that psychology pursue the PERMA model: positive emotion, engagement, good relationships, meaning, and accomplishment. These are the pillars of positive psychology.

Fast-forward to 2015. Positive psychology, to my surprise, has now become popular. Very substantial grant funding has come from private foundations, such as the John Templeton, Bill and Melinda Gates, and Robert Wood Johnson foundations, but not from the U.S. government, whose focus is still mental illness, not mental health. From 1998 to 2015, several milestones occurred. Positive psychology became the most popular undergraduate course at Harvard University. The field of positive education sprang up, with positive psychology pervading the curriculum in hundreds of schools around the world (Seligman et al. 2009). The field of positive health arose, with the Robert Wood Johnson Foundation supporting research on protective factors rather than risk factors for cardiovascular disease (University of Pennsylvania 2014). The field of positive neuroscience developed, with funding available for researchers to look at the neuroscience not of disease but of well-being (University of Pennsylvania 2014). The U.S. States Army decided to teach positive psychology to the entire corps in an attempt to create an army that is psychologically fit as well as physically fit (Seligman and Matthews 2011).

One domain lagged behind: the clinic. Clinical psychologists did not leap forward to embrace the notion that therapy should, in addition to relieving misery, build PERMA. As a result, Tayyab Rashid and I did a considerable amount of pilot work on positive psychotherapy. We created a 14-session manual in which positive interventions were delivered systematically (Rashid and Seligman 2015). We found that positive psychotherapy did at least as well as drugs and cognitive therapy for severe depression, possibly better. Also, Rick Summers, George Vaillant, and I gave a joint seminar on positive psychoanalysis. The main takeaway (at least for me) was about termination: it would be premature to terminate treatment when the patient was relatively "conflict free"; the skills of PERMA should be taught to the patient before termination.

My hope is that this volume will be the start of the assimilation of positive psychology into the mainstream of the science and practice of psychiatry. From my point of view, positive interventions should be a supplement—not a replacement—to all therapy. The scientific understanding of well-being should supplement, not replace, the scientific understanding of suffering. My highest hope is that the mission of psychiatry will broaden from just the alleviation of misery to the building of well-being. Well-being is the birthright of every human being.

References

Rashid T, Seligman MEP: Positive Psychotherapy. New York, Oxford University Press, 2015

Seligman MEP: Flourish: A Visionary New Understanding of Happiness and Well-Being. New York, Free Press, 2011

Seligman ME, Csikszentmihalyi M: Positive psychology: an introduction. Am Psychol 55(1):5–14, 2000 11392865

Seligman MEP, Matthews MD (eds): Comprehensive soldier fitness. Am Psychol 66(1):1–86, 2011 21219041

Seligman MEP, Gillham J, Reivich K, et al: Positive education: positive psychology and positive interventions. Oxf Rev Educ 35:293–311, 2009

University of Pennsylvania: Authentic happiness. 2014. Available at: https://www.authentichappiness.sas.upenn.edu/learn/positivehealth. Accessed August 20, 2014.

Acknowledgments

We thank a number of people for their invaluable help in making this book a reality. We are most grateful for the outstanding administrative assistance of Sandra Dorsey. We enjoyed a wonderful partnership with the publisher, American Psychiatric Publishing, specifically Rebecca Rinehart, Robert Hales, M.D., John McDuffie, and Bessie Jones. We are indebted to each and every author and coauthor for her or his superb contribution. Last but not least, this book would not have been possible if not for the inspiration provided by our patients and their family members.

Introduction: What Is Positive Psychiatry?

DILIP V. JESTE, M.D.

BARTON W. PALMER, PH.D.

> Health is a state of complete physical, mental and
> social well-being and not merely the absence of
> disease or infirmity.
>
> World Health Organization (1946)

Efforts to reduce the suffering caused by mental and physical illnesses are noble and exceptionally important endeavors. However, although those goals are an essential component of psychiatric practice, education, and research, they are not sufficient. The job of mental health professionals is incomplete if they are focused exclusively on controlling the symptoms of illness. Mental health is not defined by the mere reduction or even elimination of mental illnesses. In accord with the above-cited World Health Organization definition

This work was supported, in part, by National Institutes of Health grants R01 MH099987, R01 MH094151, and T32 MH019934 and by the University of California, San Diego Center for Healthy Aging and Sam and Rose Stein Institute for Research on Aging.

of health, the goals of psychiatry should include not only addressing mental illness but also actively promoting well-being in people with or at high risk for mental or physical illnesses.

As detailed throughout this volume, a growing body of research strongly suggests that positive psychosocial factors (PPSFs) such as resilience, optimism, and social engagement are associated with objectively measurable better outcomes, including lower morbidity and greater longevity, as well as with equally important subjective positive outcomes such as well-being. Rather surprisingly, most of the existing research on positive traits, positive social factors, and other positive outcomes has been conducted outside the field of psychiatry and, perhaps of even greater importance, has had relatively little influence on everyday psychiatric practice. Thus, despite the progressive accumulation of empirical data supporting the critical role of PPSFs in overall mental and physical health, clinical psychiatric practice and training remain primarily restricted to diagnosis and treatment of mental illnesses, whereas psychiatric research focuses mainly on elucidating the underlying psychopathology and neuropathology and ameliorative interventions to treat and prevent relapses of mental illnesses. With the notable exception of pioneers such as George Vaillant, Dan Blazer, and C. Robert Cloninger, psychiatrists have generally considered positive mental health constructs to be too vague for routine clinical practice or serious scientific inquiry within the field of psychiatry. The premise of this volume is that the time has come to make these positive mental health concepts a central component of psychiatric practice, education, and research.

Definition of Positive Psychiatry

Psychiatry has been defined as "a branch of medicine that deals with the science and practice of treating mental, emotional, or behavioral disorders especially as originating in endogenous causes or resulting from faulty interpersonal relationships" (Merriam-Webster 2003). However, we believe that psychiatry should not be defined primarily in terms of the types of illnesses treated (i.e., mental illnesses); instead, psychiatry should be defined by the unique skill sets (i.e., assessment and modification of thinking, feeling, and behavior) of psychiatrists and other mental health experts that may be applied to a much broader range of individuals, such as those with mental or physical illnesses as well as those who are at high risk for developing those disorders. A comparison may be made with interventional radiology, which is not defined by the types of patients seen but rather by the unique skill set of the specialists.

Positive psychiatry then may be defined as the science and practice of psychiatry that seeks to understand and promote well-being through assessments and interventions aimed at enhancing PPSFs among people who have or are at high risk for developing mental or physical illnesses. These PPSFs have an impact not only on mental health but also on physical health. Numerous studies have shown that resilience, optimism, and social engagement are associated not only with better emotional functioning but also with increases in longevity and better physical and cognitive functioning. Table 1–1 summarizes salient differences between traditional psychiatry and positive psychiatry. These differences aside, it is important to emphasize that positive psychiatry is not meant to replace the traditional model of psychiatry; rather, it is intended to complement and enrich "psychiatry as usual," expanding its primary focus from pathology to health and from treating symptoms to enhancing well-being. Positive psychiatry is also not a specific population-focused subspecialty (such as child psychiatry, geriatric psychiatry, and addiction psychiatry); rather, it is an approach to psychiatry as a whole and is comparable to psychodynamic psychiatry or biological psychiatry. This emphasis is not intended to downplay the vital need for improving the diagnosis and treatment of psychopathology, nor do we imply that the rest of psychiatry is negative. (That implication would be analogous to saying that biological psychiatry implies that the rest of psychiatry is nonbiological.) Nonetheless, it may be noted that the considerable amount of existing data on the relationship between PPSFs and improved health and well-being has had minimal impact on the clinical practice of, training for, or research in psychiatry. Indeed, PPSFs are rarely even mentioned in psychiatric textbooks or empirical reports (Vaillant 2008).

Historical Background

The concepts and motives of positive psychiatry are not new. They probably date back at least a century to William James. In his 1906 presidential address to the American Philosophical Association, James, a psychologist and physician by training, argued for a new approach that would research and apply the psychological principles underlying the success of "mind-cure" (the mind cure movement focused on the purported healing power of positive emotions and beliefs) (Duclow and James 2002; Froh 2004). These views were, however, largely ignored until the mid–twentieth century when Maslow and colleagues developed humanistic psychology, which is concerned with understanding healthy, creative individuals, their aspirations, and their growth (Gable and Haidt 2005). Although they were written in reference to the field of psychology, Maslow's observations appear remarkably relevant to contemporary psychiatry:

> The science of psychology has been far more successful on the negative than on the positive side. It has revealed to us much about man's shortcomings, his illness…but little about his potentialities, his virtues, his achievable aspirations, or his full psychological height. It is as if psychology has voluntarily restricted it-

Table 1–1.   Main differences between traditional psychiatry and positive
                 psychiatry

Variable	Traditional psychiatry	Positive psychiatry
Targeted patients	Those with mental illnesses	Those with, or at high risk for developing, mental or physical illnesses
Assessment focus	Psychopathology	Positive attributes and strengths
Research focus	Risk factors, neuropathology	Protective factors, neuroplasticity
Treatment goal	Symptom relief and relapse prevention	Recovery, increased well-being, successful aging, posttraumatic growth
Main treatments	Medications and, generally, short-term psychotherapies for symptom relief and relapse prevention	Psychosocial and behavioral (and, increasingly, biological) interventions to enhance positive attributes
Prevention	Largely ignored	Important focus across the life span

self to only half its rightful jurisdiction, and that, the darker, meaner half. (quoted by Alex Linley et al. [2006, p. 5])

In the 1970s and 1980s, some researchers also showed early interest in the topic of happiness (e.g., Fordyce 1983, 1988). However, positive psychiatry's most immediate lineage is the positive psychology movement that emerged in the mid-to late 1990s.

In his 1998 presidential address to the American Psychological Association, Martin E. P. Seligman promoted the need for a positive psychology as

a reoriented science that emphasizes the understanding and building of the most positive qualities of an individual: optimism, courage, work ethic, future-mindedness, interpersonal skill, the capacity for pleasure and insight, and social responsibility. It's my belief that since the end of World War II, psychology has moved too far away from its original roots, which were to make the lives of all people more fulfilling and productive, and too much toward the important, but not all-important, area of curing mental illness.... It concentrates on repairing damage within a disease model of human functioning. Such almost exclusive attention to pathology neglects the flourishing individual and the thriving community.... When we became solely a healing profession, we forgot our larger mission: that of making the lives of all people better. (Seligman 1999, pp. 559–561)

Since then, positive psychology has become an international movement as evidenced by growth of active organizations such as the European Network for Positive Psychology (www.enpp.eu) and the International Positive Psychology Association (www.ippanetwork.org). Further details about key historical aspects of positive psychiatry are provided in the chapters authored or coauthored by two of its early founding parents, George Vaillant and Dan Blazer. In Chapter 3, "Resilience and Posttraumatic Growth," Vaillant includes a discussion of historical resistance to positive emotions and related constructs in psychiatry; in Chapter 4, "Positive Social Psychiatry," Blazer, along with his colleague Warren A. Kinghorn, describes one of its "false starts" in the social psychiatry movement. The history of the mental health recovery movement is also detailed in Chapter 5, "Recovery in Mental Illnesses."

Need for Positive Psychiatry

Despite its popularity in the lay media, positive psychology has had little impact on psychiatric clinical care, training, or education. One of us (D.V.J.), in his presidential address to the American Psychiatric Association, stated,

> I believe that psychiatry's mission will expand beyond reducing symptoms in people with mental illness.... The goal will be not just to improve psychopathology but also to help our patients grow, flourish, develop, and be more satisfied with their lives.... Psychiatry is the most appropriate of all the medical specialties to promote these positive traits in people with mental illnesses as well as in those with physical illnesses. More than any other medical specialty, psychiatry focuses on interventions aimed at behavior change. (Jeste 2012, p. 1028)

The concepts of positive psychiatry are inspired by those of positive psychology. These two fields are not competitors but rather allies, overlapping in their concepts and goals, although each also has unique areas of emphasis that reflect the larger traditional fields from which each sprang; each has the potential to inform and complement the other. One key component of positive psychiatry is that psychiatry, as a branch of medicine, remains focused on its application to patient populations, particularly those with or at high risk for mental illnesses as well as physical illnesses. The bulk of empirical research within the field of positive psychology has been focused on nonpatient samples, although some studies have examined positive interventions in people with mental illnesses (see Chapter 8, "Positive Psychotherapeutic and Behavioral Interventions"). Whereas most branches of academic psychology (i.e., other than the applied subfields of clinical, counseling, and educational psychology) and neuroscience target "normal" mental, social, and/or brain functioning, clinical psychiatry is almost exclusively concerned with mental illnesses and physical illnesses that have psychosocial concomitants.

Another key component of positive psychiatry is the goal for the field to be ultimately grounded in understanding the neurobiological underpinnings of PPSFs such as resilience, wisdom, and optimism (cf. Bangen et al. 2014; Jeste and Harris 2010; Meeks and Jeste 2009). Although that neurobiological understanding is presently quite limited, positive psychiatry seeks to develop pharmacological and other biological, as well as psychosocial, interventions to promote PPSFs and positive outcomes and to foster understanding of the neurobiological mechanisms that mediate effects of interventions (see Chapter 13, "Biology of Positive Psychiatry"). In short, positive psychiatry encompasses the constructs central to positive psychology but is differentiated by its focus on bringing these constructs into the clinical practice of those treating psychiatric or physical disorders, as well as the goal for positive psychiatry to be ultimately rooted in biology.

One additional pragmatic purpose in promoting positive psychiatry is more internal to psychiatry. With burgeoning public health and prevention programs, medicine has witnessed a paradigm shift from pathology to health and from caring for individual patients to enhancing the health of communities through preventive measures (National Prevention Council 2011). A similar mind-set is needed in psychiatry. Positive psychiatry has the potential to reinvigorate the field, improve patient outcomes, reduce health care costs, and attract high-quality trainees to psychiatry.

Overview of Chapters

This volume provides a summary of the core concepts of positive psychiatry and their practical applications and is also intended to help guide researchers and clinicians in further developing the field. The remainder of the volume is organized into four parts: 1) positive psychosocial factors, 2) positive outcomes, 3) interventions in positive psychiatry, and 4) special topics in positive psychiatry. As with most such organizational schemes, the divisions among these four parts are at least partially arbitrary and artificial, yet they have some heuristic value. For example, the presentations of PPSFs in Part I include some descriptions of positive outcomes such as those emphasized in Part II and vice versa; however, these part divisions are provided to help guide and direct readers to the chapters that most directly deal with the themes of each part. In addition to dealing with conceptual issues and providing an overview of empirical evidence, many of the chapters within each of these parts illustrate key points through one or more clinical vignettes and end with a selected number of clinical key points and suggested readings. A summary and guide to the contents of each part follows.

Part I: Positive Psychosocial Factors

In Chapter 2, "Positive Psychological Traits," Martin et al. introduce a range of person-centered positive traits, including optimism, wisdom, personal mastery, perceived self-efficacy, coping, creativity, conscientiousness, spirituality, and religiosity. The authors provide an overview of the definition(s) for each trait, including discussion of nuances and controversies in defining the constructs, such as those for which precise definitions remain elusive, and the degree to which the constructs are stable traits or potentially mutable. Overlaps and interactions occur among these constructs. The authors also provide an overview of empirical literature linking each trait to positive outcomes such as physical health and/or well-being, as well as describing clinical implications for the practice of positive psychiatry.

In Chapter 3, Vaillant hones his discussion more specifically on the topic of resilience and the potential for posttraumatic growth. Vaillant discusses three broad sources of, or routes to, resilience and posttraumatic growth: 1) external (social, medical, and community) support, 2) internal conscious strategies, and 3) involuntary mental mechanisms, including adaptive and maladaptive coping. He also traces historical developments in (and resistance to) the study of such positive emotions and related psychological constructs.

In Chapter 4, Blazer and Kinghorn focus on positive social psychiatry. They note that the bulk of the literature on positive psychology has focused on the positive subjective experiences and positive traits of individuals, with considerably less attention paid to study and application at the level of communities and institutions. They note that a similar focus on the individual characterizes contemporary psychiatry, such as the DSM's emphasis on the functioning of the individual. In contrast, in the 1950s through the 1970s, there was an active social psychiatry movement. Blazer and Kinghorn review the development of that movement and how it may inform the inclusion of positive social traits and units of analyses within positive psychiatry.

Part II: Positive Outcomes

Chapters 5–7 in Part II focus more specifically on the nature of positive outcomes and their measurement. Because the health outcomes are covered in reasonable detail in Chapter 2 in Part I, the emphasis in Part II is on more subjective aspects in terms of recovery and well-being.

In Chapter 5, Rufener et al. discuss the concept of recovery. This concept reflects the earlier discussion regarding the unique aspects of positive psychiatry because recovery has an inherently clinical focus; its meaning arises in the context of mental or physical disorders. The authors describe the history of the recovery movement, definitions and models of the concept, and principles and practices that characterize recovery-oriented care. They also address issues of measuring and operationalizing recovery.

Kaplan and Smith (Chapter 6) and Bech (Chapter 7) discuss the central issues of positive psychiatry: quality of life and well-being. In Chapter 6, "What Is Well-Being?," Kaplan and Smith review two different conceptual approaches. The first approach, growing from the tradition of health status measurement from the 1960s and 1970s, tends to focus on the effects of disease or disability on the individual's social role, community, and physical functioning, as well as (in some cases) on subjective quality of life. The other approach uses decision theory to weight the different dimensions of health, subjective function states, preferences for these states, morbidity, and mortality in order to provide a single expression of health status. These authors also consider specific measures and methods deriving from these approaches.

In Chapter 7, "Clinical Assessments of Positive Mental Health," Bech also considers measurement of well-being with several key scales of well-being and personality scales and addresses a number of scaling and psychometric issues, such as construct and predictive validity. In addition, he discusses the relation of well-being to ill-being; that is, are these concepts polar opposites of a single dimension or distinct dimensions? A key emphasis of this chapter is on describing scales that can be completed by clinicians, patients, and family or caregivers—that is, scales that can be applied to clinical practice.

Part III: Interventions in Positive Psychiatry

After a discussion of the nature of PPSFs (Part I) and the importance of positive outcomes such as recovery and well-being (Part II), the obvious follow-up question is whether these PPSFs and outcomes are amenable to intervention. This topic is the focus of Part III. With the exception of the discussion by Lavretsky and Varteresian in Chapter 10, "Complementary, Alternative, and Integrative Medicine Interventions," most of the interventions described in Chapters 8–12 focus on psychosocial and psychotherapeutic interventions. Given the importance of a neurobiological perspective in positive psychiatry, it should be noted that we do not view the focus on psychosocial interventions as being incompatible with a biological perspective. That is, behavioral, cognitive, and environmental interventions affect biology—and, by the same token, biological (e.g., psychopharmacological) interventions may have a behavioral impact, at least partly, through the placebo effect. The issue of neurobiological underpinnings is considered in Part IV (Chapter 13). Even though no pharmacological (or other directly biologically targeted) interventions are presently approved for fostering positive psychosocial traits, developing safe and effective interventions to target these constructs is one of the longer-term goals of positive psychiatry.

In Chapter 8, Parks and colleagues emphasize psychotherapeutic approaches to integrating positive psychiatric interventions into treatment. As the authors note, positive psychological interventions have generally been developed and tested in nonclinical samples but "have the potential to enrich the lives of individuals struggling with a range of physical and mental health conditions." This chapter provides an overview of the potential applications of such interventions to specific clinical populations. Some of the intervention activities include savoring experiences, gratitude exercises, practicing acts of kindness, pursuing meaning and hope, identifying and using one's strengths, and building compassion for oneself and others. The authors then illustrate adaptations of such interventions to schizophrenia, suicidality, smoking cessation, and chronic pain.

In Chapter 9, "Positivity in Supportive and Psychodynamic Therapy," Summers and Lord focus on the enhancement of positive mental health in the context of supportive and psychodynamic psychotherapies. Key messages in Chapter 9 include the dual presence of positive and negative emotions, the application of positive mental health principles in fostering patients' positive emotions and experiences, the contrast with traditional models of supportive psychotherapy, and insights into how positive mental health concepts can inform traditional psychoanalytic and psychodynamic notions of therapeutic alliance, working through, and termination. For example, in regard to supportive psychotherapy, a key part of the message of Summers and Lord is that a positive psychiatric supportive intervention "involve[s] supporting what is already working for the person, rather than helping him or her explore and change his or her defensive structure." Importantly, these authors also describe the application of positive mental health to multiple levels of medical education.

An exponential growth of interest in complementary, alternative, and integrative medicine (CAIM) (Barnes et al. 2008) has occurred in the last few decades. In Chapter 10, Lavretsky and Varteresian provide an overview of CAIM for treatment of mood and cognitive disorders among older adults. Some of the forms of CAIM that they consider include biologically based agents, such as herbal supplements, mind-body techniques (such as yoga, Tai Chi, and meditation), and alternative medical systems, including acupuncture and traditional Chinese medicine. Lavretsky and Varteresian appropriately stress the dearth of rigorous scientific data to support the efficacy of integrative therapies in mood and cognitive disorders in younger adults and the near absence of such data in older adults.

In Chapter 11, "Preventive Interventions," Bell provides a detailed overview of the principles and application of prevention methods. His overview includes community field principles and their application, as well as specific examples of prevention efforts. Some of the examples include prevention efforts focused on children and adolescents (e.g., fetal alcohol syndrome, antisocial behavior and delinquency, trauma- and stress-related disorders, special education, juvenile justice, and child protective services). Bell then considers prevention efforts for adults at the individual and group levels, with specific examples including trauma- and stress-related disorders, first-episode psychosis, postpartum and late-life depression, and dementia. He places a strong emphasis on the role of society in maintaining these efforts, and thus Chapter 11 is a natural companion to Chapter 4 on positive social psychiatry in Part I.

In Chapter 12, "Integrating Positive Psychiatry Into Clinical Practice," Boardman and Doraiswamy offer a pragmatic focus on integrating positive psychiatry interventions into everyday clinical practice. These interventions include those seeking to foster resilience, gratitude, prosocial activities, writing about signature strengths, and lifestyle activities (such as physical activity, meditation and yoga, sleep improvement, nutrition), as well as mindfulness-based interventions. The authors then describe development of treatment plans and tailoring interventions for specific disorders. They also emphasize the importance of engagement— viewing patients not as "passive recipients of an intervention strategy that is predetermined by their doctor, [but rather] engaging patients as 'active seekers of health.'"

Part IV: Special Topics in Positive Psychiatry

The final part of this volume contains four chapters that discuss important topics within positive psychiatry that did not fit naturally within any of the preceding divisions. In Chapter 13, Moore et al. review neurobiological substrates of PPSFs and outcomes. Their overview includes examining published data regarding neurocircuitry on the basis of brain imaging and other research in relation to PPSFs such as empathy, resilience, optimism, and creativity. The heritability and genetics of PPSFs are also considered, as well as possible blood- and saliva-based biomarkers. Moore et al. also clarify the research agenda needed for the growth of positive psychiatry as a biologically grounded field.

In Chapter 14, "Positive Child Psychiatry," Rettew discusses the application of positive psychiatry to child psychiatry in practice and education. Rettew's emphasis is on pragmatic ways that positive psychiatry can be incorporated into practice. The relevance of positive psychiatry to child and adolescent psychiatry seems obvious yet is underused in practice. Some of the specific components considered include the importance of temperament and self-regulation skills, nutrition, physical activity and participation in sports, limiting screen (television and computer) time while increasing reading, and parenting styles or strategies. He also describes the importance of community, mindfulness practices, exposure to music and the arts, and attention to sleep hygiene. Rettew further describes strategies to talk with families about wellness and health promotion. He closes with a discussion of incorporating positive psychiatry into professional education and training (see also Chapter 9).

In Chapter 15, "Positive Geriatric and Cultural Psychiatry," Marquine et al. consider the issue of population diversity in positive psychiatry in terms of older adults and ethnic and racial minorities. One of the key concepts in their discussion of older adults is that of successful psychosocial aging (cf. Depp and Jeste 2006; Jeste et al. 2013). Despite the association of aging with increased medical comorbidity, older adults tend to report higher levels of subjective well-being than younger adults do, and a majority view themselves as aging successfully. The discussion of positive psychiatry among ethnic minorities includes an overview of the mixed findings in regard to well-being among Hispanics and potential confounding factors, as well as research on mental health outcomes and well-being among African Americans and research on key predictors of well-being or life satisfaction within this group.

In Chapter 16, "Bioethics of Positive Psychiatry," Singh describes bioethical considerations and cautions for positive psychiatry. Singh reviews four commonly recognized fundamental bioethical principles (i.e., beneficence, nonmaleficence, autonomy, and justice) and describes the application of these principles to positive psychiatry via a series of vignettes. For example, promotion of optimism and resilience, if overdone, could result in neglect of important warning signs, suggesting a need for moderation. Singh proposes that promoting resilience (where the intention is in accord with the principle of beneficence) without clarifying its potential downsides could result in maleficence.

Limitations of the Concept of Positive Psychiatry

The preceding overview and the chapters that follow provide a general description of many key components of positive psychiatry. However, it is obvious that much more research on PPSFs and positive interventions is warranted in psychiatry and neuroscience. We also need practical ways of assessing the traits in clinical and nonclinical populations. One may appropriately object to the notion that optimism should be universally promoted through biological or other interventions. Indeed, Stein (2012) cautions that although there is consensus about the need to treat many physical and mental disorders, "there is less agreement about what constitutes positive mental health, and about which clinical interventions may be efficacious and cost-effective" (p. 108). Larger funding agencies tend to be oriented toward illnesses, so the ability to generate data on positive outcomes may be limited. No clinical mandate exists to define these constructs (in contrast to coding of illnesses such as depression), which slows the progress in the field. Empirical data are required to answer these questions. There is also the potential for adverse effects of positive psychological interventions (Sergeant and Mongrain 2011). For example, in an Internet study of more than 750 volunteers, participants who were described as "needy" felt reduced self-esteem following gratitude and exercises that involved listening to uplifting music. Therefore, choosing the right intervention—the match between patient characteristics and specific interventions—is an important consideration for clinical practice. Indeed, some authors believe that well-being should not be defined by hedonic feelings (positive emotions such as pleasure, contentment, and joy) but rather by promoting eudaemonic experience such as self-actualization and meaning (Delle Fave et al. 2011).

Suggestions for Further Research

Empirical psychiatric and neuroscience research in positive psychiatry is a recent phenomenon. There is tremendous potential for further progress. The first step should be better operationalization and assessment of positive psychosocial outcomes and PPSFs, using measures with at least adequate psychometric properties. The interactions of various constructs also warrant attention; as noted by Cloninger (2012), equivalent personality traits may lead to distinct health outcomes, whereas distinct personality traits can result in similar health outcomes. Additionally, it would be helpful to develop a strength index for an individual on the basis of his or her PPSFs; this index could be considered alongside commonly used risk indices such as the Framingham Risk Score for cardiovascular risk or scales for assessing suicide risk. Investigations to understand the neurobiology underlying PPSFs are critical for conceptualizing, creating, and testing novel interventions to enhance the positive traits and positive outcomes (see Chapter 13).

As mental health professionals, we recognize the importance of PPSFs and strategies for enhancing them not only in psychiatric patients but also in general health care settings. Such an emphasis is the basis for positive psychiatry, which strives to optimize health outcomes by promoting PPSFs. By strengthening the development of positive traits though psychotherapeutic, behavioral, social, and biological interventions, positive psychiatry has the potential to improve health outcomes and reduce morbidity as well as mortality. It should become an increasingly important approach to enhancing the general well-being of individuals and communities alike, thereby decreasing the general costs of health care.

Emerging Picture of Positive Psychiatry

Under the umbrella of positive psychiatry, clinicians, educators, and scientists would have rather different roles from what they have today. As discussed in Chapter 12, psychiatrists could integrate positive psychiatry into their practice in practical ways. Thus, clinicians would evaluate not just the symptoms and diagnoses but also the levels of well-being and PPSFs among their patients and would employ psychotherapeutic and behavioral (and, following additional research, more biological) interventions to enhance those traits, focusing on positive outcomes such as improved well-being, low level of perceived stress, successful aging, posttraumatic growth, and recovery. They would also train their counterparts outside mental health in implementing similar interventions in people who have or are at high risk for physical illnesses. With greater emphasis on positive outcomes, attributes, and strengths, the stigma against mental illness may be reduced. Such reduction in stigma should also help in attracting more health care professionals and trainees to psychiatry. Finally, researchers would focus on identifying and then seeking to modify biopsychosocial factors or processes underlying PPSFs.

If effective interventions to strengthen the PPSFs were provided to all psychiatric patients, mental health professionals could see a significant increase in the number of seriously mentally ill adults who achieve recovery (see Chapter 5). Similarly, through well-designed and implemented preventive strategies, positive psychiatry has the potential to improve health outcomes and reduce morbidity as well as mortality in the population at large (see Chapter 11). Thus, instead of being narrowly defined as a medical subspecialty restricted to management of mental illnesses, psychiatry of the future could develop into a core component of the overall health care system. Clearly, much more work is needed to make positive psychiatry a norm in psychiatric practice, but it is time to start that process.

Summary

Psychiatry has traditionally been defined and practiced as a branch of medicine focused on diagnosis and treatment of mental illnesses. The time is ripe to expand this definition to include the concept of positive psychiatry. *Positive psychiatry* may be defined as the science and practice of psychiatry that seeks to understand and promote well-being through assessment and interventions involving positive psychosocial attributes in people who have or are at high risk for developing mental or physical illnesses. Many of the concepts incorporated in positive psychiatry are not new, and many were particularly catalyzed by the rise of positive psychology beginning in the mid to late 1990s; however, they remain largely outside mainstream psychiatry. Components of positive psychiatry include PPSFs, which include traits and environmental, social, and community factors; positive outcomes (such as recovery and subjective well-being); neurobiology; and interventions. We believe that positive outcomes and PPSF constructs are amenable to systematic measurement and biopsychosocial study and have important implications for recipients of health care services in terms of overall well-being. Promising empirical data suggest that positive traits may be improved through psychosocial and biological interventions. Because psychiatry is a branch of medicine rooted in biology, clinicians and researchers are well poised to provide major contributions to the positive mental health movement, thereby affecting the overall health care system.

Clinical Key Points

- Positive psychiatry is the science and practice of psychiatry that seeks to understand and promote well-being through assessment and interventions aimed at enhancing positive psychosocial factors (PPSFs) among people who have or are at high risk for developing mental or physical illnesses.

- The concept of positive psychiatry is not new, but contemporary psychiatric research and practice have remained focused on pathology and symptoms, rather than expanding and building the positive aspects of patients' mental and social functioning.

- Although inspired by positive psychology, positive psychiatry focuses on patients rather than the healthy population and aims to uncover the neurobiological substrates of PPSFs, with the goal of developing not only psychosocial but also biologically based interventions.

- The goal of positive psychiatry is not to replace but to expand the field of general psychiatry from pathology to health and from treating symptoms to actively enhancing well-being among mental health and medical patients.

- Positive psychiatry has its own limitations, and many relevant important questions remain unanswered and require systematic empirical research, but several aspects of positive psychiatry can already be implemented in everyday practice.

References

Alex Linley P, Joseph S, Harrington S, Wood AM: Positive psychology: past, present, and (possible) future. J Posit Psychol 1:3–16, 2006
Bangen KJ, Bergheim M, Kaup AR, et al: Brains of optimistic older adults respond less to fearful faces. J Neuropsychiatry Clin Neurosci 26(2):155–163, 2014 24275797
Barnes PM, Bloom B, Nahin RL: Complementary and alternative medicine use among adults and children: United States, 2007. Natl Health Stat Rep 12(12):1–23, 2008 19361005
Cloninger CR: Healthy personality development and well-being. World Psychiatry 11(2):103–104, 2012 22654938

Delle Fave A, Brdar I, Freire T, et al: The eudaimonic and hedonic components of happiness: qualitative and quantitative findings. Soc Indic Res 100:185–207, 2011

Depp CA, Jeste DV: Definitions and predictors of successful aging: a comprehensive review of larger quantitative studies. Am J Geriatr Psychiatry 14(1):6–20, 2006 16407577

Duclow DF, James W: Mind-cure, and the religion of healthy-mindedness. J Relig Health 41:45–46, 2002

Fordyce MW: A program to increase happiness—further-studies. J Couns Psychol 30:483–498, 1983

Fordyce M: A review of research on the happiness measures: a sixty second index of happiness and mental health. Soc Indic Res 20:355–381, 1988

Froh JJ: The history of positive psychology: truth be told. NYS Psychol 16:20, 2004

Gable SL, Haidt J: What (and why) is Positive Psychology? Rev Gen Psychol 9:103–110, 2005

Jeste DV: Response to the presidential addresses. Am J Psychiatry 169(10):1027–1029, 2012 23032381

Jeste DV, Harris JC: Wisdom—a neuroscience perspective. JAMA 304(14):1602–1603, 2010 20940386

Jeste DV, Savla GN, Thompson WK, et al: Association between older age and more successful aging: critical role of resilience and depression. Am J Psychiatry 170(2):188–196, 2013 23223917

Meeks TW, Jeste DV: Neurobiology of wisdom: a literature overview. Arch Gen Psychiatry 66(4):355–365, 2009 19349305

Merriam-Webster: Medical Dictionary. 2003. Available at: http://www.merriam-webster.com/medlineplus/Psychiatry. Accessed August 21, 2014.

National Prevention Council: National Prevention Strategy: America's plan for better health and wellness. June 2011. Available at: http://www.surgeongeneral.gov/initiatives/prevention/strategy/report.pdf. Accessed August 21, 2014.

Seligman MEP: The president's address. Am Psychol 54:559–562, 1999

Sergeant S, Mongrain M: Are positive psychology exercises helpful for people with depressive personality styles? J Posit Psychol 6:260–272, 2011

Stein DJ: Positive mental health: a note of caution. World Psychiatry 11(2):107–109, 2012 22654942

Vaillant GE: Positive emotions, spirituality and the practice of psychiatry. Mens Sana Monogr 6(1):48–62, 2008 22013350

World Health Organization: WHO definition of Health. 1946. Available at: http://www.who.int/about/definition/en/print.html. Accessed August 21, 2014.

Suggested Readings

Carr A: Positive mental health: a research agenda. World Psychiatry 11(2):100, 2012 22654935

Dreger S, Buck C, Bolte G: Material, psychosocial and sociodemographic determinants are associated with positive mental health in Europe: a cross-sectional study. BMJ Open 4(5):e005095, 2014 24871540

Fava GA: The clinical role of psychological well-being. World Psychiatry 11(2):102–103, 2012 22654937

Jeste DV, Savla GN, Thompson WK, et al: Association between older age and more successful aging: critical role of resilience and depression. Am J Psychiatry 170(2):188–196, 2013 23223917

Keyes CLM (ed): Mental Well-Being: International Contributions to the Study of Positive Mental Health. New York, Springer, 2013

Palmer BW, Martin AS, Depp C, et al: Wellness within illness: happiness in schizophrenia. Schizophr Res 159(1):151–156, 2014 25153363

Vahia IV, Depp CA, Palmer BW, et al: Correlates of spirituality in older women. Aging Ment Health 15(1):97–102, 2011 20924814

PART I

POSITIVE PSYCHOSOCIAL FACTORS

2

Positive Psychological Traits

A'VERRIA SIRKIN MARTIN, PH.D.

ALEXANDREA L. HARMELL, M.S.

BRENT T. MAUSBACH, PH.D.

A growing body of literature strongly suggests that positive psychological traits (PPTs) such as optimism, wisdom, personal mastery, perceived self-efficacy, coping, creativity, conscientiousness, and spirituality and religiosity are associated with better physical and psychological health outcomes. (Note that in several chapters in the book, the term *positive psychosocial factors,* or PPSFs, has been used; this term refers to PPTs plus positive social or environmental factors.) Several longitudinal studies have noted that individuals who report higher levels of PPTs tend to live healthier lives (e.g., Vahia et al. 2011a). In addition, numerous studies highlight the association between PPTs and reduced mortality (Depp et al. 2013; Vahia et al. 2011a). Developed through the positive psychology movement, which focuses on the circumstances and processes that yield successful and optimal functioning in individuals, groups, and institutions (Gable and Haidt 2005), PPTs focus on attributes that determine

This work was supported, in part, by National Institutes of Health grant T32 MH019934 and by the University of California, San Diego Center for Healthy Aging and Sam and Rose Stein Institute for Research on Aging.

healthy outcomes and greater functioning in the face of normative transitions and adversities. Social scientists, including positive psychologists and psychiatrists, have long been interested in how individuals have the capacity to shape outcomes such as chronic and mental illness. Accordingly, social scientists are motivated to discover the best of what individuals can accomplish with regard to their own development and that of others (Baltes and Staudinger 2000).

In this chapter, we discuss eight PPTs: optimism, wisdom, personal mastery, perceived self-efficacy, coping, creativity, conscientiousness, and spirituality and religiosity. For each one, we provide a definition, discuss research linking the specific PPT to health, and discuss the clinical implications of the specific PPT and potential interventions. Our intent is to provide an overview of each of these traits. Despite the vast number of PPTs noted in the literature, we focus on these eight PPTs because they 1) are frequently cited in the literature, 2) are significant to positive psychiatry, and 3) are not covered in great detail elsewhere in this volume.

Optimism

What Is Optimism?

Broadly defined, *optimism* reflects the extent to which individuals expect favorable outcomes to occur. Research on optimism and its wide-ranging impact on health has flourished, largely because of the recognition that individual variability within this construct can have clinically meaningful implications. However, despite a surge in interest, operationalizing optimism remains challenging. For example, it is possible for a person to demonstrate a more optimistic outlook in some areas (e.g., relationship with spouse or friends) than in others (e.g., financial prospects). Moreover, a person's sense of optimism likely shifts as time unfolds. Thus, the stability of the construct has often been called into question. The general consensus among most researchers and clinicians is to view optimism as a relative trait that has some fluctuations over extended periods of time and is partially dependent on the particular circumstance. The heritability of optimism is estimated to be around 25% (Plomin et al. 1992), which is lower than that of most other "personality traits" but is significant nonetheless. Besides stability, another issue that has arisen in defining optimism is whether the construct should be viewed as the opposite end of a single dimension with pessimism or if it, instead, should be parsed into two independent dimensions, with one dimension specifically pertaining to optimism and the other specifically pertaining to pessimism. Regardless of the precise stability or dimensionality of the construct, studies continue to amass suggesting the importance of optimism and its strong link with both psychological and physical well-being.

Relationship Between Optimism and Health

Accumulating research suggests that higher rates of optimism (as assessed via self-report questionnaires) play a protective and positive role in both physical and psychological health. A meta-analysis of 83 studies on optimism reported significant relationships between optimism and physical outcomes, including cardiovascular outcomes, physiological markers (including immune function), cancer outcomes, outcomes related to pregnancy, physical symptoms, pain, and mortality rates (Rasmussen et al. 2009). Another study, using a large and nationally representative sample of 6,044 American adults older than 50, found that each unit increase on an optimism measure ranging from 3 to 18 was associated with a 9% reduced risk of stroke over a 2-year follow-up event (Kim et al. 2011). The exact mechanisms underlying these findings remain unclear. However, individuals who report higher levels of optimism may be less reactive to life stressors, thereby reducing physiological response to new presenting problems, ultimately causing less wear and tear on their bodies over the span of years.

Similar to the physical health benefits, psychological health benefits have also been reported in optimism research. A study by Giltay et al. (2006) found that a low level of optimism was an important and independent predictor of cumulative depression symptoms in elderly men over a 15-year follow-up. This finding appears to be consistent with a growing body of evidence showing an association between higher levels of optimism and lower levels of depression. Because characterization of depression includes having overly pessimistic thoughts and negative ruminative thinking styles, the case may be that individuals who report higher levels of optimism focus their attention more on positive cues while simultaneously filtering out negative cues. Ultimately, this selective filtering system may result in an enhancement of one's mood.

Clinical Implications and Interventions

Several underlying factors may contribute to one's currently reported level of optimism. For example, the extent to which exposure to adversity might influence optimism is unknown. It is reasonable to suspect that experiencing a multitude of stressful experiences can result in a decrease in optimism. In contrast, it may also be plausible that coping with adversity and having the ability to overcome problems that appear to be insurmountable may increase optimism for future events. Interestingly, extant literature on optimism is beginning to highlight the idea that the number and quality of positive or negative events a person experiences is not as important as the way these events are interpreted. For example, individuals who report higher levels of optimism typically differ in their attribution styles or how they explain the events in their lives compared with those who report lower levels of optimism. Although individuals with higher levels of optimism attribute successful outcomes to more internal and stable factors ("this positive outcome occurred because I am competent"), those with lower levels of optimism typically show the reverse pattern and attribute successful outcomes to more external, temporary causes ("this positive outcome occurred because of luck"). The reverse pattern is also seen in unsuccessful outcomes; individuals with higher levels of optimism will attribute unsuccessful outcomes to more external, temporary causes, and those with lower levels of optimism will attribute them to internal and stable factors. Optimism may also be affected by other mechanisms, including one's attitude and coping style. It has been suggested that people who report higher levels of optimism tend to approach situations and put forth full effort into making a situation turn out favorably. Alternatively, people who report lower levels of optimism tend to avoid situations more or give up sooner because they believe that they are likely to have a negative outcome, irrespective of the amount of effort they put forth.

Although optimism is generally viewed as a trait, intervention strategies to enhance one's optimism are certainly possible. Optimism may be cultivated by teaching individuals how to dispute pessimistic beliefs as well as ways to alter their focus from more negative stimuli to more neutral or positive stimuli. Additionally, cognitive-behavioral strategies that aim to change a person's negative view of himself or herself or the world may prove to be fruitful in intervention programs. Moreover, providing individuals with the tools that will allow them to more effectively deal with stress (e.g., relaxation and breathing exercises, cognitive reappraisals) will also likely be beneficial. Notably, few intervention studies specifically focus on enhancing optimism. Considering the extensive physical and psychological benefits that seem to be related to higher optimism, future research in this area is warranted to help enable individuals to live a more fulfilling and healthier life.

Wisdom

What Is Wisdom?

Within a historical context, wisdom is deeply rooted in philosophy and religion. Philosophically, wisdom has been understood as the thoughtful application of knowledge, whereas world religions perceive wisdom as a virtue. Although ancient cultures varied in their exact definitions of wisdom (for Greeks, *wisdom* was defined by rationality, whereas early Indian and Chinese thinkers emphasized emotional balance), there was overlap among several features, including thoughtful decision making, compassion, altruism, and insight (Meeks and Jeste 2009). Wisdom is undoubtedly a multifaceted concept with numerous subcomponents. Although no one established definition of wisdom currently exists, a number of subcomponents are commonly cited. They include prosocial attitudes and behaviors such as compassion, empathy, and altruism; social decision making and general knowledge of life; emotional regulation; reflection and self-understanding; tolerance of different value systems; acknowledgment of and dealing effectively with uncertainty and ambiguous situations; openness; spirituality; and a sense of humor (Bangen et al. 2013; Meeks and Jeste 2009). The intersection between these subcomponents can be appreciated in their utility for both the self (e.g., increased well-being) and others (e.g., creating better relationships and focusing on the greater good). As eloquently stated by Baltes and Staudinger (2000), wisdom "include[s] knowledge and judgment about the meaning and conduct of life and the orchestration of human development toward excellence while attending conjointly to personal and collective well-being" (p. 122). This overlap between subcomponents makes wisdom a compellingly complex PPT worth examining.

Historically, the interest in wisdom has been evident in disciplines such as philosophy and religious studies; however, in the last four decades, vast progress has been made in the empirical study of wisdom as it applies to human development, psychology and psychiatry, successful aging, and personal growth (Baltes and Staudinger 2000; Bangen et al. 2013). Given the complexity of wisdom, measuring this construct has presented ongoing challenges. To date, there are a number of acceptable (valid and reliable) measures for wisdom. Bangen et al. (2013) recently reviewed assessment instruments for wisdom and found nine appropriate measures. These measures were interview-based or self-report questionnaires or a hybrid of interview-based and self-report questionnaires. The measures that demonstrated substantial strengths included the Three-Dimensional Wisdom Scale, the Wisdom Development Scale, and the Self-Assessed Wisdom Scale (SAWS), along with the measures associated with the Berlin Wisdom Paradigm Studies.

Research has suggested that wisdom, to some extent, is a stable trait within an individual; however, it can also be shaped by experiences and learning (Bangen et al. 2013). For example, in one report from the Berlin Wisdom Paradigm Studies (N=125), wisdom-related performance in adults was predicted by intelligence (e.g., fluid intelligence, crystallized intelligence), the personality-intelligence interface (e.g., creativity, cognitive style, social intelligence), personality traits (e.g., personal growth, openness to experience), and life experience (e.g., general life experience, professional experience) (Baltes and Staudinger 2000). It has been hypothesized that because of accumulated life experiences, wisdom increases with age, and it is likely that age-related wisdom would provide an evolutionary advantage to humans (Jeste and Harris 2010). However, despite this common belief, the association between wisdom and age has not been consistently supported in empirical study (Baltes and Staudinger 2000; Jeste and Harris 2010). It has been noted that significant overlap exists between wisdom and other PPTs, such as resilience and social cognition, which share some of the previously mentioned subcomponents. However, wisdom is distinct and includes a multidimensionality not seen within these other traits.

Relationship Between Wisdom and Health

There is evidence relating wisdom to better physical health, as well as enhanced quality of life in older adults (Bangen et al. 2013). In older adults, wisdom may increase an individual's ability to survive and thrive in the face of declining health. Correspondingly, wisdom in younger adults may deliver a fitness advantage that provides a counterbalance to the loss of fertility in older age (Jeste and Harris 2010). In addition, wisdom contributes to successful personal and social functioning (Meeks and Jeste 2009). This increase in personal functioning may be maintained by increased reflection and self-understanding, as well as the ability to deal effectively with uncertainty. Additionally, increased social function could be in direct relation to higher levels of prosocial attitudes and behaviors, including compassion, empathy, and altruism.

Despite some initial evidence that wisdom may be linked to well-being as individuals age, how wisdom is directly related to various physical or mental illnesses is unclear. Certain disorders (e.g., variant of frontotemporal lobar degeneration, autism spectrum disorders, antisocial personality disorder) may help explain the biological basis of wisdom because these disorders typically include loss of some compassion and empathy. Furthering our knowledge of these underlying neurobiological mechanisms may be useful for developing rehabilitative intervention programs with the goal of enhancing wisdom (Meeks and Jeste 2009).

Clinical Implications and Interventions

Wisdom functions both individually and relationally. The literature has suggested that social collaboration increases wisdom-related performance. Participants who discussed a problem with a significant other before responding individually or had a dialogue with a person of their choice performed better overall on wisdom performance tasks (Baltes and Staudinger 2000). This result may suggest the importance of interactive relationships in the ongoing development of wisdom and a possible site for intervention. Increasing the subcomponents related to wisdom (i.e., prosocial attitudes, dealing effectively with uncertainty, emotional regulation) can increase general levels of wisdom and optimize human development both individually and collectively. With a focus on interactive relationships as well as subcomponents of wisdom, community-based intergenerational programs, in which schoolchildren are mentored by older adult volunteers, may benefit society while simultaneously supporting increased wisdom (Jeste and Harris 2010).

Although wisdom cannot be improved through medication intervention, there is a belief that it can be enhanced through intervention. However, to the best of our knowledge, only one intervention directly targets wisdom. *Wisdom therapy,* based on the Berlin Wisdom Project's research, may promote an individual's ability to process challenging life events through multiple perspectives. The goal of this intervention is to enhance several subcomponents of wisdom such as acceptance of uncertainty and flexible thinking, thereby increasing general wisdom (Bangen et al. 2013). In addition, cognitive rehabilitation techniques intended to improve executive functioning and cognitive flexibility may have an impact on wisdom. Undoubtedly, the development of wisdom from childhood to late adulthood is an important component for increased functioning throughout the life span (Baltes and Staudinger 2000). Further study of wisdom should be conducted to fully comprehend the mechanisms of change and potential entry points for intervention.

Personal Mastery

What Is Personal Mastery?

Personal mastery is another PPT that has garnered significant attention. Personal mastery, which reflects a tendency toward feeling that life circumstances are under one's control, overlaps to some extent with other PPTs, such as self-efficacy, locus of control, and optimism. Self-efficacy is differentiated from personal mastery by its emphasis on one's perceived ability to execute actions that are required to deal with specific circumstances (e.g., self-efficacy for solving math problems). Mastery reflects general expectations about personal coping resources versus confidence in performing specific behaviors. Also highly related, locus of control is a construct whereby individuals perceive whether life circumstances are under their control or are due to external, chance circumstances. Earlier conceptualizations of locus of control used a forced-choice assessment method, implying that individuals were either internal or external in their perceptions of control. In this sense, personal mastery is distinguished from locus of control in that individuals low in mastery are not assumed to believe that circumstances are due to chance or external forces. More recently, internal and external loci of control have been considered to be separate domains, whereby individuals can vary along both scales simultaneously. In this sense, personal mastery is closely related to internal locus of control. Finally, although both high personal mastery and high optimism reflect a tendency toward positive expectancies, personal mastery differs from optimism in that it is more reflective of one's expectations of being personally effective in achieving desired outcomes. Individuals high in personal mastery feel that they have a sense of control over both their future and their life circumstances. Having low personal mastery, in contrast, can translate into feelings of helplessness and powerlessness over circumstances. According to a well-known *transactional model* of stress posited by Lazarus and Folkman (1984), the interaction between external environmental stresses and internal resources can influence health outcomes. Thus, it is not necessarily the level of stress but, instead, an individual's belief about how well he or she is able to cope with it that results in health morbidity. Personal mastery can be considered one of the few internal resource factors delineated in the transactional model; therefore, it has the potential to modify certain aspects of an individual's health trajectory.

Relationship Between Personal Mastery and Health

Overall, high levels of personal mastery have been found to attenuate or lessen some of the deleterious effects of stress. A systematic review of 32 studies examined the effect of mastery on outcomes in a wide variety of different populations. The authors of this review article reported an association between mastery and better cardiometabolic health and reduced risk for disease and/or death (Roepke and Grant 2011). Another review article (Harmell et al. 2011) cited several different studies from the dementia family caregiving literature. These articles reported that higher levels of personal mastery in dementia caregivers were related to reduced norepinephrine reactivity to stressors and increased β_2-adrenergic receptor sensitivity (this latter finding has been associated with improved immune system functioning). The authors of this review concluded that stronger control beliefs (i.e., greater levels of mastery) may aid in reducing physiological responses to stress and may serve as a resilience factor for better health in the dementia caregiver population.

Clinical Implications and Interventions

Personal mastery seems to have many downstream health benefits. This correlation is likely related to the fact that those who view themselves as capable of coping with problems also view themselves as being more capable of controlling problems. The significance behind feeling more in control over one's circumstance in life cannot be understated because it can have profound effects on not only psychological processes such as one's mood but also physiological processes such as one's physiological response to acute and chronic stress. Individuals with higher levels of personal mastery may be more likely to view their health as controllable and, as a result, may exercise more, eat healthier, use health care services more often, and have improved medication management. Individuals low in personal mastery may feel that their health is outside of the purview of their control and may be less likely to engage in these proactive positive health behaviors.

Given the identification of personal mastery as a potential buffer from the negative ramifications of stress, interventions targeting increased mastery may be of paramount importance. However, to date, these interventions have been limited. One question that remains to be addressed is whether personal mastery is a dynamic, changing construct that can, in fact, be altered. Some evidence suggests that cognitive-behavioral interventions that include changing appraisals (positive self-talk) and increasing pleasurable activities may result in an increased sense of control (Coon et al. 2003). However, whether these results generalize to long-lasting alterations in personal mastery and the health benefits that seem to come as a result has yet to be determined. In caregiver populations, skill-based interventions where caregivers can learn and practice how to better manage stressful life circumstances related to their caregiving responsibilities may be a good avenue to explore. For individuals diagnosed with HIV, targeting personal mastery and coping skills may be of greater importance than targeting stressors directly. Improving personal mastery and coping skills may be achieved through coping effectiveness training, cognitive-behavioral stress management, and direct psychotherapy. Moreover, it is further recommended that interventions targeting mastery be examined in a variety of different populations to help determine in what patient population and under which specific circumstances high mastery seems to be the most beneficial.

Perceived Self-Efficacy

What Is Perceived Self-Efficacy?

Perceived self-efficacy is a positive psychological construct closely related to personal mastery, but it has a more specific and definitive meaning. Perceived self-efficacy in relation to life stressors refers to an individual's perceived confidence in his or her ability to activate specific coping strategies to overcome life challenges and to influence outcomes by his or her actions. Thus, perceived self-efficacy involves a dual process consisting of appraisal of whether an outcome is controllable via coping and an estimation of whether an individual feels equipped to carry out the necessary coping strategy to manage the stressor. Perceived self-efficacy beliefs are thought to influence whether an individual thinks in self-promoting or self-debilitating ways. Additionally, perceived self-efficacy can influence whether problems appear to be manageable or overwhelming. Coping self-efficacy is a specific form of perceived self-efficacy that exclusively relates to the extent to which an individual believes he or she can carry out specific coping behaviors necessary to cope with a challenge (e.g., stop unpleasant thoughts, seek out social support). Throughout the literature, coping self-efficacy seems to be the most researched form of self-efficacy.

Relationship Between Perceived Self-Efficacy and Health

Emerging evidence shows that higher levels of perceived self-efficacy may have psychological and physiological advantages. For example, coping self-efficacy has been shown to have a protective effect on the relationship between caregiving stress and the proinflammatory marker cytokine interleukin–6 (IL-6), a risk factor for cardiovascular disease (Mausbach et al. 2011), as well as reduced resting blood pressure and significantly lower cumulative health risk. A negative relationship between perceived self-efficacy and both physical and mental health has also been reported in Alzheimer's caregivers. In other words, caregivers who reported higher levels of perceived self-efficacy also reported fewer depressive and physical health symptoms (Fortinsky et al. 2002).

Clinical Implications and Interventions

The mechanisms involved in the connection between perceived self-efficacy and positive health outcomes may stem from the strong involvement of perceived self-efficacy in cognitive, affective, and behavioral processes. For example, whereas an individual high in perceived self-efficacy may view a stressful experience as something to be mastered and take action, an individual low in perceived self-efficacy may ruminate on past failures, become depressed, and lose confidence in his or her ability to take constructive action. The direct and/or indirect result of not taking constructive action may lead to more enduring negative cognitions and even less confidence in the ability to take constructive action in the future. Accordingly, low or high perceived self-efficacy may create a self-perpetuating cycle, leading to decreased or increased perceived self-efficacy, respectively, when an individual is faced with future stressors. Therefore, clinicians and researchers may be able to use an assessment of perceived self-efficacy beliefs to identify the individuals most at risk for psychological and physical comorbidity.

Several approaches to increasing perceived self-efficacy have been reported. Most of these interventions target positive appraisals and teach specific coping strategies. One dementia caregiver study conducted a randomized trial to increase perceived self-efficacy and found the treatment condition to be successful (Coon et al. 2003). Another intervention study found that higher perceived self-efficacy improved physical functioning after coronary artery bypass graft surgery in patients with ischemic heart failure (Barnason et al. 2003). These findings provide support for the thought that perceived self-efficacy may be a malleable construct that can be implemented as a target for therapeutic interventions. Additionally, these intervention studies illustrate that increasing perceived self-efficacy may be a worthwhile goal because it can lead not only to behavior change but ultimately to positive health outcomes. The following vignette describes how perceived self-efficacy is relevant to clinical assessment and treatment.

Clinical Vignette

Elizabeth is in her late 70s and cares for her husband with Alzheimer's disease. She is responsible for dressing him, bathing him, feeding him, and reminding him when it is time to take his medications. His condition is getting progressively worse, and her caregiver role is becoming more and more time-consuming. On top of providing care for her husband, Elizabeth is also trying to manage her own medical issues, including hypertension, high cholesterol, type 1 diabetes, and ulcerative colitis. She is in charge of all of her and her husband's finances and asks her daughter for help only when she feels it is absolutely necessary. Considering the many tasks that Elizabeth is responsible for, it is important to gauge her confidence level in facing these daily tasks as well as her belief in her ability to cope with these tasks.

Assessing Perceived Self-Efficacy

It is important to assess for perceived self-efficacy because higher levels of perceived self-efficacy have been shown to have protective effects against the negative impact of caregiver stress. In addition, increasing levels of perceived self-efficacy may reduce resting blood pressure and significantly lower cumulative health risk.

Self-efficacy can be assessed with one of several self-report questionnaires. For example, the General Perceived Self-Efficacy Scale (Schwarzer and Jerusalem 1995) consists of 10 items rated on a four-point Likert scale. Higher scores are indicative of greater confidence in coping in a wide variety of demanding situations. Sample statements include the following:

- I can always manage to solve difficult problems if I try hard enough.
- It is easy for me to stick to my plans and accomplish my goals.
- I can remain calm when facing difficulties because I can rely on my coping abilities.
- When I am confronted with a problem, I can usually find several solutions.

In addition to administration of one or more self-efficacy self-report questionnaires, it is strongly recommended that clinicians conduct an in-person interview using an effective problem-solving approach. The clinician can ask the patient to consider problems that he or she needs to address; the patient then brainstorms a variety of solutions, and the clinician asks the patient to determine the solution he or she feels the *most* confident about putting into effect (i.e., self-efficacy). The clinician could then prioritize this action for clinical intervention.

Increasing Perceived Self-Efficacy
On the basis of the assessment, the clinician can

- Target the strategy that the patient feels most confident putting into effect while simultaneously working to bolster other areas the patient feels less confident in pursuing.
- Provide education and coping strategies that are specific to solving a particular task or problem.
- Have a trainer or someone similar to the patient demonstrate the skill: social modeling.
- Role-play the solution with the patient and process the interaction.

Action

As with any treatment plan, psychoeducation surrounding the patient's particular stressors is incredibly important. In the case of Elizabeth, the clinician should provide her with information about her husband's health as well as tips on how to manage her own health care issues. Intervention should target teaching the patient positive appraisals (e.g., help redirect the patient's focus from past failures to past successes) as well as specific coping strategies such as training Elizabeth to think about multiple solutions to a problem and developing a strategy for coping with specific stressors. For example, if bathing her husband daily seems overwhelming to Elizabeth, perhaps bathing him every other day would reduce caregiver burden and increase her confidence in this particular domain.

Problem-Focused Coping

What Is Coping?

As noted in the previous section, coping is closely related to perceived self-efficacy. Specifically, *coping* is defined as an attempt (cognitive or behavioral) to manage situations that are considered stressful to an individual. A variety of coping strategies should be considered in accordance with the ability of each strategy to influence possible outcomes (Roesch et al. 2005). These strategies fall within two types of coping that are prevalent in the literature: emotion focused and problem focused. Emotion-focused coping is an internal process, whereby the individual manages his or her emotional stress and internal demands. Strategies involved in emotion-focused coping include distancing, self-control, escape avoidance, and positive reappraisal. Problem-focused coping aims to control stressors externally and decreases conflict within the individual's environment. Strategies related to problem-focused coping include managing external aspects of a stressor, accepting responsibility, planful problem solving, and seeking instrumental support. Another commonly used taxonomy for coping includes approach versus avoidance coping. Approach coping includes strategies such as active coping, optimism, coping self-efficacy, seeking information, guidance and support, positive reappraisal, and problem solving. In contrast, avoidance coping includes strategies such as passive coping, wishful thinking, denial, behavioral and/or mental disengagement, helplessness, self-blame, alcohol and/or drug use, threat minimization, and distancing and distraction (Duangdao and Roesch 2008; Roesch et al. 2005).

Relationship Between Coping and Health

Individuals who directly confront their illness using active instrumental approach coping report psychological and physical benefits (Roesch et al. 2005). Problem-focused coping has been linked to better emotional status, metabolic control, and better adjustment in chronically ill individuals. Focusing directly on the issue appears to reduce the internalization of the problem by making the problem external to the self and surmountable. Correspondingly, approach coping is related to better adjustment, and avoidance coping is related to poorer adjustment, in individuals with chronic illness (Duangdao and Roesch 2008; Roesch et al. 2005). For example, individuals who use active coping strategies—planning, seeking information and support, remaining optimistic, learned self-control, and adherence to medical routines—report lower levels of depression and anxiety, as well as a better ability to control glucose levels (Roesch et al. 2005). In samples of chronically ill individuals, emotion-focused coping has been linked to poor adjustment and adherence to health regimens and outcome. Consequently, actively and effectively coping with life stressors is fundamental for maintaining physical and psychological health.

Clinical Implications and Interventions

Increased levels of problem-focused and approach coping appear to be linked to healthier outcomes. Therefore, interventions should be aimed at increasing active coping methods, encouraging adaptive coping, and discouraging maladaptive coping strategies. Several coping skills training programs are grounded in Bandura's notions of self-efficacy, such as developing the individual as the agent for change. These training programs contain modules for communication, conflict resolution, social problem solving, and cognitive-behavioral modification (Roesch et al. 2005). The goals of coping skills training programs are to increase constructive behaviors that improve self-management and, in turn, to increase overall quality of life, increase treatment adherence, and reduce possible medical complications. Intervention strategies outlined in the "Perceived Self-Efficacy" section are also deemed appropriate for increasing positive coping.

Creativity

What Is Creativity?

Creativity has been at the forefront of psychology in the United States for decades, with more than 10,000 papers related to creativity from a psychological
perspective being written in the last 10 years. Because of the vast body of literature, the question of the exact definition of creativity remains under debate. Generally, creativity can be considered to be one's ability to produce novel, unique
artistry, ideas, or insights that are useful or valuable (Davis 2009). Two types of creativity are most commonly noted in the literature: "big C" creativity, which suggests eminent creative abilities that are innate, and "little c" creativity, which
constitutes everyday creativity that is developed and functional in nature. Creativity inspires more flexibility in thinking, such as the ability to evaluate situations and develop solutions to problems.

Relationship Between Creativity and Health

Creativity has been linked to successful adaption to daily life and increased well-
being. Older adults who participate in the arts—dance, expressive writing, music, theater, and visual arts—are noted as having improved physical health, cognitive health, mental health, and quality of life. For example, in a recent review
of participatory art wellness studies, Noice et al. (2014) reported that older adults
who take part in dance demonstrate greater balance and gait, improved resting
heart rate, and better cognitive performance. Similarly, individuals who perform expressive writing tasks show decreased depression, improved processing
speed, and enhanced self-concept over time (Noice et al. 2014).

An ongoing debate concerns the relationship between creativity and mental
health pathologies (i.e., schizophrenia, psychosis). There is evidence that creative
thinking is sensitive to mood, yet there has been some disagreement as to the direction of the relationship. In a meta-analysis of the relationship between creativity and mood, Davis (2009) found that compared with neutral and/or negative
moods, positive moods appeared to increase creative performance. In addition,
mood attributions, mood intensity, and characteristics of the creative task appeared to affect overall creativity.

Clinical Implications and Interventions

Fostering a more positive mood may enhance creativity, promoting originality,
flexibility, fluency, and improved health. A number of types of approaches have
been used to foster creativity, such as provisioning of effective incentives, identification and acquisition of requisite expertise, optimization of climate and cul-

ture, effective structuring of group interactions, and training to enhance creativity. Creative training has been the preferred method and has been used in a variety of settings such as business, education, and medicine. Creative training is diverse in its application across programs; 172 techniques or instructional methods have been identified. In a meta-analysis of 70 creativity training programs, Scott et al. (2004) revealed that the studied programs contributed to increased divergent thinking, problem solving, and performance and more positive attitudes and behaviors. Specifically, programs that incorporated a cognitive approach appeared to be the most positively related to study outcome success.

Another area of intervention for creativity is active participation in the arts. Increasing an individual's participation in the arts has the ability to increase health in all domains. In one example of a participatory art intervention, the researchers randomly assigned depressed older adults to receive private ballroom dance lessons for 8 weeks and, following the intervention, found an increase in self-efficacy and a decrease in hopelessness in this group compared with a wait-listed control group (Haboush et al. 2006). Arts participation is naturally motivating, provides social support through group arts instruction, and is stimulating to the participant. Although the current literature discusses dance, expressive writing, music, theater, and visual arts (Noice et al. 2014), a number of other participatory art avenues, such as drawing and painting, other types of writing, and photography, may also prove to be beneficial to individual well-being.

Clinical Vignette

Ivy is in her mid-50s and has recently been diagnosed with major depressive disorder. Within her assessment, she reports that she is feeling isolated, has few close relationships, and has a negative self-concept. In addition, she is mostly homebound with limited interaction.

Ivy's treating mental health professional is struck by her level of isolation, which is increasing her depression. Her clinician also notes that she has difficulty making decisions and often cannot generate any potential solutions. Her clinician decides to assess Ivy's creativity on two levels: creative thinking and participation in creative activity.

Assessing Creativity

Creativity can be assessed with a clinical interview. Specifically, the interview would include questions about the patient's ability to evaluate situations and develop solutions to problems. The clinician wants to understand if the patient can develop unique and novel ideas. In addition, the clinician can assess the patient's participation in creative endeavors, such as the arts. Sample questions include the following:

- When you encounter a problem, how easy is it for you to find a solution?

- What steps do you typically take in order to evaluate a situation and develop solutions?
- If you were to consider one problem you are currently facing, what are possible solutions to that problem?
- Do you participate in any types of art (i.e., writing, dancing, painting, photography)?
- Is there any type of art that feels complementary to your personality?

Enhancing Creativity

From a clinical perspective, evidence shows that fostering a more positive mood may enhance creativity, promoting originality, flexibility, fluency, and improved health. Consequently, it may be important to focus on increasing the patient's mood before beginning any creativity training. Cognitive-behavioral therapy that incorporates strategies for generating new ideas, finding solutions to problems, and developing flexible thinking may be one strategy for enhancing creative thinking. Alternatively, another strategy may be to increase the amount of time a patient spends participating in the arts (i.e., writing, dancing, painting, photography). Assessing an individual patient's interest in various participatory arts and encouraging thoughtful participation may increase levels of creativity and, as a result, affect overall health.

Action

Ivy demonstrated difficulty pinpointing any specific problem and was unwilling to consider solutions to the problem. In addition, she does not participate in any creative activities but notes that she absolutely loves to paint. On the basis of this feedback, the clinician develops a plan for brief cognitive-behavioral therapy that focuses on maladaptive thoughts and idea generation. In addition, Ivy and her clinician consider ways to incorporate painting back into her life. Specifically, her clinician would like her to take a painting class to reduce her level of social isolation.

Conscientiousness

What Is Conscientiousness?

Conscientiousness is a spectrum of personality-related constructs that are indicative of individual differences in the propensity to be hardworking, rule abiding, orderly, planful, responsible, and task and goal directed. In addition, *conscientiousness* denotes the ability to follow socially prescribed norms for impulse control and to delay gratification (Bogg and Roberts 2004; Roberts et al. 2014). Taken as a whole, conscientiousness has been identified as an independent construct with the introduction of the Big Five taxonomy of traits, which classifies personality traits into five domains: extraversion, agreeableness, conscientiousness, emotional stability, and openness to experience (Bogg and Roberts 2004). From this point of view, the Big Five dimension of conscientiousness is defined as a family of six interrelated traits or facets that reflect one's level of industriousness, order, self-control, responsibility, traditionalism, and virtue (Chapman et al. 2014). Conscientiousness has been found to be directly related to a number of major areas of life, and positive aging has been noted as a crucial predictor of life span health (i.e., physical health, cognitive health, mental health). Furthermore, conscientiousness plays a role in work outcomes, income, occupational attainment and leadership, and predicting marital stability over time (Roberts et al. 2014).

The most common method for measuring conscientiousness is through self-report measures, although these self-reports can be augmented through observer ratings reported by friends and/or family members. In addition, some researchers use "objective" measures that are less susceptible to biases, such as experimentally derived measures or implicit approaches (Roberts et al. 2014). Conscientiousness is characteristically measured via self-report using subscales of larger personality inventories that reflect estimates of specific behaviors, feelings, and thoughts. The wide range of global personality trait scales includes, but is not limited to, measures such as the 16 Personality Factor Questionnaire, the Adjective Checklist, the Big Five Inventory, the Minnesota Multiphasic Personality Inventory, the Multidimensional Personality Questionnaire, and the NEO Personality Inventory (Bogg and Roberts 2004). Objective measures of conscientiousness include projective tests, such as the picture story exercise or the Thematic Apperception Test, and standardized laboratory-based computerized experimental tasks that directly measure specific behaviors (e.g., impulsive decision making, inattention, and disinhibition).

Relationship Between Conscientiousness and Health

Conscientiousness appears to have an effect on health outcomes through its relationship with social environmental factors such as work and marriage and through its association with health-related behaviors. Social environmental factors that are frequently associated with higher levels of conscientiousness include divorce (negatively related) and number of children (positively related) (Chapman et al. 2014). Social environmental factors such as socioeconomic status, family, and religiosity may also have a direct relationship with levels of conscientiousness. Bogg and Roberts (2004) conducted a meta-analysis of conscientiousness-related traits—order, self-control, responsibility, industriousness, traditionalism, and virtue—as they relate to the health-related behaviors that contribute to mortality in the United States (tobacco use, diet and activity patterns, excessive alcohol use, violence, risky sexual behavior, risky driving, suicide, and drug use). Data were retrieved, and 194 studies were quantitatively synthesized. The six conscientiousness-related traits significantly predicted each of the risky health-related behaviors, with the largest predictive relationship found between conscientiousness-related traits and the behavioral domain of drug use $(r=-0.28)$. Of note, correlations ranged from -0.12 to -0.25 for the behavioral domains of suicide, unhealthy eating, risky sex, tobacco use, excessive alcohol use, risky driving, and violence. Of the six conscientiousness-related traits, self-control and traditionalism most consistently predicted health behaviors, although responsibility and virtue were also associated with the majority of the health-related domains. Industriousness and order appeared to have the smallest associations with the health-related domains. Overall, this study established the important relationship between conscientiousness and notable health-related behaviors.

Conscientiousness is also important to consider in the development of clinical treatment interventions because it affects the patient's overall adherence to treatment such as attending appointments and taking medicines as prescribed. For example, dialysis patients who report lower levels of conscientiousness may benefit from structured and supervised interventions, whereas patients reporting higher levels of conscientiousness may find less structured interventions in which they maintain a sense of personal control more beneficial (Chapman et al. 2014). Consequently, consideration of individual conscientiousness levels may be valuable in developing effective and personalized clinical treatment interventions.

Clinical Implications and Interventions

Although classical thought suggested that personality traits such as conscientiousness are fixed, research over the last decade has demonstrated that personality is more adaptable than was previously thought (Chapman et al. 2014). Psychotherapy is the suggested entry point for interventions that increase levels of conscientiousness. Psychotherapy affects personality change through the modification of personality processes. To increase levels of conscientiousness, therapy should target specific personality processes related to conscientiousness (e.g., self-control, order, responsibility) so that patients can make an effort to alter the natural set point or default mode of functioning for these specific processes. When planning an intervention to increase levels of conscientiousness, the clinician must consider the underlying constructs or causal chain as the target for intervention. For example, to increase reported levels of conscientiousness, the clinician or interventionist should focus on mechanisms that increase self-monitoring and self-regulation (Chapman et al. 2014). This bottom-up model of personality change provides corrective experiences that modify the overall functioning of conscientiousness (Chapman et al. 2014). Ultimately, therapy needs to be personalized on the basis of individual needs; the effectiveness of therapy may be dictated by the amount of therapy received.

A number of studies reported increased conscientiousness as a result of psychotherapy. For example, using a yearlong mindfulness intervention with primary care physicians, researchers demonstrated an increase in conscientiousness ($d=0.29$), with changes maintained at 3-month follow-up (Krasner et al. 2009). Another study demonstrated improvements in conscientiousness in traumatized women after 16 weeks of generic therapy or interpersonal therapy (see Chapman et al. 2014).

Therapy at the family level may also be advantageous in increasing individual levels of conscientiousness. For instance, spouses who demonstrate higher levels of conscientiousness may moderate the health risks of individuals with lower levels of conscientiousness (Chapman et al. 2014), illustrating the indirect effect experience through family transmission. This correlation is also evident in peer relationships and neighborhood environments. For example, high-risk behaviors such as smoking are frequently transmitted through extrafamilial social networks. Consequently, altering group attitudes may increase conscientiousness by steering individuals toward increasingly adaptive tendencies. In one study, suicide awareness was disseminated within a school network using the influential members of the system to leverage change (Chapman et al. 2014). This type of social network intervention could be applied in most social environments, such as in the workplace to increase self-directedness or in retirement communities to increase physical goal setting.

Spirituality and Religiosity

What Are Spirituality and Religiosity?

Spirituality and religiosity are multifaceted constructs that are challenging to define because of differences in perspectives, underlying assumptions, and measurement within the relevant empirical literature. Currently, conceptual definitions of spirituality and religiosity vary widely, ranging from subjective human experience to organized formal institutions. Religion is an important fixture in many people's lives, with 96% of adults reporting that they believe in God and 72% noting that religion is the most important influence in their personal lives (Ano and Vasconcelles 2005). The definition of religion has evolved over time to be more indicative of a fixed system of ideologies and is no longer closely associated with the dynamic, existential personal journey. Spirituality commonly refers to a transcendent relationship with an entity that is beyond physical, psychological, or social dimensions of life. Furthermore, spirituality is often linked to the existential journey for purpose and meaning (Sawatzky et al. 2005). Some recognize spirituality as a personal or subjective experience of religiosity.

In the last two decades, a trend toward polarization of spirituality and religiosity has developed, with spirituality being identified with personal, subjective, emotional transcendent expression and religion being identified as more institutional, authoritarian, and nonexpressive (Koenig et al. 2012). However, another view, put forth by Hill and Pargament (2003), suggests that spirituality and religion should represent dependent constructs because both spirituality and religiosity are focused on the sacred (i.e., God, transcendence, ultimate reality), which distinguishes them from other phenomena. Given this view, one of the most difficult challenges for a researcher of spirituality and religiosity is attempting to define and objectively measure the meaning of "the sacred" within this context. The two scales most widely used to measure these constructs in health research are the Multidimensional Measurement of Religiousness/Spirituality (MMRS; Fetzer 2003) and the Brief Multidimensional Measurement of Religiousness/Spirituality (BMMRS; Piedmont et al. 2006). Within the MMRS, the key domains of religiousness and spirituality that are measured are daily spiritual experiences, meaning, values, beliefs, forgiveness, private religious practices, religious and spiritual coping, religious support, religious and spiritual history, commitment, organizational religiousness, and religious preferences. In contrast, the BMMRS is a shortened, 38-item version that uses select questions from each of the domains in the MMRS to broadly measure spirituality and religiosity.

Relationship Between Spirituality and Religiosity and Health

A body of literature suggests that spirituality and religiosity have beneficial effects on health (Hackney and Sanders 2003; Hill and Pargament 2003; Sawatzky et al. 2005). This relationship appears to be multidimensional and to affect biological, psychological, and social health. Spirituality and religiosity have been linked to a number of positive health outcomes, including lower rates of depression, better quality of life, increased longevity, lower mortality due to positive health practices, faster recovery from illness, higher self-esteem, and better cognitive function (Powell et al. 2003; Vahia et al. 2011b). In a literature review, Seeman et al. (2003) reported evidence that stronger spirituality and religiosity were associated with a variety of health outcomes such as better lipid profiles, lower blood pressure, and better immune function.

A meta-analysis reported a significant positive relationship between spirituality and perceived quality of life, including well-being and life satisfaction (Sawatzky et al. 2005). In addition, religion has been associated with decreased psychological distress, increased life satisfaction, and increased self-actualization

(Hackney and Sanders 2003). This relationship may be due to the protective mechanism of spirituality and religiosity on health and/or to its moderating effects on those who are affected by disease and disability (Powell et al. 2003).

Clinical Implications and Interventions

In the health care industry, there is increased recognition that spirituality and religiosity can have a profound influence on health outcomes. Spirituality and religiosity appear to increase one's ability to cope successfully with life's stressful events through a shared community and internal strength. Vahia et al. (2011b) found that individuals who reported the strongest levels of spirituality also had higher levels of resilience. This finding highlights the protective nature of spirituality and religiosity when coping with negative life events and normative life transitions. Positive religious coping strategies (e.g., forgiveness, seeking support, religious focus, spiritual connection) have previously been related to positive psychological adjustment (i.e., acceptance, emotional well-being, happiness, purpose, resilience) in people who are experiencing a stressful life event. In contrast, negative religious coping strategies (e.g., spiritual disconnect, interpersonal religious discontent, pleading for direct intercession) are frequently associated with negative health outcomes (Ano and Vasconcelles 2005). There is currently an increased focus on integrating spirituality and/or religiosity into therapeutic practice by guiding patients to increase features of their spirituality and/or religiosity that are beneficial while deemphasizing aspects that could potentially be harmful. Focusing on aspects of spirituality and religiosity such as personal devotion has the potential to lead to positive results regardless of the clinical target (Hackney and Sanders 2003). Furthermore, the addition of mind-body interventions such as meditation and relaxation may increase physiological and/or functional health in patient populations (Seeman et al. 2003).

Summary

We have provided an overview of several PPTs—optimism, wisdom, personal mastery, perceived self-efficacy, coping, creativity, conscientiousness, and spirituality and religiosity—that are relevant to positive psychiatry. In this chapter, we have noted the reciprocal relationship between these PPTs and physical and mental health outcomes. Targeting these PPTs using the noted interventions can enhance well-being and life satisfaction at the individual and systemic levels. Although there has been great progress in research related to each of these PPTs, there is substantial need for additional research to understand the underlying mechanisms and specific aims for clinical intervention.

Clinical Key Points

- Optimism may be enhanced by teaching individuals how to dispute pessimistic beliefs as well as ways to alter their focus from more negative stimuli to more neutral or positive stimuli. Moreover, providing individuals with the tools that will allow them to more effectively deal with stress (e.g., relaxation and breathing exercises, cognitive reappraisals) will also likely be beneficial.

- Wisdom is related to better physical health and quality of life in older adults. Encouraging interactive relationships with family, friends, and/or strangers may enhance levels of wisdom through interaction.

- Overall, high levels of personal mastery (i.e., a tendency toward feeling that life circumstances are under one's control) have been found to attenuate or lessen some of the deleterious effects of stress. Personal mastery has been shown to be increased through cognitive-behavioral interventions that include changing appraisals (positive self-talk) and increasing pleasurable activities.

- Assessment of low or high self-efficacy beliefs can be used as a way to identify the individuals most at risk for psychological and physical comorbidity. Furthermore, self-efficacy may be a malleable construct that can be implemented as a target for therapeutic interventions through teaching positive appraisals and specific problem-focused coping strategies.

- Creativity has been positively linked to physical, mental, and cognitive health. It is possible to target creativity through participatory art interventions. Promoting inclusion in arts such as dance, expressive writing, and theater may decrease the deleterious effects of aging and increase self-concept.

References

Ano GG, Vasconcelles EB: Religious coping and psychological adjustment to stress: a meta-analysis. J Clin Psychol 61(4):461–480, 2005 15503316

Baltes PB, Staudinger UM: Wisdom: a metaheuristic (pragmatic) to orchestrate mind and virtue toward excellence. Am Psychol 55(1):122–136, 2000 11392856

Bangen KJ, Meeks TW, Jeste DV: Defining and assessing wisdom: a review of the literature. Am J Geriatr Psychiatry 21(12):1254–1266, 2013 23597933

Barnason S, Zimmerman L, Nieveen J, et al: Impact of a home communication intervention for coronary artery bypass graft patients with ischemic heart failure on self-efficacy, coronary disease risk factor modification, and functioning. Heart Lung 32(3):147–158, 2003 12827099

Bogg T, Roberts BW: Conscientiousness and health-related behaviors: a meta-analysis of the leading behavioral contributors to mortality. Psychol Bull 130(6):887–919, 2004 15535742

Chapman BP, Hampson S, Clarkin J: Personality-informed interventions for healthy aging: conclusions from a National Institute on Aging work group. Dev Psychol 50(5):1426–1441, 2014 23978300

Coon DW, Thompson L, Steffen A, et al: Anger and depression management: psychoeducational skill training interventions for women caregivers of a relative with dementia. Gerontologist 43(5):678–689, 2003 14570964

Davis MA: Understanding the relationship between mood and creativity: a meta-analysis. Organ Behav Hum Decis Process 108:25–38, 2009

Depp CA, Martin AS, Jeste DV: Successful aging: implications for psychiatry. Focus 11:3–14, 2013

Duangdao KM, Roesch SC: Coping with diabetes in adulthood: a meta-analysis. J Behav Med 31(4):291–300, 2008 18493847

Fetzer I: Multidimensional measurement of Religiousness/Spirituality for Use in Health Research: A Report of the Fetzer Institute/National Institute on Aging Working Group. Kalamazoo, MI, John E Fetzer Institute, 2003

Fortinsky RH, Kercher K, Burant CJ: Measurement and correlates of family caregiver self-efficacy for managing dementia. Aging Ment Health 6(2):153–160, 2002 12028884

Gable SL, Haidt J: What (and why) is Positive Psychology? Rev Gen Psychol 9:103–110, 2005

Giltay EJ, Zitman FG, Kromhout D: Dispositional optimism and the risk of depressive symptoms during 15 years of follow-up: the Zutphen Elderly Study. J Affect Disord 91(1):45–52, 2006 16443281

Hackney CH, Sanders GS: Religiosity and mental health: a meta-analysis of recent studies. J Sci Study Relig 42:43–55, 2003

Haboush A, Floyd M, Caron J, et al: Ballroom dance lessons for geriatric depression: an exploratory study. The Arts in Psychotherapy 33(2):89–97, 2006

Harmell AL, Chattillion EA, Roepke SK, Mausbach BT: A review of the psychobiology of dementia caregiving: a focus on resilience factors. Current Psychiatry Reports 13(3):219–224, 2011 21312008

Hill PC, Pargament KI: Advances in the conceptualization and measurement of religion and spirituality: implications for physical and mental health research. Am Psychol 58(1):64–74, 2003 12674819

Jeste DV, Harris JC: Wisdom—a neuroscience perspective. JAMA 304(14):1602–1603, 2010 20940386

Kim ES, Park N, Peterson C: Dispositional optimism protects older adults from stroke: the Health and Retirement Study. Stroke 42(10):2855–2859, 2011 21778446

Koenig HG, King DE, Carson VB: Handbook of Religion and Health, 2nd Edition. New York, Oxford University Press, 2012

Krasner MS, Epstein RM, Beckman H, et al: Association of an educational program in mindful communication with burnout, empathy, and attitudes among primary care physicians. JAMA 302(12):1284–1293, 2009 19773563

Lazarus RS, Folkman S: Stress, Appraisal, and Coping. New York, Springer, 1984

Mausbach BT, von Känel R, Roepke SK, et al: Self-efficacy buffers the relationship between dementia caregiving stress and circulating concentrations of the pro-inflammatory cytokine interleukin-6. Am J Geriatr Psychiatry 19(1):64–71, 2011 20808097

Meeks TW, Jeste DV: Neurobiology of wisdom: a literature overview. Arch Gen Psychiatry 66(4):355–365, 2009 19349305

Noice T, Noice H, Kramer AF: Participatory arts for older adults: a review of benefits and challenges. Gerontologist 54(5):741–753, 2014 24336875

Piedmont RL, Mapa AT, Williams JE: A factor analysis of the Fetzer/NIA Brief Multidimensional Measure of Religiousness/Spirituality (MMRS). Research in the Social Scientific Study of Religion 17:177, 2006

Plomin R, Scheier MF, Bergeman CS, et al: Optimism, pessimism and mental health: a twin/adoption analysis. Pers Individ Dif 13:921–930, 1992

Powell LH, Shahabi L, Thoresen CE: Religion and spirituality: linkages to physical health. Am Psychol 58(1):36–52, 2003 12674817

Rasmussen HN, Scheier MF, Greenhouse JB: Optimism and physical health: a meta-analytic review. Ann Behav Med 37(3):239–256, 2009 19711142

Roberts BW, Lejuez C, Krueger RF, et al: What is conscientiousness and how can it be assessed? Dev Psychol 50(5):1315–1330, 2014 23276130

Roepke SK, Grant I: Toward a more complete understanding of the effects of personal mastery on cardiometabolic health. Health Psychol 30(5):615–632, 2011 21534674

Roesch SC, Adams L, Hines A, et al: Coping with prostate cancer: a meta-analytic review. J Behav Med 28(3):281–293, 2005 16015462

Sawatzky R, Ratner PA, Chiu L: A meta-analysis of the relationship between spirituality and quality of life. Soc Indic Res 72:153–188, 2005

Schwarzer R. Jerusalem M: Generalized self-efficacy scale. Measures in health psychology: a user's portfolio. Causal and Control Beliefs 1:35–37, 1995

Scott G, Leritz LE, Mumford MD: The effectiveness of creativity training: a quantitative review. Creat Res J 16:361–388, 2004

Seeman TE, Dubin LF, Seeman M: Religiosity/spirituality and health: a critical review of the evidence for biological pathways. Am Psychol 58(1):53–63, 2003 12674818

Vahia IV, Chattillion E, Kavirajan H, Depp CA: Psychological protective factors across the lifespan: implications for psychiatry. Psychiatr Clin North Am 34(1):231–248, 2011a 21333850

Vahia IV, Depp CA, Palmer BW, et al: Correlates of spirituality in older women. Aging Ment Health 15(1):97–102, 2011b 20924814

Suggested Cross-References

Optimism is discussed in Chapter 13 ("Biology of Positive Psychiatry"). Self-efficacy is discussed in Chapter 11 ("Preventive Interventions"). Coping is discussed in Chapter 3 ("Resilience and Posttraumatic Growth"). Spirituality is discussed in Chapter 10 ("Complementary, Alternative, and Integrative Medicine Interventions") and Chapter 13.

Suggested Readings

Depp CA, Martin AS, Jeste DV: Successful aging: implications for psychiatry. Focus 11:3–14, 2013

Harmell AL, Chattillion EA, Roepke SK, Mausbach BT: A review of the psycho-biology of dementia caregiving: a focus on resilience factors. Curr Psychiatry Rep 13(3):219–224, 2011 21312008

Jeste DV, Palmer BW: A call for a new positive psychiatry of ageing. Br J Psychiatry 202:81–83, 2013 23377203

Snyder CR, Lopez SJ (eds): Handbook of Positive Psychology. New York, Oxford University Press, 2002

Stein Institute for Research on Aging Web site. Available at: aging@ucsd.edu.

Vahia IV, Chattillion E, Kavirajan H, Depp CA: Psychological protective factors across the lifespan: implications for psychiatry. Psychiatr Clin North Am 34(1):231–248, 2011 21333850

3

Resilience and Posttraumatic Growth

GEORGE E. VAILLANT, M.D.

Lord, make me an instrument of your peace;
Where there is hatred, let me sow **love;**
Where there is injury, let me sow **forgiveness;**
Where there is doubt, let me sow **faith;**
Where there is despair, let me give **hope;**
Where there is sadness, let me give **joy.**
O Master, grant that I may not so much to seek
compassion but to **give compassion....**

"The Peace Prayer of St. Francis,"
attributed to Father Esther Becquerel (1912)

In human lives, discontinuities are of two sorts. The first sort of discontinuity is tragic: the promising youth ends up surprisingly dysfunctional; the already vulnerable but loving mother loses her only child as a result of leukemia. From this first sort of discontinuity we learn little that we did not already know. We all know that Humpty Dumpty can fall off a wall and be shattered beyond repair. The second sort of discontinuity has more to teach us: the traumatized veteran becomes a loving and creative success, and the child who seemed to have no clear chance in life actually turns out quite well. We have much to learn from once fragmented "Humpty Dumpties" who, 10—or even 40—years later, become whole.

45

At the heart of recovery from disadvantage and trauma is the concept of resilience. The term *resilience* is preferred over the popular—but unempathic—term *invulnerability*. In no way does the eventual survival and recovery of resilient youth convey invulnerability. Indeed, Emmy Werner, the intellectual mother of one of the great longitudinal studies of child development (Werner and Smith 1982), has called such mended Humpty Dumpties "vulnerable but invincible." Another empathic term that exceeds resilience is *posttraumatic growth*—a term more relevant to this book because it conveys alchemy of the human spirit. The concept of posttraumatic growth exemplifies a basic principle of positive psychology—to strive not for a return from −5 to 0, but for a return from −5 to +5.

Unfortunately, in their laudable quest to relieve human suffering, both psychiatrists and psychologists have been little interested in enabling such positive transformations. Instead, the traditional focus of both psychiatry and psychology has been directed toward curing pathology rather than toward enhancing what is normal. However, in the last 15 years, in contrast to psychiatrists, psychologists have made laudable efforts to develop a *positive psychology* based on sound theory and empirical investigation. The goal is to produce positive mental health, not merely to alleviate mental illness (Seligman 2002). A key aspect of positive psychology is the emphasis on empirical evidence. The goal is to replace the woolly world of Abraham Maslow's "humanism," Esalen's "self-transformation," and Norman Vincent Peale's "power of positive thinking" with evidence-based positive transformation. Much of the evidence-based content of this chapter is drawn from positive psychologists as well as from the Harvard Study of Adult Development (Vaillant 2002). This latter study is based on a collection of three seven-decade-long prospective studies of Harvard graduates, disadvantaged inner-city Bostonian youths, and a subgroup of gifted California women from Lewis Terman's study.

Resilience and Positive Transformation

Three broad classes describe ways to seek resilience and positive transformation. In the first class are the ways in which an individual elicits help from appropriate others, namely, seeking social, medical, and community support (see Chapter 4, "Positive Social Psychiatry"). The second class consists of conscious strategies that people intentionally use to make the best of a bad situation (Lazarus and Folkman 1984), which range from cognitive-behavioral therapies in the clinical realm to damage control rehearsals on naval vessels. The third class consists of involuntary mental mechanisms that distort or modulate our perception of internal and external reality to reduce subjective distress. For caregivers, the most critical of these inner sources of resilience are positive emotions and involuntary mental coping mechanisms. The internal and external sources of resilience and positive transformation are summarized in Table 3–1.

Table 3–1. Potential sources of resilience

External and cognitive sources of resilience

Social support

    The helping community

    Warm childhood environment

Sociobiological good luck

    Absence of risk factors (social and genetic)

    Historical moment, timing, and/or context

    Social attractiveness

    High IQ

Cognitive (i.e., conscious) strategies

    Attributional style

    Cognitive therapy

Positive psychological traits: inward focused

Independent traits

    Childhood temperament

    Emotional intelligence

    Passing normal developmental milestones, ages 0–80

    Selective age-dependent memory

Independent traits facilitated by positive psychotherapy

    Positive emotions

    Empathic involuntary coping mechanisms

Definition of Terms

Clear description and discussion of the phenomena of positive psychological traits can be difficult because of semantic issues. The term *resilience* can be used in many different ways with only partial overlap in meaning. However, within the context of positive psychology or psychiatry, the term conveys both the capacity to be "bent without breaking" and the capacity, "once bent, to spring back." In this vein, Werner and Smith (1982) offered a concise and useful definition of *resilience*: "the self-righting tendencies within the human organism." This sense of resilience is analogous to the physiological concept of *homeostasis*. A phenomenon beyond simple "springing back" is positive transformation; the best term for the latter appears to be *posttraumatic growth*. By way of analogy, if one loses one's shoes, one's soles become harder and resistant to corns.

Sources of Resilience

Similar to other constructs such as intelligence or athletic ability, resilience is a multidimensional concept. There are as many ways of being resilient as there are ways of being intelligent or athletic. Table 3–1 lists 14 widely cited potential sources of resilience, although none of these operates entirely independent of the others. The focus of the current chapter is on the last two sources of resilience listed in Table 3–1, that is, positive emotions (Vaillant 2008) and involuntary coping mechanisms (Vaillant 1993). (Note that my use of the metaphor *mechanism* is for semantic convenience; the terms *style* and *trait* would be equally appropriate. In a literal sense, neither the brain nor the mind consists of mechanisms.)

Some investigators see resilience as simply a balance sheet of the relative absence of risk factors and the relative presence of protective factors (Werner and Smith 1982). Under this model, given sufficient environmental insults (e.g., neonatal complications, an alcoholic mother, and poor schools), anyone would fail. However, as noted by Rutter (1986), the notion that adverse experiences inevitably lead to lasting damage to personality "structure" has little empirical support. My own work (Vaillant 2012) confirms Rutter's findings; that is, findings from my research suggest that the things that go right in one's life, rather than the things that go wrong, are primarily what shape one's future. Admittedly, the illnesses of alcoholism and major genetic mental illness can overwhelm the things that go right. Consider the man who was blessed with intelligence, a warm family, a Harvard education, and superb health. Still, for much of his life, he lived alone and sometimes homeless in Key West, Florida. He was alienated from his wife and children and slept with his dog in the back of a station wagon. Why? All his life he had felt vulnerable, and his gradual development of both alcoholism and bipolar illness left him not resilient but rather overwhelmed by life.

Sometimes resilience seems as if it results from a system of fate designed by Rube Goldberg, Dr. Seuss, or chaos theory. Good deeds backfire; mistakes are rewarded. For want of a nail, the battle is lost, and by missing the plane, a life is saved. Sometimes a chance experience can change a person's life. But, to paraphrase Louis Pasteur, in producing resilience and posttraumatic growth, chance favors interpersonal warmth and mature egos, or, put in the context of this chapter, chance favors positive emotions and adaptive involuntary coping mechanisms.

In this chapter, I consider people who initially lacked the three broad categories of protective factors for stress resistance summarized by Masten and Garmezy (1985): 1) self-esteem and a positive social orientation, 2) family cohesion, and 3) the availability of an external support system that encouraged and supported their social skills. However, they became successful, loving, and generative. Why? As Rutter points out, resilience is more than just an algebraic sum of risk and protective factors. Resilience reflects the inner traits summarized in Table 3–1.

External and Cognitive Traits for Resilience

Table 3–1 includes a list of eight related external and cognitive sources of resilience. Thus, it is possible to conceive of resilience as one's capacity to employ appropriate *voluntary* coping strategies. In this view, resilience is nothing more than the application of intelligence, street smarts, planfulness, social supports, and education. However, in the Harvard Study of Adult Development, some of the inner-city men with minimal education fared better in life than the brilliant (mean IQ of 150). From whence did their resilience spring?

To account for such exceptions, cognitive psychologists have noted the importance of attributional style to resilience. In this context, *attributional* refers to how an individual regards his or her own responsibility versus external responsibility for the good and bad events that befall him or her (similar to the concept of *locus of control*). When an individual gets an A on a math exam, does he or she feel that it was a mistake? Likewise, just as detrimental, does he or she believe that the A was a unique event and that it will never happen again? Or does the individual take credit for the A in math and believe that the success will generalize to spelling as well and that he or she will probably continue to do well in math? A resilient attributional style for a person with diabetes would be to *think,* "I am a normal person with a disease called diabetes (a limited, not global, problem), which I have the power to treat (responsibility) with daily self-injections of insulin (controllability)." A vulnerable attributional style would be to think, "I am a hopeless diabetic (globally defective) with an incurable affliction (helpless) that will lead to inevitable impotence and blindness (hopeless)."

Positive Inward-Focused Traits for Resilience

Positive psychology is concerned less with mere survival after multiple risk factors and more with positive transformation and well-being. It is not enough that vulnerable orphans survive the refugee camp; they must learn to run and laugh and feel joy as well. Indeed, only a minority of people exposed to traumatic events develop long-standing psychiatric disorders, whereas according to Linley and Joseph (2004), estimates of the prevalence of growth among people who have experienced trauma tend to range from sizeable minorities (30%–40%) to majorities (60%–80%).

The importance of *inward-focused psychological traits* (childhood temperament, emotional intelligence, passing typical developmental milestones, positive emotion, and involuntary coping mechanisms) for resilience is illustrated by the example of a participant in the Harvard Study of Adult Development, Butch, who grew up in one of the most dismal families in the study. His IQ was only 60. To master such handicaps, Butch's extraordinary ability to deploy stoicism (suppression, hardiness, or grit), *an adaptive involuntary coping mechanism,* and the *positive emotion* of gratitude, instead of resentment, seemed particularly germane.

Clinical Vignette

Life granted Butch few external sources of resilience. All his life, Butch's parents had been on welfare, and they had lived in a "blighted" three-story wooden tenement. The mother's father was illiterate, and the neighbors saw the entire Patriarcha family as feebleminded. The mother herself had been charged with alcohol abuse and assault and battery. Her house was described in a police report as "dirty," with a "filthy floor." Butch's father not only was an alcoholic but also was so badly disabled that he could hardly walk. He had made at least one suicide attempt and had received multiple court summons for child neglect and nonsupport. When he was at home, he shared a bed with Butch.

Between ages 6 and 10, Butch had three skull fractures. The psychiatrist described his physical appearance as "untidy, filthy looking…with stooped shoulders" and noted that he was "obviously very dull" and had a speech impediment. At age 17, he was still in the seventh grade with the reading ability of an 8-year-old. As for his bodily health, Butch had a cleft palate, a wandering left eye, and rickets. By age 18, he had lost all his teeth. Butch had no demonstrated athletic skills. With difficulty, he finally gained entrance into the U.S. Army only to spend a month sequestered in the brig. His army psychiatric classification was "feebleminded."

Somehow in this Pandora's chest of horrors, if Butch did not find hope, he found the involuntary adaptive mechanism called *suppression* (American Psychiatric Association 1994), sometimes called *grit* and sometimes referred to as *hardiness*. When he was 14, the psychiatrist did not fully realize the value of the lifesaving fact that Butch was "a fairly placid fellow who is content to plod along." Despite the negative reinforcement of repeated failures, he stuck with school until he was 18 (the positive emotion of *hope*). Perhaps it was also noteworthy that during all the years that he failed to progress in reading, fell four grades behind at school, and was relegated to special classes, he, nevertheless, took elaborate jigsaw puzzles out of the library and painstakingly assembled them.

Up to the point of his marriage at age 25 (developmental milestone of *intimacy*), Butch's only real accomplishments as a teenager had been to attend church and the Boy's Club and, as an adult, to work regularly for a trucking company. For the next 35 years, he continued to work for the same Cleveland trucking firm (developmental milestone of *career consolidation*). He took pride in and was grateful (*positive emotion*) for being assigned to the higher-paying graveyard shift on the loading dock. Having spent his entire childhood on welfare, by age 50 Butch was proud to be making almost $40 an hour (in 2007 dollars). He could now take his family to Florida in the winter and to a Maine cottage in the summer. In contrast to the shabby house in which he grew up, Butch took pride in the fact that he had fixed up and painted the inside of his well-cared-for apartment, still ensconced within an externally shabby tenement.

By age 47, Butch not only had worked for the same company for 25 years but had remained attached to the same network of close friends (*positive emotion*). His oldest friend went back to boyhood, and he was godfather to that friend's child. To offset his lack of fathering, he worked hard volunteering for the Boy

Scouts (*the* involuntary coping style of *altruism*). One of his sons became an Eagle Scout, another source of pride. Because Butch worked nights, he would nap while his sons were in school so that he could play with them when they came home (*generativity*, another developmental milestone). By age 50 when he was interviewed, Butch still nagged his sons to make sure they did their homework. He had paid tuition to send his children to parochial school. Both his sons graduated from high school and entered skilled trades.

When Butch was 50, the interviewer, blind to his childhood intelligence tests, summed him up as follows: "Butch and his wife were quite honestly interested in the study. Their questions seemed unusually sensitive to the subtleties and significance of studying adult development. In the same way, both of them seemed to be able to grasp the intent of the interview questions without much explanation and responded as openly as they could" (*emotional intelligence*). Butch had survived his childhood with considerable productive energy. With virtually no support from schools or from luck, he sustained his curiosity and human responses to the world and to people. He presented himself with dignity. He did not apologize for his education or his speech, although he knew he had paid a high price for both (*emotional intelligence*). He and his wife were able to give freely to their family and to their community and seemed to enjoy doing so.

Butch had used neither rose-colored glasses nor denial. Instead, as a stoic and a master of suppression (*involuntary coping*), he simply never missed noting the silver linings in the clouds of life. As he grew older, Butch's coping style included being able to remember the past as a little better than it was (*selective memory*), which contributed to his sense of gratitude (*positive emotion*). Although he could recall having had to go to work and bring all the money back to his mother, Butch said that he sometimes wished that he was back in his childhood. He remembered his schoolwork as being very hard and recalled having to attend special speech classes; nevertheless, he remembered school as a task at which he had worked every day and had liked. He dealt with his bad moods by saying nothing to anyone. Then, as the day went by, "I work myself out of my cranky mood." Butch never seemed to quit anything he started.

Butch's wife was clearly more intellectually gifted than her husband, and he was grateful, not resentful, of the fact that his wife looked after him. Of his wife, he said, "She's a wonderful woman. I couldn't have met anyone better." She "takes care of me," and "she would do anything that I asked her to do." He also stayed close to his family of origin. Since his parents died, Butch had become the family patriarch (developmental milestone of *keeper of the meaning*). During one of the study interviews, his sister called long-distance from Boston to ask her brother for help. He might not have done as well as his classmates on intelligence tests, but within the relatively less intelligent Patriarcha family, he had always been a smart fellow who could solve puzzles.

As an aside, Butch was a poster child for the most important internal psychological trait that there is, one that cannot be shoehorned into Table 3–1 and is an unfamiliar concept except in psychoanalytic discourse: the ability to take love in.

Positive Emotions

Historical Development

The significance of emotions in human experience has been recognized since ancient times, but often, emotions have been seen as a weakness not an asset. By the time of the Enlightenment, emotions were increasingly viewed as best ignored altogether. Since the Enlightenment, emotions, especially positive emotions, have been difficult for academicians to appreciate. In their lengthy and influential nineteenth-century textbooks, which founded scientific psychology, Wilhelm Wundt and William James each allotted a single chapter—and a somewhat disdainful one at that—to the emotions. By the time that modern physicists had discovered quantum mechanics, biologists still knew very little about human emotional life. In 1933, psychologist Max Meyer (1933), founder of the Psychology Department at the University of Missouri and a former mentee of theoretical physicist Max Planck, prophesized, "Why introduce into science an unneeded term, such as emotion, when there are already scientific terms for everything we have to describe?...In 1950 American psychologists will smile at both these terms [will and emotion] as curiosities of the past" (p. 300). As Meyer predicted, a decade after the invention of the atomic bomb, Burrhus F. Skinner (1953), a brilliant and most rational psychologist, still dismissively proclaimed, "The 'emotions' are excellent examples of the fictional causes to which we commonly attribute behavior" (p. 160).

By the end of the nineteenth century, Sigmund Freud's appreciation of the likelihood that distortion of emotions via unconscious mechanisms led to psychopathology again made emotion a respectable focus for medical attention. However, for the next 100 years that focus remained on only the negative emotions. For example, the index of the twenty-first-century *Comprehensive Textbook of Psychiatry* (Sadock et al. 2005) directs the interested reader to thousands of lines on the terms *depression* and *anxiety* and hundreds of lines on *fear, shame, anger, hatred,* and *guilt*. However, the index shows only five lines on *hope*, one on *joy*, and none on *awe, love, compassion, forgiveness, faith,* or *gratitude*.

Cortical Versus Limbic Positive Emotions

The 20-item Positive and Negative Affect Schedule (PANAS) is still the most frequently used academic measure of positive emotion. The terms in the following list from the PANAS are very cognitive (cortical not limbic):

- Cheerful
- Relaxed
- Happy
- Attentive
- Delighted
- Joyful
- Surprised
- Inspired
- Excited

- Proud
- Lively
- Alert

- Enthusiastic
- Interested
- Energetic

- Confident
- Interested

This list contrasts sharply with those made by individuals not fettered by the cognitive shackles of the Enlightenment and thus able to freely access limbic reality. The following list of "Fruits of the Spirit" was compiled by a first-century evangelist (*Saint Paul's Letter to the Galatians* 5:22–23):

- Love
- Faith
- Compassion

- Grace
- Peace
- Hope

- Joy
- Gentleness
- Fulfillment

The next list, called "The Secret of Happiness," was compiled by a very bright 8-year-old girl traveling home from a funeral:

- Love
- Help
- Together
- Give

- Share
- Heart
- Feel
- Picture

- Kindness
- Friends
- Forgive

(When queried by her mother, the girl explained that *picture* meant "what is going on in another person's mind," in short, empathy.)

As an example of how recent our post-Enlightenment understanding of human emotion is, consider that *empathy* (not in the 8-year-old's vocabulary) was also not found in the 1940 20-volume *Oxford English Dictionary* and that the phenomenon of infantile autism was not discovered until 1943 by a Johns Hopkins child psychiatrist, Leo Kanner—in his own son. Today, the congenital lack of empathy and difficulties of attachment present in childhood autism affect roughly 1% of the population and can be recognized by any competent pediatrician.

It was not until 1945–1950 that psychoanalyst and ethologist John Bowlby first convinced physicians that orphans needed tactile affection as much as food and convinced psychiatrists that humans learn love through touch, eye contact, and attachment, not through gratification of lust and hunger. Indeed, nonsexual love (i.e., attachment) did not become a tangible biological reality for psychologists until the late 1950s after Harry Harlow's objective findings in rhesus monkeys.

Adaptive Role of Positive and Negative Emotions

Love, hope, joy, forgiveness, compassion, faith (meaning limbic basic trust and not cortical religious ideology), awe, and gratitude are the important positive emotions addressed in this chapter. I omit from the list four other positive emotions—excitement, contentment, mirth, and a sense of mastery—because we can feel these latter four emotions alone on a desert island. In sharp contrast, the eight positive emotions that I have selected all involve human connection. None of the eight are all about the self. All should be part of a clinician's therapeutic repertoire. Clinicians should learn to "hear," empathize, and reinforce them.

Negative emotions such as fear, grief, lust, and anger are also inborn and are of tremendous importance. Negative emotions are often crucial for survival, but only in time present. The positive emotions are more expansive and help us broaden and build (Fredrickson 2001). They widen our tolerance, expand our moral compass, and enhance our creativity. They help us survive in time future. Careful experiments document that whereas negative emotions narrow attention and cause us to miss the forest for the trees, positive emotions, especially joy, make thought patterns more flexible, creative, integrative, and efficient (Isen et al. 1991).

The effect of positive emotion on the autonomic (visceral) nervous system has much in common with the relaxation response to meditation popularized by Harvard professor of medicine, Herbert Benson (1996). In contrast to the metabolic and cardiac arousal that the fight-or-flight response of negative emotion induces in our *sympathetic* autonomic nervous system, positive emotion via our *parasympathetic* nervous system reduces basal metabolism, blood pressure, heart rate, respiratory rate, and muscle tension.

In order to illustrate the transmutation of pain into positive emotion, consider the following empirical examples of the power of emergent positive emotion. In an ongoing Web-based survey of 24 positive character "strengths," two well-known psychologists, Christopher Peterson and Martin Seligman, charted the effect of the September 11, 2001, terrorist attacks. Peterson and Seligman (2003) compared the self-reported character strengths of 529 Web respondents in the 2 months before the event with the self-reported character strengths of 490 Web respondents in the 2 months after the 9/11 World Trade Center bombing. The salience of cognitive strengths, such as prudence, curiosity, bravery, self-control, and wisdom, did not change significantly. Six strengths that are more emotional in nature increased the most—all significantly. These strengths were gratitude, hope, kindness, love, spirituality, and teamwork.

Historical Resistance to Positive Emotions

Although open to the negative emotions, psychiatry has had even more difficulty than psychology in accepting the positive emotions. In academic writing, use of positive emotions has become "politically incorrect." For example, Alcoholics Anonymous's (AA) eleventh-step prayer of "Faith, Hope and Love," presented in the epigraph ("The Peace Prayer of St. Francis"), or AA's schmaltzy slogans "develop an attitude of gratitude" and "fake it 'til you make it" are enough to make psychodynamically trained counselors' skin crawl, until the counselors consider the evidence-based science that demonstrates AA's dependence on fostering positive emotions works very significantly better than psychotherapy (Vaillant 2005).

Although he deserves credit for putting emotions on the medical map, Freud intellectualized love by calling it *libido* and confusing it with lust. Nowhere in the 24 volumes of his collected writings did he mention "joy." To keep tender passions at bay, psychoanalysis is still often conducted without eye contact. By lumping three positive emotions (contentment, excitement, and joy) together as *pleasure*, Freud obscured our ability to build a satisfactory theory of affects. In a letter to Freud, the novelist Romaine Rolland suggested that the "oceanic feeling" associated with joy was not a cognitive belief in God, but a major emotion (Jones 1995, p. 87). The brilliant Princeton psychologist Sylvan Tomkins (1962) pointed out that dynamic psychology, in general, and Freud, in particular, had each tended "to limit themselves to the ramifications of the affects of fear and anger and to the hypothalamic drives of sex and hunger" (p. 396). Thus, Tomkins had to remind psychologists—had to remind us all—that we cannot understand human beings unless we understand love and joy and how they come to be. Tomkins suggests that joy often binds us to people who have first produced and then reduced pain. Certainly, without the pain of farewell, there can be no joy in reunion. Without the pain of disapproval, there can be no joy in forgiveness. Thus, just as hope, love, forgiveness, and compassion are all connected with suffering, so too is joy. Terrible things happen in life, and positive emotions do not *deny* them. Tomkins goes on to suggest that implicit in Freudian theory "is a hidden—indeed rather puritan—value judgment that the early communion between mother and child is to be transcended in development. . . . This we take to be a blindness to the enduring positive and universal values for human beings. It reflects a puritanical prejudice against dependency per se and an insensitivity for a type of communion in which separateness is transcended through complete mutuality" (Tomkins 1962, p. 421).

In short, love and joy are scary—at least to academics. On the one hand, they make us feel both vulnerable and not in control. On the other hand, both Freud and Marx failed to understand that love and joy, the soothing processes inherent in spiritual and/or human communion, are a major source of the very community building that they both held dear and that pleasure is not the same as joy. For example, joy is not a substitute for sex, but sex is very often a substitute for joy. More important, joy and pleasure differ because we can be tickled only in a relationship; we can masturbate anytime we choose.

Interaction With Social and Interpersonal Constructs

Rather than dismissing the positive emotions as Pollyanna denial, the task of coaches, counselors, and clinicians is to help "hold" patients as they wrestle with the vulnerability of experiencing and "containing" love and joy, just as they have helped their clients experience and contain grief and rage. In other words, if social supports are important to resilience, their effect is complexly mediated. First, social supports not only must be present but also must be recognized and then internalized. Social experience is not just what happens to you; it is what you do with what happens to you. Just as part of the skill of a good football running back is the ability to find existing blockers, part of resilience is the ability to identify and take in the positive emotions within one's interpersonal matrix. In addition, resilience is often the ability not only to identify but also to bond with the one good family member, teacher, or neighbor within a matrix of disappointing ones. Such bonding involves reciprocity. In tracing how vulnerable poor children in Kauai became effective adults, Emmy Werner (Werner and Smith 1982) stressed the importance of being a "cuddly" child who elicits predominantly positive responses from the environment and who manifests skill at recruiting substitute parents. Such good fortune often depends on a temperamental match, or what Thomas and Chess (1984) called "goodness of fit." However, as the life of actress Marilyn Monroe sadly illustrated, being cuddly is not enough. One must be able to take in the love that one is given.

At the Universities of Michigan and North Carolina, Barbara Fredrickson and her coworkers did the most important work in demonstrating that the positive emotions and their effect on both vagal (parasympathetic) tone and interpersonal relations play an intrinsic role in both biological and mental health. Citing their own work and that of others, they demonstrated that "compared with people in affectively neutral control conditions, people randomly assigned to experience positive emotion show greater social engagement, social inclusiveness... self disclosure, interpersonal trust and compassion" (Kok et al. 2013, p. 1124).

In the Harvard Study of Adult Development, a fortunate choice of mates was often lifesaving to the resilience of men who, up to that point, had experienced poor success in recruiting love, but only if they "metabolized it" (in other words, took the love in). As Harry Harlow demonstrated through his follow-up on monkeys raised with inanimate mothers made from wire and terry cloth, one cannot mature without social supports, and as the studies of autism and schizophrenia demonstrate, one cannot mature if one does not absorb the love that is offered. I suspect that the capacity to appreciate what is good and nourishing in available social supports is the limbic counterpart of an optimistic style of cognitive attribution and appraisal. Of course, the process of metabolizing social supports is far subtler. Clinicians can teach people *ideas*. They can teach someone to view a glass as half full rather than half empty; they can teach people to have positive attributions. However, how to teach people the ability to treat an onrush of love as a gift, and not a threat, is a more daunting task.

To treat the experience of being loved as if it were a gift and neither a danger nor a right, people sometimes need help to be able to recognize and absorb those who love them now and to remember those who loved them in the past. Just as some people regard a Rockefeller or a Rothschild trust fund as a destabilizing burden, some people are panicked by love.

Indeed, love, hope, and faith or trust are inextricably entwined. How can a child caught in the middle of a divorce or an exam failure or a child languishing in a refugee camp remember that once things used to be better? How can he or she continue to have faith that "this too shall pass"? Hope and faith (by which I mean basic trust not a religious ideology) are, after all, very simple words, but they encompass an essential facet of resilience. It is no accident that hope has been viewed, from the days of Pandora, as the psychic balm on which resilience depends. The induction and support of positive emotion should play a major role in any psychotherapy.

Involuntary Coping Mechanisms

When faced with unmanageable stress, a person can cope in three quite different ways to avoid being overwhelmed: he or she can 1) employ prerehearsed cognitive coping strategies that permit conscious and voluntary mastery of his or her problems (e.g., applying a tourniquet to a bleeding arm), 2) turn to social supports for help (e.g., going to the emergency room), or 3) deploy involuntary biological mechanisms (e.g., clotting his or her own blood). Similarly, involuntary mental mechanisms, analogous to involuntary physical responses, reflect the ways that the brain alters inner and outer reality to reduce stress. Another word for this process is *homeostasis*. However, homeostasis does not capture the full power of posttraumatic growth. For example, Mother Theresa, who had a miserable childhood and agonizing internal doubts about her own faith, won the Nobel Prize for helping others through a posttraumatic use of *altruism* that was more than merely voluntary.

Although such involuntary behavior may strike observers as pathological or at least peculiar (hanging out with lepers is not most people's idea of a day at the beach), such involuntary behaviors are often creative, healthy, comforting, empathic, and lifesaving. However, although they relieve the individual's distress, some involuntary mental mechanisms, analogous to autoimmune diseases, are generally maladaptive: the compulsive dissociation of the addict, the projection of the paranoid bigot, and the somatizations of the angry help-rejecting complainer. Other involuntary mental mechanisms that may distort inner and outer reality are empathic and adaptive: the sublimation of a depressed Beethoven putting music to Schiller's "Ode to Joy" in the Ninth Symphony, the suppression and stoicism of Butch, and the humor of successful comics with miserable childhoods (e.g., Marilyn Monroe and Charlie Chaplin). Abraham Lincoln and Nelson Mandela, both men with traumatic pasts, used humor to transform the world, and they represent stunning examples of posttraumatic growth.

Adaptive Versus Maladaptive Involuntary Mechanisms

I have used three diverse 70-year prospective studies of lives—Lewis Terman's gifted women (Holahan and Sears 1995), the Gluecks' nondelinquent inner city men (Glueck and Glueck 1968), and the college men from the Harvard Study of Adult Development (Vaillant 1977)—to separate maladaptive, narcissistic, involuntary mechanisms from adaptive, empathic mechanisms. Using consensus definitions from the literature, I selected, first by hypothesis and then by empirical study (Vaillant 1993), five mechanisms that appeared to be adaptive in all three cohorts: humor, altruism, sublimation, anticipation, and suppression. The older psychoanalytic term *adaptive defense* and its synonyms *healthy denial* and *positive illusions* can have two connotations. The first is transformative (turning lead into gold), and the second is mundane (making the best out of a bad situation). Whether such a psychological healing response is seen as miraculous or merely a patch-up job depends on point of view; for example, is optimal wound healing the extraordinary result of fibroblast migration and the delicate involuntary ballet of platelets, thromboplastin, factor VII, and other ingredients in the serum (neither too much nor too little) that permits blood to clot or *just* a survival mechanism leaving a scar? Each adaptive or healthy mechanism involves the ballet of keeping idea and affect, subject and object, conscience and reality clearly in mind, if not in awareness, while simultaneously attenuating the mental conflict.

Involuntary coping mechanisms affect modes of feeling, thought, or behavior and are relatively unconscious. They arise in response to perceptions of psychic danger or conflict, unexpected change in the internal or external environment, or cognitive dissonance (American Psychiatric Association 1994). They obscure or diminish stressful mental representations that, if unmitigated, would give rise to depression or anxiety. They can alter perception of any or all of the following: *subject* (self), *object* (other person), *idea*, or *emotion*. In addition, these mechanisms dampen awareness of and response to sudden changes in reality, in emotions and desires, in conscience, and in relationships with people. Involuntary coping mechanisms can keep emotions within bearable limits during sudden changes in emotional life, such as the death of a loved one. They can deflect or deny sudden increases in biological drives, such as heightened sexual awareness and aggression during adolescence. Such mechanisms also give individuals a period of respite to master changes in self-image that cannot be immediately integrated. Examples of such changes might be puberty, an amputation, or even a promotion. Involuntary coping mechanisms can mitigate inevitable crises of conscience (e.g., placing a parent in a nursing home). Finally, defenses enable individuals to attenuate unresolved conflicts with important people, living or dead.

Similar to physiological homeostasis but in contrast to so-called cognitive coping strategies, involuntary coping mechanisms are usually deployed outside of awareness. As with hypnosis, the use of involuntary coping mechanisms compromises other facets of cognition.

Behavioral cases, obtained through multidecade longitudinal observation, have made it possible for the Harvard Study of Adult Development to devise a reliable rating of adaptive versus maladaptive involuntary mechanisms—a scientific safeguard not possible in psychoanalytic studies. By contrasting the involuntary coping styles of the longitudinally studied inner-city men, of the Terman women, and of the Harvard men (Vaillant 1993), the study reached several surprising conclusions. The relative adaptiveness of coping style was not the product of social class, IQ, gender, or education. For example, the 70 inner city men who manifested the most adaptive coping mechanisms were just as likely as the 73 men with the least adaptive mechanisms to have come from welfare families in social class V. In contrast, in midlife, only 1% of the men with the most adaptive coping mechanisms but 21% of the men with the least mature defenses were still in social class V. In short, deployment of adaptive coping mechanisms helped to catalyze escape from poverty.

Conscious Versus Unconscious Coping

Involuntary mental mechanisms raise the whole problem of "conscious" versus "unconscious," ingenious versus weird, coping versus "defensive" behavior. When Freud first recognized the phenomenon of what he was to label "defenses," he himself had difficulty believing that behavior, as seemingly purposeful and as subject to interpretation, could be unconscious. The debate continues, but I hope the following example clarifies the debate a little.

After I had participated in the Harvard Study of Adult Development for 30 years, an internist told me, with vividness and enthusiasm, about his hobby: growing tissue cultures in his basement. With still more interest and enthusiasm, he told me that the cells from one culture came from a lesion on his mother's leg. The physician viewed his hobby as unremarkable; outsiders saw growing one's mother in the basement as bizarre. I have yet to describe his hobby to an audience without laughter (perhaps transforming their negative emotion of horror) sweeping the room. At the end of the interview, the internist revealed—in the most matter-of-fact way—that his mother had died only 3 weeks earlier! Knowing from prior longitudinal study that he had been very attached to her, I asked how he had coped with his grief. His conscious explanation was that he used altruism; he had spent his time comforting his father. Behaviorally, however, he had been tending a tissue culture with the enthusiasm and warmth usually allotted to real people and had just described the recent death of a beloved person with the blandness usually allotted to tissue cultures. In other words, a grown child's very real love was displaced from his deceased mother and reattached to a tissue culture, an example of the coping mechanism of displacement. Twenty-five years later when I asked about his unusual hobby, he did not remember it at all!

Involuntary coping mechanisms involve far more than simple neglect or repression of reality. They reflect integrated dynamic psychological processes. Like their physiological analogues of involuntary response to tissue injury (redness, heat, pain, and swelling), they reflect healthy, often highly coordinated responses to stress rather than a deficit state or learned voluntary adaptation. Thus, involuntary coping mechanisms have more in common with an opossum involuntarily but skillfully playing dead than with either the biological paralysis of polio or the consciously controlled evasive maneuvers of a football halfback.

Involuntary Coping Mechanisms as Pathology Versus Adaptation

Implicit in Sigmund Freud's original concept of *abwehr,* or defense, was the conviction that the patient's idiosyncratic unconscious response to stress shapes psychopathology. However, just as physicians no longer classify a cough as a disease but as an adaptive involuntary mechanism for coping with respiratory obstruction, clinicians must learn to respond to involuntary adaptive mechanisms not as denial to be interpreted but as a sometimes healthy response to be facilitated. Beethoven's impulsive commitment to put joy to music in the Ninth Symphony probably did him more good than all the cognitive therapy in the world.

All styles of involuntary coping are effective in denying or defusing conflict and in "repressing" or minimizing stress, but the mechanisms differ greatly in the severity of the psychiatric diagnoses assigned to their users, and like emotions, they lie along a continuum from self-centered to empathic. Just as negative emotions are all about the self and positive emotions are all about the other, the most adaptive mechanisms (humor, sublimation, suppression, anticipation, altruism) are relatively selfless, whereas the most maladaptive mechanisms (projection, fantasy, dissociation, passive aggression, hypochondriasis, and acting out), although equally effective in mitigating anxiety and depression, are narcissistic and irritating to others.

Construct Limitations

It should be noted that there are real drawbacks to the concept of adaptive involuntary coping mechanisms. Our definitions of such mechanisms are vague, overlapping, and ambiguous. Everybody has a different name for them. Like the study of personality types, for which Gordon Allport discovered 30,000 labels, the study of coping mechanisms (or shall we call them "defenses" or "positive illusions" or "hardiness"?) lacks a stable nomenclature. A review by Beutel (1988) listed 37 labels used by 17 psychoanalytically oriented catalogers of defenses; worse yet, reasonable consensus was reached for only 5 of the 37 defenses listed by Beutel. In 1986, within 50 miles of San Francisco, six competing, nonoverlapping nomenclatures for involuntary coping mechanisms were in use. Each nomenclature was used by a distinguished investigator of stress.

On the one hand, involuntary coping mechanisms, like positive emotions, can be formulated as crisis-driven dynamic processes; on the other hand, coping mechanisms, like positive emotions, can be regarded as stable character traits. Is snow a once in a lifetime "crisis" or a stable characteristic of winter? Clearly, snow is often one or the other or both. Sometimes coping mechanisms are situation specific, and sometimes they are generalizable. In most cases, paranoid (using projection) individuals are narcissistic and unpleasant, but during the Battle of Britain they made wonderful airplane spotters.

From the beginning, coping mechanisms posed a problem for experimental psychology. First, clinicians have as much difficulty accepting involuntary adaptive coping mechanisms as they do accepting positive emotions. Both violate the clinician's wish to remain in control.

Second, no clear line separates symptoms of brain disease and unconscious coping processes. For example, sometimes one's obsessions are due to genetic factors alleviated by selective serotonin reuptake inhibitors; sometimes obsessions are efforts at conflict resolution via intellectualization, displacement, and reaction formation; and sometimes they are both. In addition, behaviors associated with involuntary coping can arise from sources other than conflict. For example, altruism can result from conscious gratitude and empathy as well as from conflict.

Additional Comments on Involuntary Coping Mechanisms

In the last 40 years, several empirical studies have suggested that it is possible to arrange defense mechanisms into a hierarchy of relative psychopathology (e.g., from projection [paranoia] to displacement [phobia] to sublimation [art]) and also to place them along a continuum of personality development (Vaillant 1977). For example, with the passage of decades, a sexually abused child's coping style could mature from *acting out* (e.g., engaging in rebellious promiscuity) to *reaction formation* (joining a convent where sex is bad and celibacy is good) to *altruism* (working as a mature middle-age nun counseling pregnant teenage mothers).

Common to everyday life are the relatively maladaptive involuntary behaviors found in adolescence, immature adults, and individuals with personality disorders. They externalize responsibility and cause individuals with personality disorders to appear to refuse help. Such coping styles are narcissistic; they are often traits rather than momentary states and are negatively correlated with mental health. They profoundly distort the affective component of human relationships. The use of involuntary styles such as projection, tantrums, and help-rejecting complaining causes more immediate suffering to others than to the user.

Maladaptive coping mechanisms rarely respond to verbal interpretation alone. They can be breached by confrontation, often by a group of supportive peers. These maladaptive styles can also be breached by improving psychological homeostasis, for example, by rendering the individual less vulnerable and lonely through empathic social support or less tired and hungry through rest and food or less intoxicated through sobriety or less adolescent through maturation.

The most common intermediate coping styles, sometimes referred to as "neurotic" or "the psychopathology of everyday life," include mechanisms such as *repression* (deleting the idea associated with a conscious emotion, e.g., forgetting a dental appointment), *intellectualization* (deleting the emotion from a conscious idea, e.g., cutting open a patient's abdomen without emotion), and *displacement* (transferring emotion to a more neutral object). In contrast to less adaptive defenses, the defenses of "neurosis" are manifested clinically by phobias, compulsions, obsessions, somatizations, and amnesias. Those who use such defenses often seek psychological help, and such behaviors respond more readily to interpretation. In addition, such styles usually cause more suffering to the user than to those in the environment.

Mature empathic involuntary adaptive coping styles still distort and alter both awareness of and emotional response to the stresses of strong emotion, conscience, relationships, and reality, but they perform these tasks gracefully and flexibly. For example, to the onlooker, the fact that the depressed, lonely, angry Beethoven put Schiller's "Ode to Joy" to music (i.e., sublimation) could reflect extraordinary denial, but this action was financially rewarding, instinctually gratifying, and perhaps lifesaving for the composer.

Adaptive or mature defenses (*altruism, sublimation, suppression, humor, anticipation*) are common among the mentally healthy and become more salient as individuals mature from adolescence to midlife (Vaillant 1977). In keeping with the conceptualization of positive psychology, the association of mature defenses with mental health remains whether health is measured by subjective happiness, psychosocial maturity, occupational success, richness and stability of relationships, or absence of psychopathology (Vaillant 1993). Individuals with brain damage (e.g., alcohol intoxication, schizophrenic relapse, multiple sclerosis) replace adaptive defenses with more maladaptive mechanisms, most notably projection.

Illustrative Examples

In keeping with positive psychology, adaptive defenses often appear just as moral to the observer as maladaptive defenses appear immoral. The prejudice of projection and the tantrums of acting out appear to others to be sins. In contrast, doing as one would be done to (altruism), "turning lemons into lemonade" (sublimation), planning for the future (anticipation), and the ability not to take one's self too seriously (humor), as well as a stiff upper lip (suppression), are the very stuff with which positive psychology should be concerned. Let me illustrate these involuntary but adaptive mechanisms one by one.

Altruism

First, let me provide an example of *altruism*. My wife, at the time 5 months pregnant, was interviewing a couple from the inner city sample of the Harvard Study of Adult Development for which the study offered no compensation. The greatest pain in the couple's life was having lost six infants because of Rh incompatibility. As my wife got up to leave, the childless woman, whose grief and envy can only be imagined, gave my wife a handsome, handmade baby sweater. The lives of everyone in the room had been suddenly enriched.

Sublimation

Clinical Vignette

Like Beethoven, Ben Bright, a participant in the Harvard Study of Adult Development, was a poster child for *sublimation*. His mother's brother had spent 2 years in a penitentiary; his father had been arrested for both larceny and alcohol abuse. When he was young, Ben grew up in a tenement without central heating, and he repeated ninth grade. At age 25, he read only tabloids and comics, and as far as the interviewer could tell, he was unable to add or multiply. At age 31, he was working as a truck driver's helper for only slightly more than the minimum wage.

On the positive side, Ben belonged to a three-generation family where everyone stayed very close. Ben's mother was a very good housekeeper, and by middle life his father had become hardworking, sober, and strict. Of her seven children, Ben was his mother's favorite. Of the 14-year-old Ben, she said, "He never plays. He goes to school, works after school; and in the summertime, he works all day." A little Calvinistic perhaps, but with an IQ of 79, he had to try harder. The adjectives that the interviewer used to describe Ben were "extroverted, adventurous, emotionally stable, conscientious, practical, *aggressive*." Ben saw both of his parents in a positive light and experienced their discipline as "firm but kindly" (Vaillant 1993).

In young adulthood, being a policeman had been Ben's dream, but he had been unable to pass the entrance exams. Instead, he began work for the San Jose Department of Recreation, and very quickly he was promoted to supervisor. At the time, Ben appeared to the interviewer as a "very virile looking man, muscular, good physical shape, appeared quite young for his age, talked easily with much candor, good eye contact, high energy level, responded to questions easily with his feelings." "He conveyed a certain excitement about playing sports and working with kids. He had self assurance, confidence and candor."

In his park job, Ben sometimes lost his temper, but he never got into physical fights. In his use of aggression, Ben illustrated sublimation. He used his anger to solve problems rather than to cause difficulty. The interviewer noted that most of his fights "seem to come from his protectiveness of his facilities or his staff." In inner-city life, the resistance of others had to be forcibly overcome but for worthy ends. He had used his assertiveness both to ensure playing-field etiquette against aggressive coaches and, at a time when he had no money, to get his son's cleft palate repaired by a sluggish urban welfare bureaucracy. Family conflicts were solved by the entire Bright family gathering like a team around the dining room table to "get it out of our system and not carry it around inside of us."

By age 60, Ben had been repeatedly promoted and was making $100,000 a year (in 2010 dollars). Because of his learning difficulties, he still had to delegate his paperwork to his wife, but as he boasted to the interviewer, "They love me because I'm rough and honest." It is interesting that two of Ben's sons have become policemen.

Another example of sublimation comes from studying college professors who participated in the Harvard Study of Adult Development. In terms of their Harvard grades and tested intellectual aptitudes, the men in the college sample with brilliant teaching careers at Stanford and Harvard were not more gifted than fellow study members teaching joylessly at mediocre institutions. Rather, too often, the less successful professors in the college cohort used displacement and isolation so compulsively that their cognitive academic interests were stripped of affect and passion. In contrast, in every facet of their lives, not just in their teaching and publishing, the successful professors were more comfortable in coloring their ideas with the pigment of emotion (Vaillant 1977). They all scored high in *sublimation*.

Anticipation

Anticipation differs in an important way from using cognitive isolation of affect and intellectualization to make soothing "lists." Anticipation involves more than just the ideational work of cognitive planning. Anticipation involves both thinking and feeling about the future. For example, consider legendary aviators such as Charles Lindbergh and Chuck Yeager. They calmly survived exciting flying careers by dealing with anxiety as Mithridates did with poison—taking a little at a time. To have underestimated danger would have been fatal. To have exaggerated danger would have been emotionally incapacitating. Thus, in contrast to Scarlett O'Hara's philosophy of "I'll think about that tomorrow," these aviators worried in advance, they made lists, and they practiced. Then, appreciating that they had prepared as well as they could, they relaxed. Like suppression and altruism, anticipation is very easy to prescribe but very difficult to do.

Humor

Everyone recognizes that *humor* makes life easier. As Freud (1905/1960) suggested, "Humor can be regarded as the highest of these defensive processes," for humor "scorns to withdraw the ideational content bearing the distressing affect from conscious attention, as repression does, and thus surmounts the automatism of defense" (p. 233). Humor permits the expression of emotion without individual discomfort and without unpleasant effects on others. Humor, like anticipation and suppression, is such a sensible coping device that it ought to be conscious, yet almost by definition, humor always surprises people. Like the other mature defenses, humor requires the same delicacy as building a house of cards— timing is everything. The safety of humor, like the safety of dreams during rapid eye movement (REM) sleep, depends on cataplexy. People see all and feel much, but they do not act. Like involuntary coping in general, humor is difficult to illustrate. Like a rainbow, humor is real but forever evades our grasp.

Professional Resistance to Involuntary Coping Constructs

When I first became involved in the Harvard Study of Adult Development, I felt sure that mastering stress with adaptive coping would play a role in men's longevity; the 50-year-old men with adaptive coping always "felt" so much better than the others. Now that the Harvard men are 90, I have found adaptive defenses transform only the perception of reality, not reality itself. Thus, adaptive defenses dramatically predicted both social support and the absence of subjective physical disability up to 30 years later, but adaptive, empathic coping defenses did not predict physical health decline (objective) when assessed by an independent internist (Vaillant 2012).

As early as 1970, involuntary defense (coping) mechanisms, popularized by psychoanalysis, appeared to be too metaphysical to empirical psychopathologists. Such mechanisms were excluded from DSM-III (American Psychiatric Association 1980) because when a select group of psychoanalysts, including me, were challenged by DSM-III's empirically grounded editors, we could not agree on their definition. Years later, as a result of interdisciplinary negotiation, involuntary coping mechanisms were included as a glossary in DSM-III-R (American Psychiatric Association 1987), and more years later still, because social scientists, only some of whom were psychoanalysts, reached consensual definitions, defenses became a clinical schema included as an optional axis for DSM-IV.

However, the argument did not stop there. Involuntary coping mechanisms have been dropped again from DSM-5 (American Psychiatric Association 2013). In the words of one clinician invited to advise the DSM-5 Task Force (Berkson 2009), "I proposed adding a dimension of 'mechanisms of defense' to the phenomenological criteria already existing in DSM-IV.... It would also be another way of looking at personality disorders.... The response of the Task Force to my proposal was patronizing, condescending, and insulting."

Are Freud's defenses and DSM-IV's coping mechanisms to be regarded as fictions in the same way that Skinner maintained that emotions could be dismissed as "fictions"? Or do we have to take the creative denial of Beethoven, the involuntary grit of Butch, and the coping behavior of the "doctor who grew his mother in the basement" seriously? The jury is still out.

Originally, building on the work of Norma Haan (1977) at Berkeley, I tried to operationalize defenses and to demonstrate their predictive validity (Vaillant 1977, 1993). Since then, experimental strategies for studying involuntary coping mechanisms have improved (Cramer 1991; Horowitz 1988; Perry et al. 2009; Vaillant 1992). However, as suggested by Phoebe Cramer's (1991) encyclopedic review of the methodology for identifying and quantifying defenses, no one has yet developed a method for assessing them that meets conventional standards for psychometric reliability. Nevertheless, it is good to remember that astronomers, by observing regular distortions of the orbits of other planets, had evidence-based certainty of Neptune's existence years before the planet was visualized by a telescope. Nevertheless, involuntary coping, no matter how ingeniously relabeled or assessed, reflects value judgments about mental process, as do process concepts in physics (e.g., forward motion and velocity). All three, velocity, forward motion, and defenses, depend on the vantage point of the observer and involve processes rather than static qualities like mass or the imagery of functional magnetic resonance imaging (fMRI). Nevertheless, if people wish to understand their own lives in time and space, process concepts are judgments worth making.

Final Thoughts

In nonconflictual situations, of course, the putative "mechanisms" of anticipation, altruism, and suppression can seem quite conscious and voluntary. In highly emotionally charged situations, however, the involuntary deployment of these mechanisms can be seen as transformative. Just try to be as funny as Nelson Mandela was to his guards on Robben Island or as stoical as Butch on purpose. Such transformative behaviors often emerge with maturation as delicate mental balancing acts rather than as a result of good advice and self-help cognitive strategies. However, in permitting, even fostering, such adaptive "denial" rather than interpreting or interfering with it, a good therapist, friend, or parent is invaluable. Outsiders can help provide a vulnerable person with the safety to try something new rather than just offer sound cognitive advice. "Holding" a person riskily replacing a maladaptive coping mechanism with an adaptive one is akin to holding Inspector Javert in the musical *Les Misérables* while he tolerated the vulnerability of gratitude toward Jean Valjean for saving his life rather than resentfully killing himself by jumping into the Seine.

Summary

In the sixteenth century, the barber surgeon Ambroise Paré famously wrote, "I dressed the wound, God healed him." Indeed, in those days wound healing was usually made worse by external intervention. During World War II, perhaps the most important surgical discovery was how to maintain electrolyte and fluid balance and thereby facilitate an individual's inner-directed capacity for wound healing. In this chapter, I have described "the self-righting tendencies within the human organism" that permit positive well-being (Werner and Smith 1982). To offer an evidence-based, if extreme, example, I compare the effectiveness of Esalen, psychopharmacology, and psychotherapy with Alcoholics Anonymous in efforts to prevent relapse to alcoholism. Esalen, a retreat in California that costs hundreds of dollars a day, offers New Age experts to guide "self-help"; there is no evidence that this self-help prevents alcoholic relapse. Similarly, despite initial enthusiasm, over the long term, there is no evidence that "magic bullets" like disulfiram, acamprosate, and LSD (in the hands of Bill W., the founder of AA) prevent sustained relapse. Dynamic psychotherapy, which gives pride of place to the negative emotions of sadness and anger and interprets "ego defenses" in order to breach the alcoholic's denial, has been equally ineffective in preventing relapse. Even cognitive-behavioral therapy, in its efforts to achieve the longed-for mirage of "moderation management," has been shown by long-term follow-up to be less effective than AA in preventing relapse, as illustrated by the evidence-based science of one of cognitive-behavioral therapy's most skilled practitioners (Miller et al. 1992).

In contrast, there is evidence-based proof of the efficacy of AA in preventing relapse and promoting posttraumatic growth. Alcoholics in stable remission (mean of 19 years) attend 20 times as many AA meetings with their "attitude of gratitude" as matched controls who remain in relapse all their lives (Vaillant 2005). AA emphasizes the alcoholic's "self-righting tendencies." Consider AA's permission for suppression—that is, abstinence rather than the popular but, over the long term, relapse-promoting wish for moderation management (Vaillant 1995). Consider the positive emotions in AA's eleventh-step prayer (showcased as this chapter's epigraph) and the gratitude, love, and joy evoked by alcoholics twelfth stepping the "still suffering alcoholic." Just like opiates, joy and love are shown by fMRI studies to activate the nucleus accumbens. In contrast to dynamic psychotherapy, AA gives permission to its members to indulge in altruism without interpretation. Consider the inevitable, lifegiving, spontaneous humor present in its meetings. An outside observer might inwardly shout "denial." Therapists, family members, and patients alike need to continue to value the external healing power of integrative medicine, of psychopharmacology, and of cognitive and psychodynamic therapy. At the same time, they must also foster the internal self-righting powers of their clients, their relatives, and themselves.

Clinical Key Points

- Important inner sources of resilience are positive emotions and involuntary mental coping mechanisms. Expressed in one sentence, the cornerstone of positive emotion is the capacity to give and receive love. Conveyed in one sentence, the cornerstone of involuntary coping is mental wound healing, or, expressed metaphorically, the involuntary psychic capacity to spin straw into gold.

- Reviewing the 40 years that I have spent on the study of development, I realized that it was the things that go *right* in our lives, rather than the things that go *wrong,* that shape our futures. This conclusion is congruent with Sir Michael Rutter's summary of his own work on resilience (Rutter 1986).

- Rather than dismissing the positive emotions as Pollyanna-like denial, the task of coaches, counselors, and clinicians is to "hold" patients while they wrestle with the vulnerability of experiencing and containing love, trust, gratitude, and joy, just as they have helped patients experience and contain grief and rage.

- Although it is an unfamiliar concept except in arcane psychoanalytic discourse, the ability to take love in is the most important internal psychological trait that there is; Butch was a poster child for this trait, even if it took him 25 years to find love.

- Just as physicians no longer classify a cough or a sneeze as pathological but as an adaptive involuntary mechanism for coping with respiratory obstruction, clinicians must learn to respond to involuntary adaptive mechanisms not as denial to be interpreted but as a healthy response to be facilitated.

References

American Psychiatric Association: Diagnostic and Statistical Manual of Mental Disorders, 3rd Edition. Washington, DC, American Psychiatric Association, 1980

American Psychiatric Association: Diagnostic and Statistical Manual of Mental Disorders, 3rd Edition, Revised. Washington, DC, American Psychiatric Association, 1987

American Psychiatric Association: Diagnostic and Statistical Manual of Mental Disorders, 4th Edition. Washington, DC, American Psychiatric Association, 1994

American Psychiatric Association: Diagnostic and Statistical Manual of Mental Disorders, 5th Edition. Arlington, VA, American Psychiatric Association, 2013

Benson H: Timeless Healing. New York, Scribners, 1996

Berkson RP: DSM-V: Mind made up? Psychiatric Times, July 16, 2009

Beutel M: Bewältigungsprozesse Bei Chronischen Erkrankungen. Weinheim, Germany, VCH Edition Medizin, 1988

Cramer P: The Development of Defense Mechanisms. New York, Springer-Verlag, 1991

Fredrickson BL: The role of positive emotions in positive psychology: the broaden-and-build theory of positive emotions. Am Psychol 56(3):218–226, 2001 11315248

Freud S: Jokes and their relation to the unconscious (1905), in The Standard Edition of the Complete Psychological Works of Sigmund Freud, Vol 8. Translated and edited by Strachey J. London, Hogarth Press, 1960, pp 9–236

Glueck S, Glueck E: Delinquents and Non-Delinquents in Perspective. Cambridge, MA, Harvard University Press, 1968

Haan N: Coping and Defending. New York, Academic Press, 1977

Holahan CK, Sears RR: The Gifted Group in Later Maturity. Stanford, CA, Stanford University Press, 1995

Horowitz MJ: Introduction to Psychodynamics: A New Synthesis. New York, Basic Books, 1988

Isen AM, Rosenzweig AS, Young MJ: The influence of positive affect on clinical problem solving. Med Decis Making 11(3):221–227, 1991 1881279

Jones JM: Affects as Process. London, Analytic Press, 1995

Kok BE, Coffey KA, Cohn MA, et al: How positive emotions build physical health: perceived positive social connections account for the upward spiral between positive emotions and vagal tone. Psychol Sci 24(7):1123–1132, 2013 23649562

Lazarus RS, Folkman S: Stress, Appraisal, and Coping. New York, Springer, 1984

Linley PA, Joseph S: Positive change following trauma and adversity: a review. J Trauma Stress 17(1):11–21, 2004 15027788

Masten AS, Garmezy N: Risk, vulnerability and protective factors in developmental psychopathology, in Advances in Clinical Child Psychology, Vol 8. Edited by Lahey BB, Kasdin AE. New York, Plenum, 1985, pp 1–52

Meyer MF: The whale among the fishes: the theory of emotions. Psychol Rev 40:292–300, 1933

Miller WR, Leckman AL, Delaney HD, Tinkcom M: Long-term follow-up of behavioral self-control training. J Stud Alcohol 53(3):249–261, 1992 1583904

Perry JC, Beck SM, Constantinides P, Foley JE: Studying change in defensive functioning in psychotherapy, using the Defense Mechanism Rating Scales: four hypotheses, four cases, in Handbook of Evidenced Based Psychodynamic Psychotherapy: Bridging the Gap Between Science and Practice. Edited by Levy RA, Ablon JS. New York, Humana Press, 2009, pp 121–153

Peterson C, Seligman ME: Character strengths before and after September 11. Psychol Sci 14(4):381–384, 2003 12807415

Rutter M: Meyerian psychobiology, personality development, and the role of life experiences. Am J Psychiatry 143(9):1077–1087, 1986 3529992

Sadock BJ, Sadock VA, Ruiz P: Comprehensive Textbook of Psychiatry, 8th Edition. Baltimore, MD, Williams & Wilkins, 2005

Seligman MEP: Authentic Happiness: Using the New Positive Psychology to Realize Your Potential for Lasting Fulfillment. New York, Free Press, 2002

Skinner BF: Science and Human Behavior. New York, Free Press, 1953

Thomas A, Chess S: Genesis and evolution of behavioral disorders: from infancy to early adult life. Am J Psychiatry 141(1):1–9, 1984 6691419

Tomkins SS: Affect Imagery Consciousness, Vol 1: The Positive Affects. New York, Springer, 1962

Vaillant GE: Adaptation to Life. Boston, MA, Little Brown, 1977

Vaillant GE: Ego Mechanisms of Defense: A Guide for Clinicians and Researchers. Washington, DC, American Psychiatric Press, 1992

Vaillant GE: Wisdom of the Ego. Cambridge, MA, Harvard University Press, 1993

Vaillant GE: Natural History of Alcoholism, Revisited. Cambridge, MA, Harvard University Press, 1995

Vaillant GE: Aging Well. Boston, MA, Little Brown, 2002

Vaillant GE: Alcoholics Anonymous: cult or cure? Aust N Z J Psychiatry 39(6):431–436, 2005 15943643

Vaillant G: Spiritual Evolution: A Scientific Defense of Faith. New York, Doubleday Broadway, 2008

Vaillant GE: Triumphs of Experience: The Men of the Harvard Grant Study. Cambridge, MA, The Belknap Press, 2012

Werner EE, Smith RS: Vulnerable but Invincible. New York, McGraw-Hill, 1982

Suggested Cross-References

Social factors are discussed in Chapter 4 ("Positive Social Psychiatry"), Chapter 5 ("Recovery in Mental Illnesses"), Chapter 11 ("Preventive Interventions"), Chapter 12 ("Integrating Positive Psychiatry Into Clinical Practice"), and Chapter 16 ("Bioethics of Positive Psychiatry"). Resilience is discussed in chapters 12 and 13 ("Biology of Positive Psychiatry"). Coping is discussed in Chapter 2 ("Positive Psychological Traits"). Positive emotions are discussed in Chapter 9 ("Positivity in Supportive and Psychodynamic Therapy").

4

Positive Social Psychiatry

DAN G. BLAZER, M.D., M.P.H., PH.D.

WARREN A. KINGHORN, M.D., TH.D.

To what extent are happiness and human flourishing social, rather than individual, phenomena? And how do healthy individuals and healthy communities and societies reciprocally enable each other? Because psychiatry and clinical psychology are organized around models of individual mental health and mental illness, these questions are often deferred to other social scientific disciplines such as sociology and organizational behavior.

Positive psychology, as it has emerged and matured over the past two decades, follows this same general trend. In the earliest days of the positive psychology movement, Seligman and Csikszentmihalyi (2000) included "positive institutions," along with positive subjective experience and positive individual traits, as a core subject of the science of positive psychology. Seligman and Csikszentmihalyi's (2000) focus on institutions "that move individuals toward better citizenship: responsibility, nurturance, altruism, civility, moderation, tolerance, and work ethic" (p. 5), follows naturally from the utopian aspirations evident in Seligman's 1998 American Psychological Association presidential address that first called for a "new science of human strengths":

> Entering a new millennium, we face a historical choice. Standing alone on the pinnacle of economic and political leadership, the United States can continue to increase its material wealth while ignoring the human needs of our people and of the people on the rest of the planet. Such a course is likely to lead to increasing

71

selfishness, alienation between the more and less fortunate, and eventually to chaos and despair....At this juncture, psychology can play an enormously important role. We can articulate a vision of the good life that is empirically sound and, at the same time, understandable and attractive. We can show the world what actions lead to well-being, to positive individuals, to flourishing communities, and to a just society. (Seligman 1999, p. 560)

As positive psychology has evolved and matured as a research discipline, contributors to the field have remained attentive to social and institutional contexts of flourishing. Many of the "character strengths and virtues" cataloged by Peterson and Seligman (2004) are clearly social, including the strengths of citizenship ("social responsibility, loyalty, teamwork"), fairness, and leadership, which collectively compose the virtue of justice. Positive psychology principles have been investigated in relation to educational systems, workplaces, and military culture (see chapters 53–56 of Lopez and Snyder's [2009] handbook for an overview), and considerable attention has been paid to prosocial emotions and behavior (Mikulincer and Shaver 2010). Furthermore, in his popular writing, Seligman proposes that the "long mission for positive psychology" should be that "by the year 2051, 51% of the people of the world will be flourishing," with implications for future geopolitical conflict (Seligman 2011, p. 240). However, within the literature of positive psychology, work on positive institutions is dwarfed by work on positive subjective experience and positive individual traits, and when individual traits are considered, they are often judged by their relationship to subjective well-being. Work on communities and institutions is often done not within positive psychology per se but within the related subdiscipline of positive organizational behavior.

If positive psychology has struggled to sustain attention to institutions and to the traits and behaviors that predict flourishing communities and institutions, such attention would seem even more of a challenge within positive psychiatry. Mental disorders, after all, are generally characterized in DSM-5 as "clinically significant disturbances in *an individual's* cognition, emotion regulation, or behavior" (American Psychiatric Association 2013, p. 20; emphasis added), and psychiatric research and practice are still organized primarily around the dyadic psychiatrist-patient encounter. Articulating a positive psychiatry that is not centered on psychopathology and disorder is itself a challenge for psychiatrists; articulating a positive *social* psychiatry would seem to be doubly so.

If this is the case, however, it was not always so. Psychiatry has not always been as individualistically oriented as it is now. Indeed, from the 1950s until the 1970s, *social psychiatry*, the study of the mental health of communities and of social correlates of mental health and mental illness, existed as a recognizable subfield within the psychiatric literature. In some ways, the mid-twentieth-century social psychiatry movement, focused on the prevention of mental illness through the cultivation of healthy communities, shared the utopian aspirations of some researchers within the modern positive psychology movement. These utopian aspirations arguably contributed to social psychiatry's marginalization within the increasingly medicalized American psychiatry of the 1970s, and we argue that this marginalization bears important lessons for any future positive psychiatry. However, the insights of mid-twentieth-century social psychiatry did not disappear; rather, they were increasingly considered in relation to the mental health of individuals, through the emergence of literature on social stressors and social support. Emerging in the aftermath of social psychiatry's prominence, these socially focused areas of inquiry no longer bore the culture-shaping aspirations of social psychiatry in its heyday; they sought to continue to explore only the impact of social environment and circumstances on individuals.

In this chapter, we consider how the history of social psychiatry might inform the articulation of positive social traits within a new field of positive psychiatry. Although the valuable literature of positive psychology ought to inform positive psychiatry, we argue that positive psychiatry should not simply involve an appropriation of the dominant themes of positive psychology into psychiatric research and practice. Psychiatry, after all, is its own discipline with its own distinct history, arising historically from the practice of attending to those who have various forms of mental and physical illness. The Greek roots of the nineteenth-century term *psychiatry* are *psyche* (mind or soul) and *iatreia* (healing); the idea that psychiatrists work with people who seek healing or curing of some kind is deeply woven into psychiatry's history and self-understanding.

Although it is logically conceivable that positive psychology might be concerned with only the promotion of happiness or flourishing, without any attention to mental and emotional suffering, it is less conceivable that positive psychiatry could ever be so. Positive psychiatry, we believe, will be credible, helpful, and sustainable to the degree that its attentiveness to happiness and flourishing emerges from the experience of attending to people and communities that are not flourishing but deeply desire health and meaning and wellness.

Attentiveness to the experience of people who suffer can and should cure positive psychiatry of any lingering utopian aspirations that psychiatric knowledge will somehow create cultures and communities where suffering is absent. However, in place of utopian aspirations, positive psychiatry can appropriate the hard-won insights of social psychiatry and its disciplinary successors, which view the health of individuals and the health of their communities as deeply integrated and interrelated. Positive psychiatry may, in fact, be an excellent medium through which to reintegrate these insights within psychiatry as a whole. In what follows, we briefly consider positive psychology's conceptualization of positive social traits and then turn to the history of social psychiatry. We conclude the chapter by proposing a conceptualization of *virtue* that is different from that proposed by Peterson and Seligman (2004) but that resonates both with the insights of social psychiatry and with Aristotle.

Positive Psychology and the Lessons of Social Psychiatry

Any investigation of social traits relevant to psychiatry must attend to the decades of research focusing on psychiatric disorders and emotional suffering embedded in social environments, particularly the social psychiatry movement, which was most prominent in the 1960s. Any such investigation must also attend to the study of social stressors and supports, which have been demonstrated through empirical research to modify the risk of psychiatric symptoms and disorders, to mediate their impact on the individual, and/or to protect the individual from other forms of stress. These studies do not seem particularly "positive," however. What might psychiatrists make of the elucidation of social traits within the positive psychology movement?

As mentioned, in the last 20 years, positive psychology has gained much traction as a response to decades of nearly exclusive focus on psychopathology within clinical psychology and psychiatry. However, the focus of psychiatry has been on the individual (individual diagnoses and therapies), and for the most part, positive psychology has also focused on the individual. The paucity of theory and research on the social environment in the positive psychology movement has been critiqued in both the professional and the popular press. For example, Gable and Haidt (2005) have critiqued positive psychology specifically for the lack of progress in research informing the development of positive institutions and communities. Seligman, for example, has performed and spawned extensive research on the ways that positive individual emotions and virtues contribute to individual happiness. Positive psychology has also demonstrated the benefit for happiness of strong family units. However, much less empirical support exists for Seligman's repeated assertions that democracy and free inquiry, for example, are causally related to happiness (Diener and Seligman 2002).

The absence of a clear evidence base regarding the mental health correlates of democracy and free inquiry renders positive psychology vulnerable to critics who charge that free inquiry and democracy, in the context of late modern capitalism, legitimize large and toxic environmental forces detrimental to the health and well-being of mere individuals (conversely, there is no body of evidence suggesting that any other sociopolitical system is a better alternative). However, even if the correlation between liberal democracy and happiness or well-being were proved beyond doubt, there is no evidence that any psychological intervention might change these macrolevel dynamics within a society. Positive psychology is therefore in a bind: not only might changing the environment be beyond the control of the mental health professions, but also it is not even clear that large-scale changes would improve mental health (Seligman 2002).

In her book *Bright-Sided,* journalist and social critic Barbara Ehrenreich (2008) takes on a variety of individual attitudes and behaviors that in her opinion presume that individuals can conquer the social environment in which they reside. Paradoxically, the impetus for these changes in behavior and attitudes is institutions. For example, she critiques evangelical Christian megachurches that preach the good news that you only have to want something to get it because God wants the believer (and the megachurch) to "prosper" as a reward for trust. Such promises ignore the realities of a tough economic environment that is out of the control of the individual. In an earlier book, Ehrenreich (2001) wrote of her own experience struggling to survive in low-wage jobs. She also critiques illness support groups for their emphasis on positive thinking as a presumed health benefit. Ehrenreich is a victim of breast cancer, and the pink ribbons emblemizing this positive attitude were especially abhorrent to her. She also challenges academia for instituting new departments of "positive psychology" and the "science of happiness," specifically targeting Seligman. Finally, she takes on large corporations for glossing over the realities of job loss and salary stagnation through pep talks and seminars on positive, individualistic approaches to career progression. What renders Ehrenreich's critique relevant to this chapter is that she largely focuses on social realities such as unemployment and suboptimal employment as well as a toxic social environment. In this context, she critiques therapeutic approaches that seek to cultivate positive emotions in individuals and yet provide little guidance on how the individual can effectively change the social environment.

In summary, critics of positive psychology have alleged that positive psychology underestimates the degree to which social environments can be unavoidably toxic and stressful, more dystopian than utopian. In this respect, these critics echo critics of social psychiatry in the 1960s and 1970s. Many psychiatrists are not aware that 60 years ago, numerous psychiatrists were attracted to what now appear to be utopian aspirations to fundamentally reconstitute social environments on the basis of psychiatric research and theory—a much more optimistic view of social change as a means to greater individual well-being. To be fair, none suggested that a utopia was possible; dystopian novels such as *Nineteen Eighty-Four* (Orwell 1948) and *Brave New World* (Huxley 1932) were still very much on everyone's minds. However, the interest of social psychiatrists in providing guidance toward a more positive social environment anticipated the broader push toward positive social change that pervaded the 1960s through movements such as the Civil Rights Movement and the Great Society. Such interests, although not utopian, were, nevertheless, most optimistic about the potential for a better society and coincided with general American social optimism leading into the 1960s.

In this chapter, we first review some of the early epidemiological studies, which were thoroughly grounded in the theory that optimal social environments enhance mental health and well-being, a key assertion of modern positive psychology. At least one study directly addressed the theoretical interconnection between positive social traits and an integrated social network in the facilitation of mental health. We then consider how, after the decline of social psychiatry as a field in the 1970s, research into social factors migrated from a focus on the social environment to a focus on individual stressors (e.g., stressful life events and daily hassles) and supports (e.g., social support). We conclude by arguing that positive psychiatry has the opportunity to draw on this research to focus not just on individuals in society but also on the health of communities.

Utopian Aspirations of Postwar Social Psychiatry

Of all the early epidemiological studies, the Stirling County Study was perhaps the most theoretically rich. The theoretical foundations of the study were presented in *My Name Is Legion* (Leighton 1959), and the core findings were given in *The Character of Danger* (Leighton et al. 1963). The motivating theory was that socially integrated communities would facilitate mental health, specifically by enhancing the development of what Leighton described as "striving sentiments." These sentiments could easily be viewed as positive social traits. He described sentiments as follows:

> Sentiments are the predominant ideas that are colored with emotion and feeling, that occur and recur more or less consistently, which govern acts and give a sense of knowing what to expect.... Sentiments therefore provide a framework in terms of which personalities may be characterized descriptively and then salient points explored and analyzed with reference to origins and determinants.... People are anchored in [a sense of] place and time. (Leighton et al. 1963, pp. 26–27)

The essential striving sentiments, according to Leighton, were physical security, sexual expression, the giving and receiving of love, spontaneity, a sense of orientation in relation to society, inclusion in a moral order, and inclusion in and of a system of values. What renders these sentiments unique from isolated personal characteristics is that they are "anchored" in the social environment; that is, they develop positively or are thwarted as a result of contingencies in the social environment. In other words, the study hypothesized that striving sentiments can flourish in socially integrated environments.

The Stirling County Study itself was an ecological study that compared the frequency of psychiatric disorder (or, more specifically, behaviors of psychiatric interest) in two socially integrated communities, a socially disintegrated community, and a mix of the two in a larger city in Nova Scotia (Leighton et al. 1963). Although emphasis was placed on the definition of social disintegration, descriptions of social integration can easily be derived by considering the inverse of the indices of social disintegration: low frequency of broken homes, strong associations within the communities, strong and competent leaders, ample opportunity for recreation, low frequency of hostility (angry outbursts), low frequency of crime and delinquency, effective lines of communication (e.g., telephone lines and roads), no recent history of disaster, overall good health, low levels of poverty, homogeneous culture, strong religious institutions, limited migration, and a slow pace of social change. The investigators did find lower frequency of behaviors of psychiatric interest in the integrated communities compared with disintegrated communities.

Five decades later, this list of indices of social integration looks almost Pollyannaish, perhaps displaying a bias toward idyllic rural communities in contrast to urban communities. That was not the intent of the investigators, who did not suggest that society could return to the small integrated communities described in the study that were selected for their contrast between integration and disintegration. However, the researchers did seek to investigate the relative frequency of psychiatric disorders in urban and rural communities—a distinction that even in that time was becoming quite difficult. They found that each social milieu expressed unique characteristics. In urban areas of developed countries, multiple communities overlap, and therefore, most individuals do not reside in a homogeneous social environment, moving from family to the workplace to social outlets to faith communities almost seamlessly. Even rural communities were beginning to mirror these urban characteristics at the time of the study. The Stirling County Study served as a model for other social psychiatry investigators, who found the characteristics developed by A.H. and D. Leighton to be attractive in some ways and overly restrictive in others.

The Stirling County Study was only one of a number of investigations into social correlates of mental health and mental illness in the 1950s and 1960s. Some social psychiatry investigators tended to idealize rural communities, hypothesizing that their tight-knit social fabric would protect against mental illness and incubate positive social traits. One such study to test these hypotheses empirically was Eaton and Weil's (1976) investigation of the Hutterites (a Christian sect resembling the Amish) in the northern Great Plains overlapping Canada and the United States. At the time of the study (1955), the small communities of Hutterites were extraordinarily stable and had been highly effective in providing cradle-to-grave support for their members. Contrary to initial hypotheses, however, psychiatric disorders were just as frequent among the Hutterites as in other communities, with the frequency of depression perhaps being even higher (at the time, prior to DSM-III (American Psychiatric Association 1980) and the rise of structured diagnostic interviews, it was very difficult to compare one study with another).

After Utopia: The Decline of Social Psychiatry and Rise of Social Stress and Social Support Research

Social psychiatry, so apparently promising in the optimistic context of postwar America in the 1950s and 1960s, saw its influence and status decline within American psychiatry in the late 1960s and 1970s (Blazer 2005). Initially weakened by its failure to demonstrate that primary prevention of mental disorders was possible by improving social conditions, it was targeted by the antipsychiatry voices of the 1960s (e.g., Thomas Szasz) and fell victim to the increasingly biological and medical focus of American psychiatry during the 1970s. In a review of social psychiatry's history, Flaherty and Astrachan (1999) reflect the profession's dominant self-narrative when they note that

> psychiatry has improved its image both within and outside the profession of medicine through rejection of the expansive and utopian promise of offering solutions to all social ills and by realigning with medicine to concentrate on nosological reliability, treatment of disease, and etiological and pathophysiological studies in neurosciences and molecular biology. (p. 39)

The decline of social psychiatry, however, did not mean the end for attentiveness to the social environment within psychiatric research. The focus, rather, shifted to the assessment of individual social stressors and social support. These literatures differed in important ways from the earlier social psychiatry literature, each marking the end of social psychiatry's utopian aspirations. First, both social support and social stressors are individual-centered concepts; they consider social factors insofar as these factors affect the experiences of individuals. Second, these constructs of stress and support were understood to be largely out of the control of the individual. Social stressors and social support can be measured and can be considered to be risks or mediators on the etiological pathway to psychiatric disorders (and positive mental health for that matter), yet the response of the individual is in the service of adaptation to a more or less intransigent social environment. These commitments to methodological individualism and to the presumptive intransigence of social environments follow naturally from the profession's loss of faith in the belief that psychiatric intervention could change social environments at a macrolevel or even a microlevel. In the post-utopian literature, positive social traits transitioned from characteristics enabling a health-producing society to characteristics that enable successful adaptation to intransigent (and sometimes hostile) social environments.

Studies on social stressors emerged from earlier studies that focused on socioeconomic status (SES). For example, Faris and Dunham (1939) found that first admission rates for most psychoses were highest in the central underresourced neighborhoods of Chicago. Like the Stirling County Study, this study was ecological. The association between individual SES and psychiatric symptoms has persisted in subsequent literature. Lorant et al. (2003), for example, found that persons with low SES were at twice the risk for incurring depression initially and experiencing persistent depression. Since the 1970s, however, researchers have generally not advocated systematic efforts to alter or change SES. Rather, in the literature, SES is assumed to be relatively static and unalterable; it is valuable primarily for identifying persons at disadvantage who might benefit from individual resources and clinical interventions. However, the development of even these resources, such as job training, has been at the periphery of psychiatric treatment.

Life stress, codified through a tabulation of stressful life events by Holmes and Rahe (1967), was found to lead to a higher risk for depressive symptoms and disease in both cross-sectional and longitudinal studies. Following Holmes' and Rahe's research, many subsequent studies have associated stressful life events with psychiatric disorders (Mazure et al. 1997). In addition, other researchers developed much more sophisticated approaches to assessing life stress, which included not only specific life events, such as the death of a spouse, but also daily hassles and chronic strain (Brown and Harris 1978; Dohrenwend 2006). These studies have focused most frequently on depression and have increasingly shown that life stress is associated with the onset, recovery or remission, relapse, and recurrence of depression. Given this emerging literature, many therapies that focus on adaptation to the environment have been developed to treat depression. Interpersonal psychotherapy, for example, is designed to assist the patient with adapting to changes in the environment or to ongoing stressors (Weissman et al. 2000). For example, the patient may be assisted with appropriate mourning in bereavement, including complicated bereavement; resolving an interpersonal struggle in a role dispute with another person; a life transition, such as mourning the loss of an old role and assuming a new one following retirement; or decreasing social isolation that results from poor social skills. Cognitive-behavioral therapy operates in a similar fashion. Modern psychotherapies such as interpersonal psychotherapy and cognitive-behavioral therapy carefully avoid any prediction that individual behaviors will improve the overall social environment; instead, they focus on the individual's adaptive negotiation with that environment.

Work in the area of social support follows a similar trend. Interest in social support originated in the recognition that social support assessment was a strong predictor of mortality in community-based populations (Berkman and Syme 1979; Blazer 1982). Social support has been considered to be a buffer for stressful life events. Furthermore, studies typically identify social support as a buffer to the effects of stressful events (George et al. 1989; Landerman et al. 1989). Social support research, however, has been plagued by its inability to demonstrate interventions that successfully enhance the social support available to individuals who need it.

These examples make it clear that psychiatry's interest in the social did not die completely in the 1970s, but rather shifted to the consideration of how (presumptively intransigent) social environments affect the mental health of individuals. Largely lost in the postutopian literature, however, were attempts to describe and articulate positive social traits that might not only enhance the ability of *individuals* to successfully negotiate their social environments but also change social environments for the better.

However, rare and promising exceptions to this general trend do exist, although they are generally sponsored within social scientific disciplines other than psychiatry. The Project on Human Development in Chicago Neighborhoods (PHDCN), for example, is an in-depth study of selected Chicago neighborhoods that seeks to map the social environmental characteristics of healthy communities (Sampson 2003, 2012). In this study, which echoes the mid-twentieth-century social psychiatry literature, the investigators found that physical and mental health were facilitated by the capacity of residents to achieve social control over their environment and to engage in collective action for the common good. They found that the strong ties among neighbors necessary for such proactive action are no longer the norm in many urban communities because friends and social support networks are not organized locally. Given this reality, the investigators proposed a "collective efficacy theory" in which they focused on the combination of working trust and shared willingness of residents to intervene in social control, a move away from reliance on personal ties. Specifically, they emphasized the importance of shared beliefs in a neighborhood's conjoint capability for action. For example, if a neighbor believed that a child was misbehaving, that neighbor needed to feel empowered to intervene without fear of retribution from the child's parents. Neighborhoods exhibiting a high collective efficacy manifested significantly lower rates of violence, which was, in turn, associated with physical and mental health outcomes in this investigation.

Reflecting prevailing assumptions about the static nature of the social environment, the PHDCN investigators noted that traditional thinking about disease has emphasized behavioral change among individuals as a means to reduce the risk for disease (e.g., smoking cessation interventions) (Sampson 2003). However, in the case of smoking, they found that environmental approaches such as taxation policies, regulation of smoking in public places, and restriction of advertising all contribute to reduction in the risky behavior of smoking (cf. Singer and Ryff 2001). We note, however, that these sorts of macrolevel approaches remain the exception rather than the rule in psychiatric research and practice, which continue to engage social environmental factors primarily to identify individuals at increased risk for mental disorder who would then be candidates for individual therapeutic interventions.

Beyond Utopia: Flourishing, Suffering, and Virtue in Positive Psychiatry

We began this chapter by referencing the prominence given to positive institutions within the early literature of positive psychology and the utopian aspirations of some of the field's prominent voices. We noted, however, that within positive psychology this focus on positive institutions has been overshadowed by the much greater attention given to positive subjective experience and positive individual traits. We then turned to psychiatry's own historical experience with utopian social thought as it was displayed in the postwar American social psychiatry movement. In this body of literature, which predates positive psychology by a half century, initial optimism and confidence about the possibility of promoting flourishing and preventing mental illness through the construction of salutogenic social environments gradually waned because successful primary-prevention interventions were elusive and psychiatrists turned increasingly to individualistic medical and biological paradigms to guide research. In the wake of social psychiatry, psychiatric researchers turned to individual-centered paradigms of social stress and social support, which assume the intransigence of social environments and the need to assist individuals with adaptive coping within these environments. We highlighted the PHDCN as an example of a more contemporary research project that continues the trajectory of social psychiatry, albeit outside of the structures and institutions of modern psychiatric research. We turn now to the key question, How should positive social traits be understood within a positive psychiatry?

In the light of the rise and fall of social psychiatry, we believe that positive psychiatry should avoid the utopian aspirations that pervaded mid-twentieth-century social psychiatry and that also punctuate the modern positive psychology literature. Such aspirations, we believe, run counter to the particular forms of wisdom inherent in psychiatry that stem from closely attending to individuals seeking healing from unwanted experience and behavior. In two centuries of practice, psychiatrists have learned that humans are beautiful, complex, resilient, and often broken beings and that social systems are rarely less complex and broken than the individuals who compose them. Efforts to shortcut the psychological dynamics of individuals by engineering social processes have always been at best marginally effective, and all utopias prove unsustainable. Furthermore, although positive psychologists are quite right to assert that flourishing has its own shape and structure and does not imply the absence or obverse of the negative (Duckworth et al. 2005), we believe that psychiatry can best discern the shape of flourishing when it stays close to the experience of those who seek healing. Positive psychiatry, even when it takes into account social structures and processes, must therefore always attend to the experience of individuals, including individuals who are in distress.

The abandonment of utopianism, however, does not justify the way that psychiatric research since the 1970s has focused almost exclusively on the mental health of individuals, with the social environment considered to be, at best, one of the many determinants of an individual's mental health. As the PHDCN study illustrates, macrolevel social factors are important in ways that exceed the descriptive capacities of these individualistically focused research paradigms.

We believe that positive psychiatry offers a very important opportunity for psychiatrists to articulate a relationship between individual and communal flourishing that does not devolve into either aspirational utopianism or pervasive individualism. We suggest that the concept of virtue, which is very important within positive psychology (Peterson and Seligman 2004), can help to clarify thinking within psychiatry about the relationship between social and individual flourishing and, therefore, about the nature of positive social traits, but only if virtue is considered in a way different from its dominant interpretation within positive psychology.

Virtue has been an important part of positive psychology since its earliest days, when Peterson and Seligman set out to develop a "manual of the sanities" that would serve as a positive *alter ego* of the DSM. Their 2004 classification, known as the VIA (Values in Action) Classification of Character Strengths, lists 24 "character strengths" organized into six categories of virtue: wisdom and knowledge, courage, humanity, justice, temperance, and transcendence (Peterson and Seligman 2004). These "big six" virtues were initially derived through expert consensus conferences, review of historical and contemporary wisdom literature across various cultural and religious traditions, and an online 240-item questionnaire known as the VIA Survey of Character Strengths. Peterson and Seligman describe virtue, rather generically, as "the core characteristics valued by moral philosophers and religious thinkers" (p. 13), and they maintain that their classification is a simple reflection of traits and strengths that are *already valued* because of their contribution to individual and social flourishing. However, Peterson and Seligman's account of virtue does not demonstrate any essential connection between the flourishing of individuals and the flourishing of their communities; positive psychology's virtues are primarily the good of individuals, even if communities benefit from their display.

However, an older account of virtue, associated with the ancient philosopher Aristotle (384–322 B.C.E.), links the individual and community in a more organic way than the dominant approach to virtue within positive psychology. Aristotle's account of virtue provides a more promising context by which to think about the relationship between individual and social flourishing because he understood the two to be part of one interconnected whole. The "master science of the good" for Aristotle was not ethics but politics, which he understood as the building and sustaining of flourishing communities (Aristotle 1999). However, to function well and to sustain themselves, political communities need the individuals who compose them to demonstrate forms of behavior that contribute to the flourishing of the community; for example, all communities need individuals who are committed to justice, who are able to confront fear when something important is at stake (courage), and who are able to restrain themselves from following every impulsive desire (self-control). Aristotle believed that when people learn to act, over time, in ways conducive to the flourishing of their communities, they find such actions easier and easier to perform; he believed that these positive forms of thinking and acting could become positive habits, which he also termed *aretai* (virtues). For Aristotle, virtues are embodied dispositions to act in ways that are conducive to flourishing. However, for Aristotle, communities and the individuals within them flourish (or languish) together; a community flourishes only when the individuals within it flourish and vice versa. Aristotle's thought contains a profoundly noncompetitive relationship between the flourishing of individuals and the flourishing of communities: each constructs the other (Aristotle 1999).

What does Aristotle, who lived more than two millennia ago, have to teach positive psychiatry about the elucidation of positive social traits? We suggest that Aristotle's virtue theory as displayed in the *Nicomachean Ethics* is functionally and pragmatically superior to the dominant VIA classification within modern positive psychology, precisely because of Aristotle's ability to link the flourishing of individuals and the flourishing of their communities into an indissociable whole. Virtues are not simply character traits that happen to be socially valued or traits that lead to the flourishing of only individuals. They are, rather, intrinsically social traits that lead to the flourishing of *both* individuals and the communities of which they are a part.

Summary

We suggest that the advent of positive psychiatry, with its increased attentiveness to traditions of wisdom that are not linked directly to medical models of disease and treatment, provides an opportunity for psychiatrists to understand positive social traits in a way that avoids both individualism and utopianism. To avoid the individualism that has characterized most psychiatric research and practice since the 1970s, psychiatrists need to reclaim the ability to view individuals and their social environments in noncompetitive ways, as Aristotle once did. Social traits, in this Aristotelian account, would not simply be individual traits that enable effective coping in demanding social environments but would also belong to communities and societies. For example, a commitment to fairness and justice could be a "trait" of a community as a whole, not only of certain individuals within it, and would both result from and enable the justice of its citizens. We believe that only this sort of noncompetitive account of the relationship between individuals and their communities, cultures, and societies can enable psychiatry to properly attend to social factors and social structures in a way that still honors the needs of individuals. In this account, social traits would be considered to be positive only if they were able to contribute to the noncompetitive flourishing of individuals and their communities together.

However, it is also very important to make certain that this turn to communal and social flourishing does not cause positive psychiatry, like social psychiatry and positive psychology before it, to lapse into forms of utopianism that will eventually undermine its credibility. We believe that this temptation will be averted only if positive psychiatry, drawing from the rich clinical traditions of psychiatry as a whole, remains closely attentive to the particular contexts of the particular individuals who approach psychiatrists for healing. Aristotle, who himself preferred empirical observation to disembodied theoretical speculation when scientific or psychological matters were at stake, can be a guide here also. For Aristotle, the virtues are always grounded in the concrete and particular realities of life, and individuals (and communities) become virtuous as they encounter obstacles to flourishing and successfully overcome them. If positive psychiatry were to ignore these concrete, particular challenges in the pursuit of some ideal of perfect mental health or perfect flourishing, it would soon lapse into unsustainable utopianism. However, if it were to fix resolutely on how individuals and communities thrive *within* these particular contexts, it could be both robustly "positive" and unquestionably and faithfully "psychiatry."

Clinical Key Points

- Psychiatry has not always been as individualistically oriented as it is now. Indeed, from the 1950s until the 1970s, social psychiatry (i.e., the study of the mental health of communities and of social correlates of mental health and mental illness) existed as a recognizable subfield within the psychiatric literature.

- Positive psychiatry will be credible, helpful, and sustainable to the degree that its attentiveness to happiness and flourishing emerges from the experience of attending to people and communities that are not flourishing but deeply desire health and meaning and wellness.

- Critics of positive psychology have alleged that positive psychology underestimates the degree to which social environments can be unavoidably toxic and stressful, more dystopian than utopian.

- Psychiatrists have learned that humans are beautiful, complex, resilient, and often broken beings and that social systems are rarely less complex and broken than the individuals who compose them. Efforts to shortcut the psychological dynamics of individuals by engineering social processes have always been, at best, marginally effective, and all utopias prove unsustainable.

* The virtues are always grounded in the concrete and particular realities of life, and individuals (and communities) become virtuous as they encounter obstacles to flourishing and successfully overcome them.

References

American Psychiatric Association: Diagnostic and Statistical Manual of Mental Disorders, 3rd Edition. Washington, DC, American Psychiatric Association, 1980

American Psychiatric Association: Diagnostic and Statistical Manual of Mental Disorders, 5th Edition. Arlington, VA, American Psychiatric Association, 2013

Aristotle: Nicomachean Ethics Translated and With an Introduction by John Ostwald. Upper Saddle River, NJ, Prentice-Hall, 1999

Berkman LF, Syme SL: Social networks, host resistance, and mortality: a nine-year follow-up study of Alameda County residents. Am J Epidemiol 109(2):186–204, 1979 425958

Blazer DG: Social support and mortality in an elderly community population. Am J Epidemiol 115(5):684–694, 1982 7081200

Blazer DG: The Age of Melancholy: Major Depression and Its Social Origins. New York, Routledge, 2005

Brown G, Harris T: Social Origins of Depression: A Study of Psychiatric Disorder in Women. New York, Free Press, 1978

Diener E, Seligman ME: Very happy people. Psychol Sci 13(1):81–84, 2002 11894851

Dohrenwend BP: Inventorying stressful life events as risk factors for psychopathology: toward resolution of the problem of intracategory variability. Psychol Bull 132(3):477–495, 2006 16719570

Duckworth AL, Steen TA, Seligman MEP: Positive psychology in clinical practice. Annu Rev Clin Psychol 1:629–651, 2005 17716102

Eaton J, Weil R: Culture and Mental Disorders. New York, Free Press, 1976

Ehrenreich B: Nickel and Dimed: On (Not) Getting By in America. New York, Metropolitan Books, 2001

Ehrenreich B: Bright-Sided: How the Relentless Promotion of Positive Thinking Has Undermined America. New York, Picador, 2008

Faris R, Dunham H: Mental Disorders in Urban Areas. Chicago, IL, University of Chicago Press, 1939

Flaherty J, Astrachan B: Social psychiatry, in Psychiatry in the New Millennium. Edited by Weissman S, Sabshin M, Eist H. Washington, DC, American Psychiatric Press, 1999, pp 39–55

Gable SL, Haidt J: What (and why) is Positive Psychology? Rev Gen Psychol 9:103–110, 2005

George LK, Blazer DG, Hughes DC, Fowler N: Social support and the outcome of major depression. Br J Psychiatry 154:478–485, 1989 2590779

Holmes TH, Rahe RH: The Social Readjustment Rating Scale. J Psychosom Res 11(2):213–218, 1967 6059863

Huxley A: Brave New World. New York, HarperCollins Publishers, 1932

Landerman R, George LK, Campbell RT, et al: Alternative models of the stress buffering hypothesis. Am J Community Psychol 17(5):625–642, 1989 2627025

Leighton AH: My Name Is Legion: Foundations for a Theory of Man in Relation to Culture. New York, Basic Books, 1959

Leighton D, Harding JS, Macklin DB, et al: The Character of Danger. New York, Basic Books, 1963

Lopez SJ, Snyder CR: The Oxford Handbook of Positive Psychology, 2nd Edition. New York, Oxford University Press, 2009

Lorant V, Deliège D, Eaton W, et al: Socioeconomic inequalities in depression: a meta-analysis. Am J Epidemiol 157(2):98–112, 2003 12522017

Mazure CM, Quinlan DM, Bowers MB Jr: Recent life stressors and biological markers in newly admitted psychotic patients. Biol Psychiatry 41(8):865–870, 1997 9099413

Mikulincer M, Shaver PR: Prosocial Motives, Emotions, and Behavior: The Better Angels of Our Nature. Washington, DC, American Psychological Association, 2010

Orwell G: Nineteen Eighty-Four. Oxford, UK, Clarendon Press, 1948

Peterson C, Seligman MEP: Character Strengths and Virtues: A Handbook and Classification. New York, Oxford University Press, 2004

Sampson RJ: The neighborhood context of well-being. Perspect Biol Med 46(3, suppl):S53–S64, 2003 14563074

Sampson RJ: Great American City: Chicago and the Enduring Neighborhood Effect. Chicago, IL, University of Chicago Press, 2012

Seligman MEP: The president's address. Am Psychol 54:559–562, 1999

Seligman MEP: Authentic Happiness: Using the New Positive Psychology to Realize Your Potential for Lasting Fulfillment. New York, Free Press, 2002

Seligman MEP: Flourish: A Visionary New Understanding of Happiness and Well-Being. New York, Free Press, 2011

Seligman ME, Csikszentmihalyi M: Positive psychology: an introduction. Am Psychol 55(1):5–14, 2000 11392865

Singer BH, Ryff CD: New Horizons in Health: An Integrative Approach. Washington, DC, National Academy of Sciences, 2001

Weissman MM, Markowitz JC, Klerman GL: Comprehensive Guide to Interpersonal Psychotherapy. New York, Basic Books, 2000

Suggested Cross-References

Social factors are discussed in Chapter 3 ("Resilience and Posttraumatic Growth"), Chapter 5 ("Recovery in Mental Illnesses"), Chapter 11 ("Preventive Interventions"), Chapter 12 ("Integrating Positive Psychiatry Into Clinical Practice"), and Chapter 16 ("Bioethics of Positive Psychiatry").

Suggested Readings

Gable SL, Haidt J: What (and why) is Positive Psychology? Rev Gen Psychol 9:103–110, 2005

Leighton AH: My Name Is Legion: Foundations for a Theory of Man in Relation to Culture. New York, Basic Books, 1959

Peterson C, Seligman MEP: Character Strengths and Virtues: A Handbook and Classification. New York, Oxford University Press, 2004

Sampson RJ: Great American City: Chicago and the Enduring Neighborhood Effect. Chicago, IL, University of Chicago Press, 2012

PART II

POSITIVE
OUTCOMES

5

Recovery in Mental Illnesses

CHRISTINE RUFENER, PH.D.

COLIN A. DEPP, PH.D.

MAJA K. GAWRONSKA, M.A.

ELYN R. SAKS, J.D., PH.D.

In the past decade, a growing variety of mental health organizations, services, and initiatives have used the term *recovery-oriented care.* The optimism embodied in the word *recovery* implies that there is a hope and capacity for improvement among people who have been substantially affected by mental health conditions, and this optimism represents a marked shift from historical conceptions of illnesses such as schizophrenia as degenerative intractable conditions. Serious scientific, consumer, and public agency effort has been directed toward defining recovery, detailing its essential ingredients, and promoting the practices and interventions that enhance its likelihood. Considerable controversy exists about how best to define recovery, *who* gets to define it; whether it is best represented as a state, a process, or an outcome; and how best to orient services to it. As opposed to many of the other concepts discussed in this volume, recovery is somewhat unique in that it is *specific* to people with illnesses and most commonly occurs in the realm of mental health and substance use conditions and treatment. Thus, the concept of recovery is important to consider in the broader context of positive psychiatry. In this chapter, we describe the history of recovery's rise to prominence, the variation in its definitions and models, and the principles and practices that exemplify recovery-oriented care.

History of Recovery

Tracing the history of psychiatry, the field has slowly evolved toward the belief that people with serious mental illnesses have the capacity to improve. In the early 1900s, the Kraepelinian depiction of schizophrenia as a "dementia praecox" was that of an earlier-onset dementia—a degenerative condition. The DSM-III description of the course of schizophrenia further specified the following: "The most common course is one of acute exacerbations with increasing residual impairment between episodes" (American Psychiatric Association 1980, p. 185). The long-term institutionalization of people with mental health conditions, which occurred up to the latter half of the twentieth century, either implicitly or explicitly endorsed the concept of assumed degeneration or lifelong diminished capacity for improvement.

Important societal events helped set the stage for the current zeitgeist of recovery. The widespread deinstitutionalization movement of the 1960s and 1970s meant that people with mental health conditions began to reside in the community and were far less removed from society. Although many legitimate criticisms have been levied about the preparedness of community-based services for people with mental health conditions from the first wave of deinstitutionalization onward, this shift did provide a door through which people with illnesses such as schizophrenia could be integrated into society.

At the same time, the rise of mental health advocacy groups and consumer survivor groups led to a new voice that helped enforce needed reforms to improve on the typical experience of being a "mental health patient." A variety of different groups were formed to address the civil rights of and stigma against people with mental health conditions, challenging practices such as involuntary commitment, physical restraints, and electroconvulsive therapy. Groups vary according to their relationship with psychiatry, from those that completely reject psychiatry to those that partner with it. Nevertheless, whether recovery occurs *in* the mental system or from it, the use of the term *recovery* became more prominent as consumers gained a stronger voice.

At the same time, research on the long-term outcomes of people with schizophrenia and other serious mental illnesses began to challenge some of the longstanding assumptions about degeneration. In the Vermont longitudinal cohort, Harding et al. (1987) found that one-half to two-thirds of a group of people with schizophrenia improved when they were assessed regularly over decades after an index hospitalization. Other longitudinal findings corroborated the finding that about 50% of people with schizophrenia experience extended periods of recovery with or without the aid of mental health services, and about one in seven are in "recovery" at any given time (Jääskeläinen et al. 2013). Longitudinal data from the aging literature led to a general consensus that average trajectories of cognitive, functional, symptom, and social function cannot be characterized as deteriorative in schizophrenia (Jeste et al. 2003) and that 10% of older adults with schizophrenia had experienced a "sustained remission" (Auslander and Jeste 2004). In addition, qualitative interviews of a sample of older adults with long-standing diagnoses of schizophrenia indicated that most felt that their symptoms and control over those symptoms had improved over the course of their lives (Shepherd et al. 2012). Thus, political, societal, and scientific viewpoints converged on the notion that schizophrenia and other serious mental illnesses are not deteriorative and that some people even seem to make dramatic improvements.

At the beginning of the twenty-first century, this paradigm shift started to be reflected at the policy level. Recovery appeared as a central concept in the report of the 2003 President's New Freedom Commission on Mental Health, which proposed the goals for an improved and more consumer-oriented mental health system and recommended a transformation that focuses on promoting recovery and building resilience. The report stated that "recovery refers to the process in which people are able to live, work, learn, and participate fully in their communities. For some individuals, recovery is the ability to live a fulfilling and productive life despite a disability. For others, recovery implies the reduction or complete remission of symptoms" (Hogan 2003). The report concluded that every person with a mental illness should be provided with hope and the possibility of improvement. However, agreement about how to define this improvement vis-à-vis recovery has been far more difficult to reach.

Current Definitions of Recovery

According to the *American Heritage Dictionary, recovery* is defined as a "return to a normal state." This succinct definition implies an outcome that can be gauged by restoration either to one's prior functioning or to a state similar to that of people who did not need to recover. In many medical diagnoses such as cancer, this definition is apt, as remission of cancer implies the absence of detectable disease. Similarly, recovery of function after an orthopedic injury indicates the capacity to return to preinjury activity.

As discussed by Bellack (2006), recovery in mental illness does not typically fit well with these standards. First, researchers and clinicians generally accept that psychiatric illnesses such as bipolar disorder or schizophrenia arise from a neurobiological diathesis and that a substantial portion of people with this neurobiological vulnerability, if not currently experiencing symptoms, are at the very least *at risk* for symptoms throughout their lives. Mounting evidence shows that premorbid dysfunction is partially present decades prior to the onset of schizophrenia, so return to premorbid function may not be a reasonable ideal either. Second, although the treatments available do modify the disease process, they are not curative for the vast majority of people with serious mental illnesses. Third, marked evidence from longitudinal studies demonstrates that even when symptoms resolve, functional disability persists. For example, Tohen found that 2 years after consumers were hospitalized for a manic episode, only 3% had not experienced a remission of the initial syndrome, but 62% experienced continued functional impairment (Tohen et al. 2000). Thus, recovery in mental illness takes on a different hue than in some other illnesses.

Several authors have attempted to operationalize the definition of recovery as an outcome, mainly focusing on schizophrenia (Table 5–1). Common among these definitions is the depiction of recovery as an outcome that can be defined by external criteria and objective indication of community participation. Moreover, the definitions contain a joint consideration of symptom attenuation, although without the need for complete absence of symptoms, and functional disability attenuation as exemplified by independent participation in instrumental and social activities. Symptom remission is thus seen as a necessary but insufficient part of recovery, which is a point of departure from the traditional focus of psychiatry (and medicine) on treating the aspects of the illness that can be observed in the clinical setting.

A parallel approach to defining recovery has grown largely out of qualitative research and subjective accounts of people with mental health problems. These definitions portray recovery as a personal process that evolves over the course of one's adaptation to the illness, occurring in stages and defined by increasing self-awareness and decreasing dependence on external supports as personal and social capital is rebuilt. A core feature of this model of recovery is its conception as a process that is deeply personal and subjectively defined. Moreover, symptom reduction is not seen as a necessary component to being in recovery, and neither are other specific objective functional indicators such as employment. One of the most widely circulated definitions of recovery that is consistent with the consumer process model is that proposed by the Substance Abuse and Mental Health Services Administration (SAMHSA) in 2011: "a process of change through which individuals improve their health and wellness, live a self-directed life, and strive to reach their full potential" (Substance Abuse and Mental Health Services Administration 2011). Embedded in this definition are elements of self-determination and self-management, without any specific mention of symptoms.

The shift away from symptom remission marks a shift from a more traditional medical model. In the view of SAMHSA, the objective of recovery-oriented treatment is to improve, to the greatest extent possible, a person's quality of life. Accordingly, a person can lead a full and meaningful life while still experiencing

Table 5–1. Selected definitions of recovery

Study	Definition
Liberman and Kopelowicz 2005	Recovery includes 1) a score less than 4 on the Brief Psychiatric Rating Scale positive and negative symptom scales, 2) if age appropriate, engagement in competitive work or its equivalent for at least half of the time over 2 years, 3) independent living as defined by lack of direct assistance with intrumental activities of daily living, and 4) at least once-weekly involvement in peer interactions outside of the family.
Torgalsbøen and Rund 2002	Recovery includes 1) not meeting criteria for a diagnosis of schizophrenia, 2) not having been hospitalized in 5 years, and 3) having a Global Assessment of Functioning scale score ≥65.
Substance Abuse and Mental Health Services Administration 2011	Recovery is "a process of change through which individuals improve their health and wellness, live a self-directed life, and strive to reach their full potential."
Substance Abuse and Mental Health Services Administration 2004	"Mental health recovery is a journey of healing and transformation enabling a person with a mental disability to live a meaningful life in the community of his or her choice while striving to achieve his or her full potential."
Anthony 1993	"Recovery is a way of living a satisfying, hopeful and contributing life even with limitations caused by the illness. Recovery involves the development of new goals, aspirations, meaning and purpose in one's life as one grows beyond the catastrophic effects of mental illness" (p. 527).

symptoms, and conversely, a person who exhibits no symptoms may be far from recovery. Recovery-oriented care focuses on a person's "roles and goals," in that treatment is individualized to help a person increase or improve his or her participation in aspects of life that are significant and gratifying. These roles and goals are not for the provider to identify but for the consumer to decide for himself or herself.

A major challenge in measuring more process-oriented definitions is that the concepts are difficult to operationalize and are subjective. However, several self-report measures have been developed to measure the consumer definition of recovery. For example, the Recovery Assessment Scale (Corrigan et al. 1999) is a 41-item, self-rated measure that includes five factors: 1) personal confidence and hope, 2) willingness to ask for help, 3) goal and success orientation, 4) reliance on others, and 5) not dominated by symptoms. Item examples include "I have a desire to succeed" and "I can handle it if I get sick again."

The Mental Health Recovery Measure (MHRM; Ralph and Kidder 2000; Young and Ensing 1999) is another example of a self-report measure. The self-rated MHRM is based on the three-phase model of recovery (Young and Ensing 1999) and covers six aspects: 1) overcoming "stuckness," 2) discovering and fostering self-empowerment, 3) learning and self-redefinition, 4) return to basic functioning, 5) striving to attain overall well-being, and 6) striving to reach new potentials (Ralph and Kidder 2000). Another measure, Self-Identified Stage of Recovery (SISR; Andresen et al. 2003), is based on the stage model of psychological recovery. SISR was designed specifically for the Australian Integrated Mental Health Initiative and consists of two parts. Part A (SISR-A) comprises five statements. Each statement corresponds to a stage of recovery: A = moratorium, B = awareness, C = preparation, D = rebuilding, and E = growth. Respondents are asked to choose the statement best representing their current recovery experience. Part B (SISR-B) includes four items corresponding to four recovery processes: hope, responsibility, identity, and meaning. Each item is rated on a six-point scale from 1 ("disagree strongly") to 6 ("agree strongly"). Finally, the Maryland Assessment of Recovery in People With Serious Mental Illness (MARS; Drapalski et al. 2012) includes 25 items reflecting the recovery domains outlined by SAMHSA: self-direction or empowerment, holistic treatment, nonlinear conception, strengths, responsibility, and hope. This self-report measure has demonstrated good internal consistency and test-retest reliability.

Much has been written about the marked discrepancies between scientific and consumer models of recovery (see Leamy et al. 2011 for a comprehensive review), varying along key dimensions about whether recovery is a process or outcome and a subjectively or objectively defined phenomenon and whether it is defined by improvement in one's capacity to manage symptoms or improvement in the symptoms themselves. It is clear that no consensus exists as to a specific definition and measurement model that might satisfy both sides of this debate. Nonetheless, there are some important similarities to note. Both consumer and scientific definitions revolve around independence with respect to both reducing reliance on service systems and making choices about one's life. Both highlight the importance of reducing the impact of the illness on one's life, and both offer a more holistic interpretation of improvement beyond symptoms to social and functional experiences. In some ways, the consumer approach is an explication of *how* individuals recover, and researcher-based models focus on *indicators* of recovery. It is clear that both sides of the debate offer important contributions to understanding recovery.

Recovery Principles

At the same time, as the field has grappled with defining what recovery means for the individual, there has been a substantial effort, largely by public health agencies such as SAMHSA, to define what constitutes recovery-focused care. In addition to providing an updated definition of recovery, SAMHSA and its community behavioral health partners established 10 defining principles that undergird recovery-oriented care (Table 5–2), and a number of practices exemplify these principles (Substance Abuse and Mental Health Services Administration 2011). Notably, these principles map to the consumer definition of recovery as outlined above.

These 10 elements of the recovery process first appeared in SAMHSA's important 2011 report, which was written to guide recovery practice in the United States: hope, strengths, individualized treatment, holistic treatment, peer support, nonlinear conception, empowerment, self-direction, respect, and responsibility (Table 5–2) (Substance Abuse and Mental Health Services Administration 2011). These principles are meant to guide providers in adapting interventions and services toward recovery orientation but are generally not prescriptive in the sense that no specific interventions are recommended. Other countries, including the United Kingdom, New Zealand, and Australia, have passed legislation endorsing that recovery model as a guiding principle of mental health services and education. Although each country has identified its own definition of recovery, these definitions overlap considerably, and the focus across all approaches is consistent: mental health services should empower individuals to achieve a meaningful and gratifying life in which they are integrated fully into a community of their choice. With regard to recovery-oriented practice, several of these terms warrant additional discussion.

Hope refers to a belief that consumers, even those with the most impactful symptoms, can make positive changes, whether that means improvements in terms of symptom reduction, improvement in daily functioning, or success in important roles (e.g., making a friend, engaging in volunteer work). To borrow from a quote commonly attributed to the American inventor Henry Ford, "Whether

Table 5–2. Substance Abuse and Mental Health Services Administration principles of recovery and examples of related practice elements

Principle	Examples of practices
Hope	Focus on a person's abilities, not disabilities.
	Share others' recovery stories to illustrate how others have overcome obstacles.
Strengths based	Ask clients about their strengths, preferences, and abilities in any assessment.
	Consider community connections that match clients' needs.
Individualized	Identify personally valued roles.
	Avoid sole reliance on manualized treatments.
Holistic	Address basic needs that may not be met: housing, finances, nutrition, exercise, and spirituality.
	Maintain community linkages to broaden available services.
Peer support	Encourage formation of mutual support groups.
	Provide paid peer training.
Nonlinear	Help clients conceptualize relapses as part of the process of recovery.
Empowerment	Provide options with regard to direction of treatment.
	Encourage clients to ask questions about their care.
Self-direction	Encourage clients to advocate for themselves within their support system or larger community.
	Assign "homework" for clients to engage in outside of direct therapeutic contact.
Respect	Ask clients for feedback regularly.
	Avoid referring to people by their diagnosis (e.g., "a schizophrenic").
Responsibility	Complete relapse prevention and/or crisis plan that outlines coping techniques that help clients manage symptoms.
	Assist clients in managing their own schedules in residential settings.

you think you can or can't—you're right." Several concepts highlight the importance of conceptualizing clients as unique individuals with *personal strengths* and abilities. A recovery-oriented practitioner helps the individual identify these strengths at the earliest stages of involvement in care and then *individualizes* the treatment to build on those strengths. Personalizing one's approach to care often means assessing for and providing *holistic* services that address a person's mental, physical, spiritual, and social health needs. The involvement of family members or other social support is seen as being critical to enhancing an individual provider's interventions. Involvement of families, for example, teaching problem-solving and stress management skills, demonstrates an investment in altering the client's environment to support improvement. Conversely, by including support systems, a provider has the potential to identify how the client's community may be interfering with the progress of the client (e.g., parents having low expectations for their child or a spouse questioning his or her partner's ability to take a step toward a goal independently) and can intervene to reduce any implicit or explicit messages of dependence or hopelessness. These support systems can and should include *peer support,* whereby consumers with shared or similar lived experiences provide mutual understanding and a sense of belonging and community.

Another principle in the SAMHSA model is that recovery is viewed as *nonlinear.* It is both typical and expected that a client will face new obstacles and challenges that may stymie growth or result in a significant setback. When providers normalize this concept at an early stage in treatment, they are contributing to a sense of *empowerment,* where the client is given trust to make his or her own decisions. Empowering a client also includes providing a client with information and resources such that he or she can make educated decisions about his or her personal needs, wants, and goals. Similarly, the recovery process should be *self-directed,* in which clients generate their personal goals on the basis of their own values and belief systems and then select treatments from a menu of choices. Autonomy and independence are encouraged and supported throughout the recovery process.

Finally, the concepts of *respect* and *responsibility* involve protecting clients' rights as independent adults so that they maintain or regain a sense of self. From a recovery framework, responsibility for one's recovery is placed in the hands of the client, not the mental health provider. A clinician cannot provide or prescribe recovery; rather, the onus is on the client to apply courage, personal strengths, and time and effort toward his or her own recovery.

Recovery-Oriented Practices

The Schizophrenia Patient Outcomes Research Team (PORT) project has produced comprehensive reviews of treatment recommendations for schizophrenia since 1998. The goal of PORT is to improve the quality of care for people with schizophrenia by reducing variations in care and promoting the adoption of evidence-based practices (Dixon et al. 2010). Toward that end, PORT publishes a list of pharmacological and psychosocial interventions that have robust empirical support for their effectiveness. Neither surprisingly nor coincidentally, the majority of the most recent psychosocial treatment recommendations contain themes of SAMHSA's recovery elements. A review of several of these individual recommendations demonstrates that recovery elements are a common thread among them.

Selected Recovery-Oriented Practices

Peer Support

Peer support is most familiar as being a core element in the treatment of—and recovery from—addictions. Alcoholics Anonymous and similar meetings create a community based on shared experiences, reduce isolation, and contribute to an overall sense of belonging. In the past several years, the concept of peer support has been increasingly applied to populations without addictions. Broadly, a *peer support provider* is someone with a current or past mental illness experience who assists others with mental illnesses. These peer support providers serve as role models in that they are individuals who have faced challenges and demonstrate coping and successes in managing their symptoms. Across populations, peers have the unique position of being able to apply their own firsthand experiences to normalize and destigmatize the experience of mental illness. They exemplify to both staff and consumers that people can and do recover from mental health challenges. National nonprofit organizations such as the National Alliance on Mental Illness and the Depression and Bipolar Support Alliance provide peer support training, in which individuals with mental health challenges can become certified as peer specialists. Peer specialists are employed by or volunteer in hospitals, community mental health clinics, county programs, and other mental health organizations. Most recently, the Department of Veterans Affairs (VA) completed a large-scale hiring initiative and hired more than 800 peer specialists to provide mentoring throughout its medical centers and community-based outpatient clinics.

Research has begun to illuminate the benefits of peer support services in mental health programs, but more research is needed to explore their active ingredients and the nature of the effect of such services on care. Training models and curricula, as well as fidelity scales and outcomes measures, are specifically needed to develop a robust evidence base for peer interventions (Davidson et al. 2006). Preliminary research has suggested that peer support may reduce the stigma of receiving mental health services and makes treatment easier and more consistently adhered to among certain populations (e.g., veterans with posttraumatic stress disorder [PTSD]) (Jain et al. 2012).

Clinical Vignette

Lieutenant "Smith's" recovery officially started in November 2004 in the storage closet of the mental health clinic at a naval air station in the eastern United States. He was in the room sobbing uncontrollably and reliving every hellish experience he had in Iraq. Fortunately, his commander at the time, who was the lead psychologist and head of the mental health department, specialized in the treatment of PTSD. The commander had Lt. Smith self-admit to the inpatient mental health ward at one of the naval medical centers. Lt. Smith was an inpatient for 2 weeks on this ward, and he was restrained six times for his own safety and the safety of the staff. By the end of the second week, Lt. Smith appeared to have developed some insight into his illness and a modest amount of acceptance of the fact that he needed help.

The next step in Lt. Smith's recovery was a day program for PTSD at another military hospital. The program was designed to be a 30-day intensive treatment program. Lt. Smith was there for 45 days. During his time with the program, he went through CBT groups and intensive one-on-one sessions with a psychologist and a psychiatrist. By the end of the program, he reported feeling that he had "a fairly decent grasp" on what it was he was going through and had a plan to deal with it.

Lt. Smith continued therapy with one of the psychologists at the naval air station for around 3.5 years. He was seen twice a week for about the first 6 months and then scaled back to once a week for about another year. Then, finally, he was seen every other week by a therapist and once every 2 months by a psychiatrist. During therapy, he went through cognitive processing therapy and some mild exposure therapy. He was also prescribed a selective serotonin reuptake inhibitor and a sleep aid that he still continues to receive. Lt. Smith recently reported that "if there is one thing that I have learned in the 9 or so years I have been in treatment, it is that PTSD is forever. I know that the things I saw and did while in country will never change and that I will never be the person I was before I went to war, but I have the ability now to process those emotions and feelings in a way that is not destructive. I can now use these experiences to help others who are struggling to find their way through recovery. That is why I work as a peer specialist at the VA, so that I can help others to achieve the sense of hope and feelings of peace and forgiveness that I have been able to find in myself. Also, it helps me to stay grounded in my own recovery and reminds me of what could be just down the road if I lapse in my own efforts to heal."

Assertive Community Treatment

Assertive community treatment (ACT) is among the most well-established interventions for significantly reducing hospitalizations and homelessness (Bond et al. 2001). ACT teams are multidisciplinary teams that provide a thorough spectrum of services to individuals with serious mental illnesses. These services include assessment, psychoeducation, and support for both clients and families; medication management; assistance with activities of daily living; and help with housing, vocational and educational goals, and socialization. Both the breadth and the depth of services provided differentiate ACT from more basic case management models. The intensity of ACT services ensures that individuals' needs are met regardless of where they stand in their own recovery, which can range from being in an acute, highly distressed state to being minimally distressed by symptoms but requiring assistance with role identity and personal goal progress. The majority of this work is done in the community, as opposed to a more traditional setting such as an outpatient mental health center, and is available 24 hours a day, 7 days a week. ACT teams support clients' individual needs and demonstrate respect for their autonomy by supplying easy access to care that is comprehensive and all-inclusive, and by providing an intervention that meets clients, quite literally, where they are. When compared with usual community care across 25 randomized controlled trials, ACT was shown to affect several important areas in the well-being of clients with serious mental illness. These areas included improvements in client engagement in services, reductions in hospitalizations, increases in housing stability, and moderate improvements in symptoms and clients' reported quality of life (Bond et al. 2001).

Supported Employment

Supported employment is a highly individualized form of vocational rehabilitation that integrates mental health treatment into the job search, attainment, and maintenance. Importantly, the model involves moving clients quickly into job placements and adheres to a philosophy of "place then train" as opposed to "train then place" and spends minimal time directly focusing on issues such as symptoms or impairments, instead emphasizing strengths (Bond 2004). Supported employment provides high levels of support throughout the entire job process and is designed to assist clients in finding jobs in the greater community, rather than placement into some type of sheltered work environment chosen by the program. Thus, it supports the premise that clients should be guided to seek a job of their choice that is intrinsically motivating, fits their sense of self, and enables them to strive toward their full potential.

The evidence base for supported employment models is well established across various settings and populations (Bond 2004). Most models share similar components that constitute the effective ingredients of the intervention. Strong evidence indicates that when supported employment is provided by a mental health treatment team and follows a rapid job search approach that connects clients to jobs based on the clients' preferences, individual strengths, and previous work experience, clients have significantly better employment outcomes. In fact, the proven effects of supported employment are more robust in the literature than the effects of other vocational program approaches (Bond et al. 2008).

Occupational engagement is seen as being quite central for many recovery processes. Certainly, in Western culture, work is a defining characteristic of one's adult identity, and lacking that piece can increase stigmatization and defeatist beliefs about one's abilities and self-worth. Work provides people with structure and a sense of focus, as well as an innately satisfying sense of accomplishment. Additionally, the workplace almost invariably includes a social element and an opportunity to interact with others in a predictable and consistent manner. Although work stressors, just like any other stressor, may exacerbate symptoms, work can also serve as a distraction or as a source of meaning and purpose.

Social Skills Training

Social skills training (SST) targets the very common deficits that individuals with serious mental illnesses have in the areas of communication, assertiveness, and general socialization (Bellack et al. 2004). Effective SST models rely on basic behavioral teaching principles, including role modeling, rehearsal, and positive feedback, to teach individuals the basic skills of initiating social contact, requesting assistance or information, and maintaining casual, familial, and intimate social relationships. SST recognizes that socialization is an inherent human want and need and provides the tools that clients need to participate fully in work, school, family, and other social settings. Moreover, these skills support clients' abilities to express their personal goals, advocate for themselves, and fortify their support systems such that they have assistance and support available to them throughout their recovery efforts.

SST has been researched across numerous studies spanning several decades. Meta-analyses have demonstrated the following: SST is particularly effective in helping clients learn new social skills, clients are able to retain their skills over time, the skills generalize to new situations outside of training sessions, and social functioning is globally improved; however, SST has limited effect on symptom severity and rehospitalization.

Individual and Group Psychotherapeutic Approaches

Psychotherapeutic approaches have been either adapted (e.g., cognitive-behavioral therapy, CBT) or developed to meet the dual goal of addressing the needs of patients with serious mental illnesses and integrating recovery-oriented components. Illness management and recovery is a psychoeducational approach that directly targets goal setting and tracking, coping with stigma, and symptom management approaches (Gingerich and Mueser 2014). Commonly used models such as CBT have been adapted for serious mental illnesses to be consistent with recovery models, for example, to include functional goal setting, monitoring, and guidance through progress on goal steps and to provide positive reinforcement for goal accomplishment. In addition, CBT for psychosis also places a strong emphasis on the establishment and maintenance of a strong, trusting therapeutic relationship, even more so than CBT for depression or anxiety (Kingdon and Turkingotn 1994). Psychodynamic approaches have also been adapted to target metacognition and self-reflection in the context of schizophrenia (Bargenquast and Schweitzer 2014). Notably, these talk therapies are part of emerging guidelines for care (Parish 2014).

Family-Based Services

Family interventions of at least 6 months in duration have been shown to lead to several valuable outcomes for both the client and the family or support system. For the client, the benefits of family services include reduced relapse rates and rehospitalization, reduced symptoms and subjective psychological distress, and improved functional and vocational status. For family members, research shows that positive outcomes include reduced distress and increased satisfaction with family relationships. Family-based therapies typically offer psychoeducation in concert with problem solving, coping techniques, and effective communication skills. Supporting the familial or support environment can contribute to a more supportive and assistive recovery environment in which both the client and the family believe that growth and positive change are possible.

Research on family psychoeducation has established a firm basis for its efficacy and effectiveness (Pilling et al. 2002). A range of positive effects have been identified, including significant reductions in relapse and rehospitalization among clients whose families received psychoeducation, with greater reductions being associated with longer psychoeducation programs. In addition, clients have been more likely to participate in supplementary programs, such as vocational rehabilitation, when their families receive psychoeducation. Finally, families report improvement in their overall well-being, which suggests that family psychoeducation creates a less distressed environment that is more conducive to recovery.

Other Recovery-Oriented Services

Other interventions exist that either emanate directly from recovery-oriented services or can be modified to embody major recovery principles. Manualized relapse prevention plans, for example, are tools that providers and clients can complete collaboratively. These plans help clients prepare for future increases of symptoms or distress by mapping out the clients' daily self-care plans, along with warning signs and triggers, and their social support, coping skills, and crisis plans. The most well known of these plans is the Wellness Recovery Action Plan, or WRAP (Copeland 1997), and SAMHSA offers a digital version called "Action Planning for Prevention and Recovery: A Self-Help Guide." These plans normalize the concept that recovery will have ups and downs and that individuals can take a proactive approach to managing their symptoms such that they can continue to remain active in their valued roles at home and in the community.

Implementation of Recovery-Oriented Practice

At first glance, it may seem particularly challenging to provide recovery-oriented services, particularly because recovery is considered a belief system and not necessarily a unitary manualized treatment. Nonetheless, basic elements of psychotherapy, such as respect and validation, goal identification, and consistent and reliable support and assistance, are all examples of recovery-oriented therapeutic behaviors. A solo practitioner, however, will find it challenging to provide the type of comprehensive assistance that is necessary to create a healthy environment conducive to recovery. Providers who spend considerable time empowering their clients to set and work toward goals may find their work undermined by other providers or by members of the client's support system whose outlooks are shaped by false or biased beliefs about the client's potential. The work of a provider is greatly facilitated by practicing within an organization that has adopted recovery principles as its guiding mission.

For a system to transition to a recovery-focused orientation, it is invaluable to have buy-in and support from leadership and, ideally, to have a recovery champion embedded in the leadership team. The VA has employed such a champion in the role of the local recovery coordinator (LRC). Required for all medical centers by the VA *Uniform Mental Health Services Handbook*, the LRC position was created "to help transform local VA mental health services to a recovery-oriented model of care, to sustain those changes, and to support further systemic change as new evidence becomes available on optimal delivery of recovery-oriented mental health care" (Department of Veterans Affairs and Veterans Health Administration 2008, p. 27). Specifically, the LRC's responsibilities include directly providing recovery-oriented services, advocating for recovery resources, and teaching and consulting with staff, veterans, and veterans' families. In addition, LRCs are typically involved with supervision or training of peer specialists who are embedded throughout the system and can be valuable agents of delivery and role models for recovery.

In the case of providers who are not part of a larger organization or health care system and who may be working out of a private or group practice, institutional change is not necessary to provide recovery-oriented services. However, such providers should enlist a support team that can provide the holistic quality necessary to foster recovery. Successful recovery programs are typically multidisciplinary in nature and include professionals who can help clients with not only their psychiatric needs but also their housing, educational, and vocational, social, and leisure needs. In the absence of such a team, nonprofit and county or state programs exist that address many or all of these important areas that help individuals live meaningful and productive lives. Consumer-run groups such as the National Alliance on Mental Illness and the Depression and Bipolar Support Alliance are two national organizations that provide starting points for consultation. Support groups, including Alcoholics Anonymous and Narcotics Anonymous, also typically have access to a variety of resources for their participants. Clubhouses are community-based centers where individuals can access comprehensive psychosocial resources in a single environment, and their focus is on increasing people's sense of belonging and active participation in the larger community. A provider can expand his or her network exponentially by connecting with one or several of these groups.

Current Limitations of Recovery-Oriented Practices

Provision of recovery-oriented care may be challenged by several factors. For example, access to community resources differs substantially by community, and most are built on grassroots efforts without substantial funding. Access to recovery-oriented care may be particularly challenging in rural settings; for example, working with outside agencies and consumer groups is time-consuming and occurs largely outside of time that is reimbursable. Certain recovery interventions, including peer support, are also not likely to be recognized as reimbursable services. Intensive and comprehensive services such as ACT are also costly and are generally available only to consumers with established need. Even though ACT teams may offset costs by reducing hospitalizations and other high-cost crisis services over time, the necessary substantial investment may be prohibitive for community mental health centers. Finally, just as tension exists about what defines recovery, no formal criteria have been established for minimum standards for the label of recovery-oriented care. Does a provider need to encompass every principle of recovery in order to be considered recovery oriented? A wide variety of instruments exist that measure recovery knowledge and attitudes of clients and providers, and a number of questionnaires address program-level measures of recovery (Campbell-Orde et al. 2005). These tools can assist providers in assessing their recovery competence and aptitude and can identify areas for growth at both the individual and systems levels.

Future Directions

The governments of the United Kingdom, Australia, New Zealand, and, more recently, the United States have explicitly endorsed a shift toward recovery-oriented services. Research to help further explicate the factors, mechanisms, and tools that promote recovery in various populations is clearly needed. Similarly, further consensus about the active ingredients of recovery-oriented practices, including those listed here, will help streamline recovery-oriented care in a way that makes these services more easily accessible and deliverable across health care systems and in independent practice. Moreover, research regarding special groups will elucidate what recovery may mean for subpopulations, including ethnic minorities, older adults, and those living in rural settings. With more robust research evidence about the benefits of providing recovery-oriented care, organizations will likely be more open to engaging in system transformation to adjust and adapt their practices. Nonetheless, clinicians may be vulnerable to an illusion, in which a person who always works predominantly with individuals in distress begins to believe that these people are representative of all of those with the same symptoms or diagnosis. Said simply, clinicians can fall into a belief that no one they see gets better, because they are not seeing the people who have moved forward in their recovery and are living full lives in the community. To buffer themselves from this bias, clinicians can seek out recovery stories from current and future clients and their families, build a resource library with an emphasis on first person accounts of recovery, and most of all, maintain a sense of hope. Only by personifying hope to clients, will providers succeed in empowering their clients to believe that recovery is possible.

Summary

Recovery-oriented practice is an approach that recognizes and emphasizes that individuals with any type of mental health condition have the capacity to live a fulfilling and satisfying life when provided with appropriate and comprehensive services and resources. The recovery model is increasingly becoming the guiding principle of mental health services across countries and states. Despite variability in the definition of recovery, as well as challenges in measuring recovery-oriented outcomes, the principles of recovery illustrate effective guidelines for adapting recovery-oriented care. Evidence-based practices for serious mental illness provide illustrative examples of how these principles can be integrated into treatment across treatment settings. Implementation of recovery practice requires a comprehensive approach that benefits from the involvement of a multidisciplinary team and/or the greater community.

Clinical Key Points

- Mounting data indicate that improvement in symptoms and functional status is common among people with serious mental illnesses.

- A consensus definition of recovery is lacking, with notable differences between scientific models, which emphasize objective outcomes, and consumer models, which emphasize subjective processes.

- The Substance Abuse and Mental Health Services Administration has provided guidance on elements of recovery-oriented care, which include hope, self-determination, and family support, among others.

- Although recovery-oriented care is not a singular practice, several evidence-based interventions exemplify recovery orientation, including assertive community treatment, supported employment, and peer support.

- Progress in implementing recovery-oriented practices will be enhanced by increasing research on effective dissemination strategies, particularly for diverse and historically underserved groups of consumers.

References

American Psychiatric Association: Diagnostic and Statistical Manual of Mental Disorders, 3rd Edition. Washington, DC, American Psychiatric Association, 1980

Andresen R, Oades L, Caputi P: The experience of recovery from schizophrenia: towards an empirically validated stage model. Aust N Z J Psychiatry 37(5):586–594, 2003 14511087

Anthony WA: Recovery from mental illness: the guiding vision of the mental health service system in the 1990s. Psychosocial Rehabilitation Journal 16:521–538, 1993

Auslander LA, Jeste DV: Sustained remission of schizophrenia among community-dwelling older outpatients. Am J Psychiatry 161(8):1490–1493, 2004 15285980

Bargenquast R, Schweitzer RD: Enhancing sense of recovery and self-reflectivity in people with schizophrenia: a pilot study of Metacognitive Narrative Psychotherapy. Psychol Psychother 87(3):338–356, 2014 24375887

Bellack AS: Scientific and consumer models of recovery in schizophrenia: concordance, contrasts, and implications. Schizophr Bull 32(3):432–442, 2006 16461575

Bellack AS, Mueser KT, Gingerich S, et al: Social Skills Training for Schizophrenia: A Step-by-Step Guide. New York, Guilford, 2004

Bond GR: Supported employment: evidence for an evidence-based practice. Psychiatr Rehabil J 27(4):345–359, 2004 15222147

Bond GR, Drake RE, Mueser KT, et al: Assertive community treatment for people with severe mental illness. Disease Management and Health Care 9:141–159, 2001

Bond GR, Drake RE, Becker DR: An update on randomized controlled trials of evidence-based supported employment. Psychiatr Rehabil J 31(4):280–290, 2008 18407876

Campbell-Orde T, Ralph RO, Kidder K, et al: A Compendium of Recovery Measures. Cambridge, MA, Human Services Research Institute, 2005

Copeland ME: Wellness Recovery Action Plan. Brattleboro, VT, Peach Press, 1997

Corrigan PW, Giffort D, Rashid F, et al: Recovery as a psychological construct. Community Ment Health J 35(3):231–239, 1999 10401893

Davidson L, Chinman M, Sells D, et al: Peer support among adults with serious mental illness: a report from the field. Schizophr Bull 32(3):443–450, 2006 16461576

Department of Veterans Affairs and Veterans Health Administration: Uniformed Mental Health Services Handbook, 2008

Drapalski AL, Medoff D, Unick GJ, et al: Assessing recovery of people with serious mental illness: development of a new scale. Psychiatr Serv 63(1):48–53, 2012 22227759

Dixon LB, Dickerson F, Bellack AS, et al; Schizophrenia Patient Outcomes Research Team (PORT): The 2009 schizophrenia PORT psychosocial treatment recommendations and summary statements. Schizophr Bull 36(1):48–70, 2010 19955389

Gingerich S, Mueser KT: Illness management and recovery, in Evidence-Based Mental Health Practice: A Textbook. Edited by Drake RE, Merrens MR, Lynde DW. New York, WW Norton, 2014, pp 395–424

Harding CM, Brooks GW, Ashikaga T, et al: The Vermont longitudinal study of persons with severe mental illness, II: long-term outcome of subjects who retrospectively met DSM-III criteria for schizophrenia. Am J Psychiatry 144(6):727–735, 1987 3591992

Hogan MF: The President's New Freedom Commission: recommendations to transform mental health care in America. Psychiatr Serv 54(11):1467–1474, 2003 14600303

Jääskeläinen E, Juola P, Hirvonen N, et al: A systematic review and meta-analysis of recovery in schizophrenia. Schizophr Bull 39(6):1296–1306, 2013 23172003

Jain S, McLean C, Rosen CS: Is there a role for peer support delivered interventions in the treatment of veterans with post-traumatic stress disorder? Mil Med 177(5):481–483, 2012 22645871

Jeste DV, Twamley EW, Eyler Zorrilla LT, et al: Aging and outcome in schizophrenia. Acta Psychiatr Scand 107(5):336–343, 2003 12752029

Kingdon DG, Turkingotn D: Cognitive-Behavioral Therapy of Schizophrenia. New York, Guilford, 1994

Leamy M, Bird V, Le Boutillier C, et al: Conceptual framework for personal recovery in mental health: systematic review and narrative synthesis. Br J Psychiatry 199(6):445–452, 2011 22130746

Liberman RP, Kopelowicz A: Recovery from schizophrenia: a concept in search of research. Psychiatr Serv 56(6):735–742, 2005 15939952

Parish C: NICE issues new guidance on treating psychosis. Ment Health Pract 17:7, 2014

Pilling S, Bebbington P, Kuipers E, et al: Psychological treatments in schizophrenia, I: meta-analysis of family intervention and cognitive behaviour therapy. Psychol Med 32(5):763–782, 2002 12171372

Ralph RO, Kidder KA: The Recovery Advisory Group: Can We Measure Recovery? A Compendium of Recovery and Recovery Related Measures. Cambridge, MA, Human Services Research Institute, 2000

Shepherd S, Depp CA, Harris G, et al: Perspectives on schizophrenia over the lifespan: a qualitative study. Schizophr Bull 38(2):295–303, 2012 20603443

Substance Abuse and Mental Health Services Administration: National Consensus Statement on Mental Health Recovery. 2004. Available at: http://store.samhsa.gov/shin/content/SMA05-4129/SMA05-4129.pdf. Accessed August 25, 2014.

Substance Abuse and Mental Health Services Administration: SAMHSA announces a working definition of "recovery" from mental disorders and substance use disorders. 2011. Available at: http://www.samhsa.gov/newsroom/press-announcements/201112220300. Accessed August 25, 2014.

Tohen M, Hennen J, Zarate CM Jr, et al: Two-year syndromal and functional recovery in 219 cases of first-episode major affective disorder with psychotic features. Am J Psychiatry 157(2):220–228, 2000 10671390

Torgalsbøen AK, Rund BR: Lessons learned from three studies of recovery from schizophrenia. Int Rev Psychiatry 14:312–317, 2002

Young SL, Ensing DS: Exploring recovery from the perspective of people with psychiatric disabilities. Psychiatr Rehabil J 22:219–231, 1999

Suggested Cross-References

Social factors are discussed in Chapter 3 ("Resilience and Posttraumatic Growth"), Chapter 4 ("Positive Social Psychiatry"), Chapter 11 ("Preventive Interventions"), Chapter 12 ("Integrating Positive Psychiatry Into Clinical Practice"), and Chapter 16 ("Bioethics of Positive Psychiatry"). Psychotherapy is discussed in Chapter 8 ("Positive Psychotherapeutic and Behavioral Interventions") and Chapter 9 ("Positivity in Supportive and Psychodynamic Therapy").

Suggested Web Sites

National Alliance on Mental Illness Web site. Available at: www.nami.org. Accessed July 14, 2014

Substance Abuse and Mental Health Services Administration Web site. Available at: http://www.samhsa.gov/recovery/. Accessed July 14, 2014.

U.S. Department of Health and Human Services Mental Health Web site. Available at: www.mentalhealth.gov. Accessed July 14, 2014.

6

What Is Well-Being?

ROBERT M. KAPLAN, PH.D.

WENDY B. SMITH, M.A., PH.D., BCB

Among all human assets, health and well-being are the most highly valued. Studies have investigated the rank order of preference for various states of being. In these exercises, there is typically little variability because virtually everyone rates health as their most desired state (Rokeach 1973). However, despite how much people value health status, the definition and measurement of health and well-being remain elusive.

Discussions of the measurement of health are often characterized by two themes. First, illness and premature death are undesirable, so at least one component of health is avoidance of serious illness and mortality. Second, the effects of illness and disability on everyday functioning and quality of life are important. Diseases and disabilities are a concern because they disrupt usual activities of daily living. For example, cancer or heart disease may shorten an individual's life expectancy and reduce that individual's capacity to engage in meaningful life activities during the time prior to death. Even relatively minor illnesses can have effects on everyday life. A common cold, for example, can interfere with social and work activities and can disrupt cognitive functioning and the ability to enjoy interactions with others. Although the common cold may disrupt life activities, it typically lasts for a relatively short time. Chronic illnesses, such as recurrent low back pain, can result in permanent disruption of enjoyable life activities. A comprehensive conceptualization of wellness must consider risk of death, reduced quality of life, and durations of health states (Brown et al. 2013).

Over the last few decades, there has been renewed interest in the measurement of patient-reported outcomes (see http://PCORI.org). Most illnesses are now evaluated in terms of their effects on usual life activities. Indicators used in common laboratory tests, such as the 16 indicators on a screening chemistry panel, are sometimes uncorrelated with life expectancy or with outcomes when viewed from the patient's perspective (Kaplan 2009). We regard these as "surrogate" measures because they may be related to clinical outcomes even though they are not outcomes in their own right. Outcome measurement requires that we capture wellness from the patient's perspective.

Many clinical studies now apply standardized measures of life quality. Figure 6–1 summarizes the number of publications under the topic of quality of life identified in PubMed between 1972 and 2012. In 1972, PubMed did not identify any publications under the quality of life key word. Over the next 40 years, the number of articles that used the quality of life keyword grew dramatically. In 2012, 1,104 articles were identified by the quality-of-life key word. The trend has continued in the most recent years. For example, in the most recent 5 years for which full data are available (2007–2012), use of this key word increased 78%. Over the last four decades, many new quality of life tools have become available. These new tools are more sophisticated in their approach to the analysis of patient-reported outcomes specific to a variety of illnesses. For example, these tools include measures specific to cancer, diabetes, and heart disease.

The recognition of quality of life as an important outcome was first stimulated by Paul Ellwood's 1988 Shattuck lecture (Ellwood 1988). Ellwood advocated for what he referred to as "a technology of patient experience." In contrast to management of symptoms, Ellwood emphasized the importance of managing patient outcomes. He saw medical care as relying on four techniques: 1) standards and guidelines that match treatments with patient desires, 2) measurement of patient well-being and functioning, 3) use of normative data to interpret patient outcomes within the context of other people, and 4) dissemination of information in ways that could influence decision makers. This approach puts the patient at the center of health care and uses patient-centered reports to offer guidance and perspective for clinical care. More recently, use of these technologies has come to be known as patient-centered outcomes research (PCOR). The use of PCOR is well represented in the Affordable Care Act and in the Patient-Centered Outcomes Research Institute (PCORI). At the center of PCOR is the measurement of outcomes from the patient perspective. Most of these measures emphasize health-related quality of life.

Definition of Health-Related Quality of Life

Numerous quality-of-life measurement systems have evolved during the last 30 years and represent various traditions in measurement. At least two different

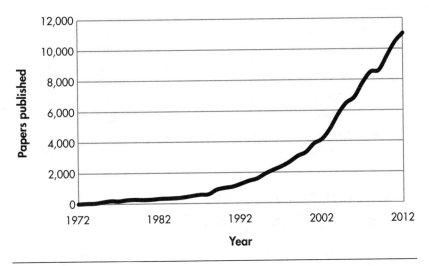

FIGURE 6–1. Papers identified in PubMed under the key word quality of life: 1972–2012.

conceptual approaches exist. One stems from the tradition of health status measurement. In the late 1960s and early 1970s, the National Center for Health Services Research (now the Agency for Healthcare Research and Quality) funded several major projects to develop general measures of health status. All of the projects were guided by the World Health Organization's definition of *health status*: "Health is a complete state of physical, mental, and social well-being and not merely absence of disease" (World Health Organization 1948). The projects resulted in a variety of assessment tools, including the Sickness Impact Profile, the Quality of Well-Being Scale, the McMaster Health Index Questionnaire, the Medical Outcomes Study 36-Item Short Form Health Survey (SF-36), and the Nottingham Health Profile (for an overview, see Centers for Disease Control and Prevention 2012). Many of the measures examine the effects of disease or disability on performance of social roles, the ability to interact in the community, and physical functioning. Some of the systems have separate components for the measurement of social and mental health. The measures also differ in the extent to which they consider subjective aspects of life quality. Most of these measures apply a psychometric approach to provide separate measures for the many different dimensions of quality of life. For example, the Sickness Impact Profile is a 136-item measure that yields 12 different scores displayed in a format similar to a Minnesota Multiphasic Personality Inventory profile.

The second approach uses decision theory and attempts to weight the different dimensions of health to provide a single expression of health status. Supporters of this approach argue that psychometric methods fail to consider that different health problems are not of equal concern. One hundred minor blisters are not the same as 100 missing limbs. In an experimental trial using the psychometric approach, one will often find that some aspects of quality of life improve, whereas others get worse. For example, a medication might increase hemoglobin but also produce greater levels of symptoms associated with renal failure (Drüeke et al. 2006). Many argue that the quality-of-life notion is the subjective evaluation of observable or objective health states. The decision-theory approach attempts to provide an overall measure of quality of life that integrates subjective function states, preferences for these states, morbidity, and mortality.

Common Methods for Measuring Quality of Life

In this chapter, we present some of the most widely used methods for measuring quality of life. Readers who are interested in more detailed reviews should consult the guide to scales and questionnaires by McDowell (2006).

Medical Outcomes Study 36-Item Short Form Health Survey

Perhaps the most commonly used psychometric outcome measure in the world today is the SF-36. The SF-36 grew out of work by the RAND Corporation and the Medical Outcomes Study. The Medical Outcomes Study attempted to develop a short, 20-item instrument known as the Short Form-20, or SF-20. However, the SF-20 did not have appropriate reliability for some dimensions. The SF-36 includes eight health concepts: physical functioning, role-physical, bodily pain, general health perceptions, vitality, social functioning, role-emotional, and mental health. The SF-36 can be either administered by a trained interviewer or self-administered.

The SF-36 has many advantages. For example, it is brief, and there is substantial evidence for its reliability and validity. The SF-36 can be machine scored and has been evaluated in large population studies. The reliability and validity of the SF-36 are well documented (Keller et al. 1999).

The SF-36 also presents some disadvantages. For example, it does not have age-specific questions, and one cannot clearly determine whether it is equally appropriate across age levels (Stewart and Ware 1992). Nevertheless, the SF-36 has become the most commonly used behavioral measure in contemporary medicine.

Patient-Reported Outcome Measurement Information System

In an effort to provide clinicians and researchers access to efficient adult- and child-reported measures of health and well-being, the National Institutes of Health funded the development of the Patient-Reported Outcome Measurement Information System (PROMIS). PROMIS instruments use modern measurement theory to assess patient-reported measures of physical and mental health and social well-being. In addition to a specific instrument to assess well-being in pediatric populations, PROMIS instruments measure general outcomes such as fatigue, physical function, depression, anxiety, and social function. Other instruments are available (see http://nihpromis.org), and additional measures are currently under development.

Major advantages of PROMIS include its ability to reduce the burden of responding to large numbers of questions and to create patient-reported outcome measures that are comparable across diseases and conditions. PROMIS tools provide clinicians with information about how various treatments might affect their patients and their patients' day-to-day functioning. Not only can the reports be used to inform treatment plans, but they can also be used by patients and physicians to improve communication.

Decision-Theory Approaches

Quality-of-life data can be used to assess the cost/utility or cost-effectiveness of health care programs. Cost studies have gained in popularity because health care costs have rapidly grown, from 4% of the GDP in 1960 to over 17% today. All health care interventions do not return equal benefit for the expended dollar. Cost studies might guide policy makers toward an optimal and equitable distribution of scarce resources. A cost-effectiveness analysis typically quantifies the benefits of a health care intervention in terms of years of life, or quality-adjusted life-years (QALYs). Cost/utility is a special use of cost-effectiveness that weights observable health states by preferences or utility judgments of quality; in cost/utility analysis, the benefits of medical care, behavioral interventions, or preventive programs are expressed in terms of well-years.

If a man dies of heart disease at age 50 and we expected him to live to age 75, then we might conclude that the disease precipitated 25 lost life-years. If 100 men died at age 50 (and also had a life expectancy of 75 years), then we might conclude that 2,500 life-years (100 men × 25 years) had been lost. Death is not the only relevant outcome of heart disease. Many adults have myocardial infarctions that leave them disabled for a long time and resulting in diminished quality of life. QALYs take into consideration such consequences. For example, a disease that reduces quality of life by one-half will take away 0.5 QALY over the course of each year. If the disease affects two people, then it will take away 1 QALY (2×0.5) over the course of each year. A medical treatment that improves quality of life by 0.2 for each of five individuals will result in the equivalent of 1 QALY if the benefit persists for 1 year. This system has the advantage of considering both benefits and side effects of programs in terms of the common QALY units.

The need to integrate mortality and quality-of-life information is clear in studies of heart disease. Consider hypertension. People with high blood pressure may live shorter lives if untreated and longer lives if treated. Thus, one benefit of treatment is to add years to life. However, for most patients, high blood pressure does not produce symptoms for many years. Conversely, the treatment for high blood pressure may cause negative side effects. If one evaluates a treatment only in terms of changes in life expectancy, then the benefits of the program will be overestimated because one has not taken side effects into consideration. On the other hand, considering only current quality of life will underestimate the treatment benefits because information on mortality is excluded. In fact, considering only current function might make the treatment look harmful because the side effects of the treatment might be worse than the symptoms of hypertension. A comprehensive measurement system takes into consideration side effects and benefits and provides an overall estimate of the benefit of treatment.

Most approaches for obtaining QALYs are similar. The approach that we prefer involves several steps. First, patients are classified according to objective levels of functioning. These levels are represented by the scales of mobility, physical activity, and social activity. Next, once observable behavioral levels of functioning have been classified, each individual is placed on the 0 to 1.0 scale of wellness, which describes where a person lies on the continuum between optimum function and death.

Some traditional measures used in medicine and public health consider only whether a person is dead or alive. In other words, all living people get the same score. However, health care professionals know that there are different levels of wellness, and these states of wellness need to be quantified. To accomplish this quantification, researchers weight the observable health states by quality ratings for the desirability of these conditions. Human value studies have been conducted to place the observable states onto a preference continuum, with an anchor of 0 for death and 1.0 for completely well. Studies have shown that the weights are highly stable over a 1-year period and are consistent across diverse groups of raters (Kaplan 1994). Finally, one must consider the duration of stay in various health states. Having a cough or a headache for 1 day is not the same as having the problem for 1 year.

This system has been used to evaluate many different health care programs. For example, it was used to demonstrate that a new medication for patients with arthritis produced an average of 0.023 QALY per year, whereas a new medication for acquired immunodeficiency syndrome (AIDS) produced nearly 0.46 of these units per year. However, the benefit of the arthritis medication may last as long as 20 years, ultimately producing 0.023×20 years = 0.46 year. The AIDS treatment produced a benefit for only 1 year, so its total effect was 0.46×1 year = 0.46 year. In other words, the general system allows the full potential benefits of these two completely different treatments to be compared (Kaplan et al. 1998).

New Approaches to the Science of Measuring Patient-Reported Outcomes

Many people feel that diagnoses in medicine can be derived exclusively from biological tests, and for many years, physicians simply ignored most of the information that was provided by their patients during clinic visits. However, it has become increasingly clear that patient reports provide the key to understanding many important illnesses and risk factors. In fact, in most cases, patients consult physicians because they experience symptoms and problems and in this way profoundly influence the delivery of health care.

Patient-reported outcomes (PROs) are defined as patients' reports about their health and circumstances surrounding their health. These measures are now recognized as a central part of health care and health care research. This recognition is for a good reason: Patients' experiences of illness drive use of the health care system, inform the use of medication, and greatly influence diagnostic decisions. What we experience as "health" is phenomenological and is often based on the experience of symptoms, such as pain, fatigue, malaise, and dozens of individual symptoms (e.g., coughs, aches, physical dysfunction). Individual interpretations of sensations are crucial in the experience of wellness and illness. The U.S. Food and Drug Administration now recognizes PRO in clinical trials (Patrick et al. 2007), and PROs are becoming critical indicators for the approval of new drugs and devices. These PROs are summarized in a report by the U.S. Food and Drug Administration (2009).

PROs are self-reports made by patients about health-related information. As such, they are susceptible to many types of bias, distortion, and error, which have been well documented by research in cognitive science and autobiographical memory. For example, when PROs ask individuals to report their symptoms over long periods of time (say, a month), many processes come into play that affect the validity and reliability of the resulting information (Patrick et al. 2007). First, fundamental limitations of memory capacity preclude the veridical recall of *some* symptom information from a lengthy period. Second, after information has been encoded into memory, certain processes enable the recall of selected information on the basis of the individual's immediate context (when a person is in a bad mood, relatively more negative memories are accessible) (Bradburn et al. 1987; Sudman et al. 1996). Third, recall is influenced by a number of cognitive heuristics, or rules of thumb, used to reconstruct past experience. One heuristic is known as the *peak-end rule* because of the greater likelihood of people reporting high-intensity experiences (e.g., severe pain) over low-intensity experiences and reporting experiences more proximal to the time of assessment (Kahneman et al. 1999; Redelmeier et al. 2003). These factors are especially relevant when experiences are difficult to remember, such as over long periods or when experiences are rapidly fluctuating. (Pain and fatigue have these qualities, which is evident when an individual tries to report pain levels for a particular day after a week or two later.) For all of these reasons, many researchers have recommended the collection of PRO data using short recall periods to minimize bias and distortion.

The development of assessments with brief recall periods (or even no recall period when the respondent is asked about immediate experience) has gone hand in hand with moving assessments out of the laboratory or clinic and into everyday life. The *experience sampling method* (ESM) and *ecological momentary assessment* (EMA) are techniques that use immediate reporting of experience in respondents' typical environments, thereby achieving a high level of data accuracy and representative design.

Early versions of momentary assessment (ESM and EMA) were based on signaling respondents via electronic pagers or wristwatch alarms to complete a pocket-size paper-and-pencil questionnaire. Typically, a series of questions about the time and date, where the person was, what he or she was doing, and who he or she was with was answered first. These questions were followed by specific content meeting the needs of a study; typically, these content questions were about affect, symptoms, or behaviors. For example, an EMA investigation of chronic pain would be likely to include questions about the severity of pain at the moment, if medications had recently been taken for the pain, how the pain was affecting functioning, and, perhaps, coping methods currently employed to deal with the pain.

Newer versions of momentary assessment protocol have been greatly enhanced with the advent of handheld computers and smart cell phones. These devices support sophisticated programs that greatly enhance the user experience of the assessment and enable implementation of complex protocols. An important component of momentary assessment is the scheduling of assessments. The early wristwatch methods were limited to whatever schedule of beeps was initially programmed into the device; beeps generated by pager systems were more flexible, but implementing more complex data collection routines was still difficult. Handheld devices can be programmed to function as autonomous data collection devices that are preprogrammed to handle a variety of circumstances that respondents may face in the real world (Shiffman 2007). One aspect of this autonomy is that the scheduling of assessments can be set by an algorithm that randomly selects moments for assessment (within preset parameters) or samples moments at set times, depending on the needs of the study design. Much more complex samplings are possible and are in the spirit of moving the laboratory into the real world because assessments can be made contingent on information other than time of day. For example, an investigator interested in how mood changes after an environmental event (e.g., marital dispute) might ask participants to self-initiate an assessment right after the event (a so-called event-driven assessment) and have the electronic diary systematically assess mood at 30-minute intervals thereafter for the next 4 hours. In this case, the environmental context is conditioning the assessment schedule, leading to a unique set of snapshots about outcomes in the real world.

Representative Design in Physiological Assessment

Knowledge of physiological states is clearly a critical source of information for preventing, identifying, and treating medical conditions. With some exceptions, collection of physiological measures has been confined to laboratory and clinic settings, and a question arises that is parallel to the one just discussed for self-reports: Are physiological measures collected in restricted settings truly representative of physiological functioning in patients' everyday lives? Unlike the field of PROs and, more generally, self-report, which has a long and rich history of research, representative design in physiological measurements is a younger field without a large body of empirical results supporting it. Therefore, there is limited literature directly on the topic of representative design with physiological measures for us to summarize here; instead, we provide an example to make the point that representative design should be a concept of interest for this domain of research and practice.

Consider the assessment of blood pressure. Many clinical decisions about the management of blood pressure are made on the basis of readings taken in an office setting. Although it has long been recommended that physicians capture blood pressure using multiple readings on multiple days (Mi et al. 2010), in practice, physicians commonly prescribe medication on the basis of a few readings or, in some cases, only a single reading. However, blood pressure varies substantially over the course of time (Mi et al. 2010). Following a circadian pattern, blood pressure surges during the morning hours and dips later in the day and tends to be lower at night (de la Sierra et al. 2009). There is considerable speculation about whether patterns of blood pressure variations throughout the circadian cycle are predictive of adverse health outcomes. For example, individuals whose blood pressure does not dip during the night might be regarded as at higher risk (Eguchi et al. 2009). However, few epidemiological studies have systematically evaluated the impact of these patterns. In fact, most of what is known about the risks of high blood pressure is based on epidemiological studies that characterize blood pressure at a few defined points in time and then follow participants prospectively to determine whether elevated blood pressure early in life results in poor health outcomes many years later (Egan et al. 2010). Many studies show that clinical-based blood pressure assessment misses much of the important variability that occurs outside the clinic. New approaches to ambulatory blood pressure assessment capture the full range of blood pressure variation that accompanies the challenges of everyday experience.

Mobile and Wireless Health

Whereas ESM and EMA methods and technology are typically (although not exclusively) used to monitor patient experience, *mobile health* (mHealth) is about using mobile computing technologies to enhance all aspects of health care, including our focus, behavioral intervention strategies. An important advance in bringing the laboratory and clinic into natural environments is the rapid development of new portable communications technologies. The revolution in technology enables studies with representative design, and ESM and EMA provide the scientific underpinnings of these developments. In fact, a direct outgrowth of EMA is an area known as *ecological momentary interventions* (EMIs). EMIs are methods intended to take interventions (usually behavioral) into the everyday lives of patients. EMIs are administered via mobile devices and are "momentary" in that they happen immediately in the natural environment (hence, the analogy with EMA). These methods have been used for interventions relevant to a range of problems, including smoking cessation, weight loss, anxiety, diabetes management, eating disorders, alcohol use, healthy eating, and physical activity (Heron and Smyth 2010).

One EMI smartphone application was designed by David Gustafson from the University of Wisconsin to reduce relapse by providing social support in real time and by using geographic information to determine types of information and support. The immediate social support is especially helpful for people in recovery after leaving a residential treatment environment and during times when it is challenging to find and attend a local meeting. The application also provides information about behavior over time (graphs that can help predict risk of relapse). Users of the application can also put in addresses of places where they have previously used drugs or alcohol or places that have high risk from other factors, and the phone will alert them when they are geographically near these areas and will provide tools to extend the reach of clinicians in real time (Center for Health Enhancement Systems Studies 2014).

Wireless and mHealth usage, which includes a range of technologies from cellular phones to wireless sensors, has developed at an exponential pace in recent years. The International Telecommunication Union (2014) estimated that about 6.9 billion cellular phones are now in use around the world and that this number will at least double (far exceeding the number of people in the world) within the next decade. China, for example, has nearly a billion wireless accounts, and the United Arab Emirates has nearly two active wireless accounts for each person in the population. Wireless communication devices have leapfrogged wired systems. Figure 6–2 shows the growth of wireless phones in relation to standard wired telephones between 2007 and 2014. About 2.3 billion people have mobile broadband access, and 55% of them are in the developing world. About 91% of U.S. adults use a mobile phone regularly. Financial resources have not hindered widespread dissemination of these technologies: the fast growing markets include economically disadvantaged African American and Hispanic users and low-income families (Zickuhr and Smith 2012). Growing evidence indicates that electronic technologies may be the best way to help low-income people change behavior (Bennett et al. 2012). The almost universal availability of cell phones means that most people are connected to a data collection and intervention apparatus, enabling the implementation of representative design as discussed in the "Representative Design in Physiological Assessment" section. Technologies are also available to collect real-time psychophysiological responses. Medical diagnosis might also undergo major changes. For example, high-resolution fiber-optic microendoscopes are small portable devices that can be used to perform cancer detection in the field. In some locations in the developing world, health workers can take images of skin problems and use cell phone technologies to beam images back to major medical centers around the world, from which they can get quick diagnosis and treatment directions.

The mHealth technologies can also help with treatment, such as chronic disease management. Smartphone applications are being developed for disease self-management for asthma, alcohol dependence, and lung cancer.

The promise of mHealth deserves serious scrutiny. The Affordable Care Act of 2010 allows providers to bill for remote monitoring beginning in 2014. Mobile technologies are likely to have a profound impact on health care and biomedical research, and health care professionals may soon be surrounded by more data than they can store, analyze, and interpret. New analysis methods may be necessary. In addition, protecting and securing the data and the privacy of the people being monitored by the devices will present serious challenges (Kaplan and Stone 2013).

Summary

Patient-reported outcomes are receiving increasing attention. The Patient-Reported Outcomes Research Institute is a public-private partnership that focuses on research from the patient's perspective. Emphasizing the patient's perspective of-

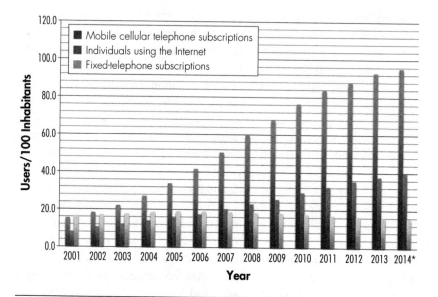

FIGURE 6–2.   Mobile wireless subscriptions in comparison to fixed telephone accounts and Internet computer users per 100 inhab-
itants worldwide: trend from 2001 to 2014.

*2014 numbers are estimates.

Source.   Data from International Telecommunication Union 2014.

ten leads to different conclusions than focusing on measures of biologic process. Significant advances in the science of patient assessment have been made in recent years, and we anticipate continued progress in this area.

Clinical Key Points

- Recognition of the importance of patient-reported experience is increasing. Many important clinical outcomes are best evaluated from the patient perspective.

- The patient perspective often leads to actions different from those of traditional approaches that emphasize biological markers.

- Measurement tools for both general and specific areas are available to assist clinicians in both the evaluation of a patient's current state and the effectiveness of particular treatment approaches.

- New mobile health technologies are being developed to increase the reach of clinicians in real time to help support patients and provide information that adds to the knowledge base.

- Efforts are under way to continue to improve how clinicians and researchers measure the important aspects of quality of life and well-being to aid in accurate diagnoses and treatment plans.

References

Bennett GG, Warner ET, Glasgow RE, et al; Be Fit, Be Well Study Investigators: Obesity treatment for socioeconomically disadvantaged patients in primary care practice. Arch Intern Med 172(7):565–574, 2012 22412073

Bradburn NM, Rips LJ, Shevell SK: Answering autobiographical questions: the impact of memory and inference on surveys. Science 236(4798):157–161, 1987 3563494

Brown DS, Jia H, Zack MM, et al: Using health-related quality of life and quality-adjusted life expectancy for effective public health surveillance and prevention. Expert Rev Pharmacoecon Outcomes Res 13(4):425–427, 2013 23977969

Center for Health Enhancement Systems Studies: Addiction CHESS Project: developing and testing a computer-based alcohol use disorder recovery system. July 1, 2014. Available at: http://chess.wisc.edu/chess/projects/AddictionChess.aspx. Accessed August 25, 2014.

Centers for Disease Control and Prevention: Health-Related Quality of Life (HRQOL). November 1, 2012. Available at: http://www.cdc.gov/hrqol/. Accessed August 25, 2014.

de la Sierra A, Redon J, Banegas JR, et al; Spanish Society of Hypertension Ambulatory Blood Pressure Monitoring Registry Investigators: Prevalence and factors associated with circadian blood pressure patterns in hypertensive patients. Hypertension 53(3):466–472, 2009 19171788

Drüeke TB, Locatelli F, Clyne N, et al; CREATE Investigators: Normalization of hemoglobin level in patients with chronic kidney disease and anemia. N Engl J Med 355(20):2071–2084, 2006 17108342

Egan BM, Zhao Y, Axon RN: US trends in prevalence, awareness, treatment, and control of hypertension, 1988–2008. JAMA 303(20):2043–2050, 2010 20501926

Eguchi K, Ishikawa J, Hoshide S, et al: Night time blood pressure variability is a strong predictor for cardiovascular events in patients with type 2 diabetes. Am J Hypertens 22(1):46–51, 2009 18833198

Ellwood PM: Shattuck lecture—outcomes management: a technology of patient experience. N Engl J Med 318(23):1549–1556, 1988 3367968

Heron KE, Smyth JM: Ecological momentary interventions: incorporating mobile technology into psychosocial and health behaviour treatments. Br J Health Psychol 15(Pt 1):1–39, 2010 19646331

International Telecommunication Union: The World Telecommunication/ICT Indicators database, 18th Edition. Geneva, Switzerland, International Telecommunications Union, 2014

Kahneman D, Diener E, Schwarz N: Well-Being: The Foundations of Hedonic Psychology. New York, Russell Sage Foundation, 1999

Kaplan RM: Value judgment in the Oregon Medicaid experiment. Med Care 32(10):975–988, 1994 7934274

Kaplan RM: Diseases, Diagnoses, and Dollars. New York, Springer, 2009

Kaplan RM, Stone AA: Bringing the laboratory and clinic to the community: mobile technologies for health promotion and disease prevention. Annu Rev Psychol 64:471–498, 2013 22994919

Kaplan RM, Ganiats TG, Sieber WJ, et al: The Quality of Well-Being Scale: critical similarities and differences with SF-36. Int J Qual Health Care 10(6):509–520, 1998 9928590

Keller SD, Ware JE Jr, Hatoum HT, et al: The SF-36 Arthritis-Specific Health Index (ASHI), II: tests of validity in four clinical trials. Med Care 37(5, suppl):MS51–MS60, 1999 10335743

McDowell I: Measuring Health: A Guide to Rating Scales and Questionnaires, 3rd Edition. Oxford, UK, Oxford University Press, 2006

Mi J, Wang T, Meng L, et al: Development of blood pressure reference standards for Chinese children. Chinese Journal of Evidence-Based Pediatric 5:4–14, 2010

Patrick DL, Burke LB, Powers JH, et al: Patient-reported outcomes to support medical product labeling claims: FDA perspective. Value Health 10 (suppl 2):S125–S137, 2007 17995471

Redelmeier DA, Katz J, Kahneman D: Memories of colonoscopy: a randomized trial. Pain 104(1–2):187–194, 2003 12855328

Rokeach M: The Nature of Human Values. New York, Free Press, 1973

Shiffman S: Designing protocols for ecological momentary assessment, in The Science of Real-Time Data Capture: Self-Reports in Health Research. Edited by Stone AA, Shiffman S, Atienza A, Nebeling L. New York, Oxford University Press, 2007, pp 27–53

Stewart AL, Ware JE (eds): Measuring Functioning and Well-Being: The Medical Outcomes Study Approach. Durham, NC, Duke University Press, 1992

Sudman S, Bradburn NM, Schwarz N: Thinking About Answers: The Application of Cognitive Processes to Survey Methodology. San Francisco, CA, Jossey-Bass, 1996

U.S. Food and Drug Administration: Guidance for industry: patient-reported outcome measures: Use in medical product development to support labeling claims, 2009. Available at: http://www.fda.gov/downloads/Drugs/GuidanceComplianceRegulatoryInformation/Guidances/UCM193282.pdf. Accessed August 25, 2014.

World Health Organization: Constitution of the World Health Organization. Geneva, Switzerland, World Health Organization, 1948

Zickuhr K, Smith A: Digital Differences. Washington, DC, Pew Charitable Trust, 2012

Suggested Cross-References

Well-being is discussed in Chapter 7 ("Clinical Assessments of Positive Mental Health"), Chapter 13 ("Biology of Positive Psychiatry"), and Chapter 15 ("Positive Geriatric and Cultural Psychiatry").

Suggested Readings

Cherepanov D, Palta M, Fryback DG, et al: Gender differences in multiple underlying dimensions of health-related quality of life are associated with sociodemographic and socioeconomic status. Med Care 49(11):1021–1030, 2011 21945974

Fryback DG, Dunham NC, Palta M, et al: US norms for six generic health-related quality-of-life indexes from the National Health Measurement study. Med Care 45(12):1162–1170, 2007 18007166

Jones CA, Pohar SL, Feeny DH, et al: Longitudinal construct validity of the Health Utilities Indices Mark 2 and Mark 3 in hip fracture. Qual Life Res 23(3):805–813, 2014 24081869

Kaplan RM: Value judgment in the Oregon Medicaid experiment. Med Care 32(10):975–988, 1994 7934274

McDowell I: Measuring Health: A Guide to Scales and Questionnaires, 3rd Edition. Oxford, UK, Oxford University Press, 2006

7

Clinical Assessments of Positive Mental Health

PER BECH, M.D., D.M.SC.

> I don't care whether it's mind or whether it's organic—it's clinical!
>
> Heinz Lehmann (1996)

The assessment of an individual's subjective dimension of positive mental health or well-being is the focal point of this chapter. For DSM-5 (American Psychiatric Association 2013), the Global Assessment of Functioning (GAF) Scale, which was an important assessment scale in DSM-IV (American Psychiatric Association 1994), was removed because of both a lack of clarity (a mixture of symptoms of illness, suicide risk, and disabilities) and poor psychometric properties. Apart from the symptomatic diagnoses of mental disorders and their suicidal risks, DSM-5 now selectively focuses on social health as measured by the World Health Organization (WHO) Disability Assessment Schedule. In other words, the clinician's assessment of an individual's well-being regarding positive mental health is lacking in DSM-5. It is not clear why the Medical Outcomes Study 36-Item Short Form Health Survey (SF-36) (Ware et al. 1994) was not adopted by DSM-5 as a measure of social, mental, and physical health.

In selecting scales measuring psychological well-being or positive mental health, the psychometric focus has been on including those scales that possess an acceptable validity or plausibility from which to draw conclusions in measurement-based care. A very simple study outside the academic laboratory of psychometrics was actually what started research in positive mental health or subjective well-being in the medical setting. This clinical study was performed by a family doctor group practice (Jachuck et al. 1982) to measure the quality of life in patients with mild to moderate hypertension treated with hypotensive drugs. Well-being was measured on a questionnaire that included mood, interest, and energy. Most important, this assessment was made not only by the family doctors but also by the patients themselves as well as by their relatives. The results showed that although all the treating family doctors found that the drug had improved the patients' well-being, only half of the patients themselves agreed, and in only one case had the relatives found an increase in the patient's well-being during the trial. A later psychoeducational intervention in patients with recurrent depressive episodes with the goal of reducing the patients' expressed emotion problems focused exclusively on the patients' relatives. This intervention resulted in a significant relapse prevention of the patients' illness (Shimazu et al. 2011).

The scales described in this chapter can be completed by the clinician, by the patients, and by the patients' significant others. The first well-being scale to be accepted by international medical journals, the Psychological General Well-Being Index (PGWB; Dupuy 1984), was actually used to discriminate between different hypotensive classes of drugs in the treatment of mild to moderate hypertension (Croog et al. 1986). Patients with cardiovascular disorders were also the subjects in the pivotal study by Garnefski et al. (2008), which was carried out to measure posttraumatic growth as a matter of positive mental health measured with the WHO-Five Well-Being Index (WHO-5) (Bech et al. 2013).

Another scale discussed in this chapter, SF-36, essentially covers the components measured by the GAF; thus, it includes dimensions of symptoms of illness and social functioning. However, the items in the SF-36 mental health subscale (Veit and Ware 1983) are based on the PGWB. Focusing on the core elements of subjective well-being as measured by scales such as PGWB and WHO-5 leads to a central research issue: this subjective dimension is very self-reflective, with many private language problems. Thus, in this dimension, the individual is communicating with himself or herself from the very moment he or she wakes up in the morning and begins perceiving and planning the day and determining whether he or she has the emotional appetite to do things. How can these existential day-to-day reflections and coping issues be measured? Studies from all over the world indicate that scales such as the PGWB and the WHO-5 actually cover a basic life perception of the dynamic state of well-being, allowing this private language to be translated into a simple communicative measure for research. Because they are disease-independent scales, they are often called generic scales for mental health.

Vaillant (2012) indicated that an overall measure of mental health focused on subjective well-being could be a single question answered on a seven-point scale ranging from delighted to terrible: "How do you feel about your life as a whole, all things considered?" According to Vaillant, this measure works with a surprising applicability. However, such an overall seven-point scale is often too crude to measure change in states of well-being because psychological well-being, when measured in the same way as "mental" blood pressure, covers at least three elements: happiness, relaxation, and mental activity.

A mental reaction to a stressor or to significant life events does not just happen. It often has a history. A clinical assessment of positive well-being thus also must take personality factors into account. For example, posttraumatic growth rather than stress is seen in connection with the fighting spirit personality factor. Therefore, in measurement-based care, states of psychological well-being and personality factors must be equally considered. When summarizing his 40 years of stress research, Selye (1974) noted that he considered stress to be an important life activator (stress without distress) that should be converted into positive mental health and not into a destructive force in the form of distress, anxiety, or depression.

Clinical Content of Well-Being Scales

In a review of well-being scales, an expert panel identified 85 self-reported health and well-being scales (Hall et al. 2011). In their protocol, the panel defined *health* as a dynamic state of complete physical, mental, and social well-being, not merely the absence of disease. Focusing on mental well-being, the panel concentrated on scales written in clear and unbiased language, without any overlap with items referring to symptoms of illness (e.g., functional disabilities or symptoms of mental disorder) or side effects of medication (e.g., psychotropic effects of drugs on memory function); that is, the panel focused on generic scales. In total, 4 of the 85 scales had a content validity of 70% or greater—that is, an adequate clinical content of general well-being (Hall et al. 2011). Among these scales, only two had clinical relevance for positive psychiatry, namely, WHO-5 (with 100% content validity) and PGWB (with 70%). Table 7–1 lists the most frequently used generic well-being scales.

Table 7–2 gives the five PGWB items and the corresponding WHO-5 items. These items cover Wundt's three components of subjective well-being. Table 7–3 provides the contrasting subjective ill-being components (Blumental 1970). A century ago, Wilhelm Wundt (1832–1920) established the first scientific laboratory for psychology in the world. During his own psychometric investigations, he found that the subjects under examination in the laboratory were able to communicate their immediate well-being versus ill-being using the three di-

Table 7–1.   Generic well-being scales

Scale	Number of items	PROQOLID[a]
Visual Analogue Scale (VAS)[b]	1	–
Satisfaction With Life (SWL)[b]	5	–
World Health Organization—Five Well-Being Index (WHO-5)[b]	5	+
Affect Balance Scale (ABS)[b]	10	+
Positive and Negative Affect Schedule (PANAS)[b]	20	–
Psychological General Well-Being Index (PGWB)[b]	22	+
Quality of Life Enjoyment and Satisfaction Questionnaire Short Form (Q-LES-Q-SF)[c]	16	+
World Health Organization Quality of Life Assessment Instrument—Brief Form (WHOQOL-BREF)[c]	26	+
Hospital Anxiety and Depression Scale (HADS)[c]	14	+

Note.   All scales listed are self-rating scales. "+" indicates that the scale in question is included in the PROQOLID database; "–" indicates that it is not included.
[a]PROQOLID database (Mapi Research Trust 2014).
[b]See McDowell 2010 for more information on these scales.
[c]See Rush et al. 2008 for more information on these scales.

alectical components happy versus unhappy, relaxed versus restless, and active versus passive (Tables 7–2 and 7–3). One of Wundt's research assistants was Emil Kraepelin (1856–1926). Using Wundt's systematic psychometric methods, Kraepelin was the first psychiatrist able to identify the major mental disorders such as schizophrenia and manic-depressive illness at the level of symptoms alone. DSM-III (American Psychiatric Association 1980) and DSM-IV were based on Krapelin's systematic approach, and so is DSM-5.

One of the well-being scales collected by the expert panel (Hall et al. 2011) is the Affect Balance Scale (ABS), which follows Wundt's approach (Bradburn 1969). The overall "balance" score in the ABS is measured by subtracting the negative score from the positive score. However, this way of measuring positive well-being has not been accepted, and the expert panel estimated that the ABS has a mere 20% content validity (Hall et al. 2011). This low ranking of the ABS is also partly because the five items measuring positive well-being and the five items measuring ill-being are scored on a dichotomized scale, where *yes* is scored 1 and *no* is scored 0. In contrast, both the WHO-5 and the PGWB have items that are all scored with six answer categories (ranging from 0 to 5), as

Table 7–2. Measuring the dynamic state of well-being using questionnaires

Wundt well-being component	PGWB questions	WHO-5 questions
Cheerful (happy)	Cheerful 5=all of the time 0=none of the time	Cheerful 5=all of the time 0=none of the time
	Interested in things 5=all of the time 0=none of the time	Interested in things 5=all of the time 0=none of the time
Relaxed (calm)	Relaxed versus high strung 5=relaxed all of the time 3=relaxed, seldom high strung 0=high strung all of the time	Relaxed 5=all of the time 0=none of the time
Active (vital)	Active versus sluggish 5=active all of the time 3=active, seldom sluggish 0=sluggish all of the time	Active 5=all of the time 0=none of the time
	Fresh and rested 5=all of the time 0=none of the time	Fresh and rested 5=all of the time 0=none of the time

Note. PGWB = Psychological General Well-Being Index; WHO-5 = World Health Organization–Five Well-Being Index.

shown in Tables 7–2 and 7 3. The PGWB, which includes items relating to both well-being and ill-being, is scored as if it were a fully positive well-being scale by converting all the negatively formulated ill-being items to positive ones; that is, for these items, the scores are reversed. Another scale reviewed by the expert panel that reverses the scores for negatively formulated ill-being (anxiety) items is the Zung Self-Rating Anxiety Scale, which received a rating of 40% content validity (Hall et al. 2011). This approach with reversed scores for negatively formulated items is clinically and psychometrically very problematic (Bech 2012).

Clinical psychometrics has frequently debated whether a simple, global scale is sufficient to measure well-being versus ill-being. In clinical trials of antidepressants, the Clinical Global Impression Scale has often been used by clinicians to assess the overall severity of an individual's depressive state. This global scale ranges from 0 (no sign of depression) to 6 (severely depressed) (Bech 2012). As concluded by Vaillant (2012), such a global scale that measures well-being often has a high degree of applicability. Another global well-being scale used in clinical trials is the Visual Analogue Scale. However, when measuring change in states of well-being in clinical trials, such global scales are less sensitive than the scales in Table 7–2 (Bech 2012).

Table 7–3.   Measuring the dynamic state of ill-being using questionnaires

Wundt ill-being component	PGWB questions	Major Depression Inventory questions
Unhappy (depressed)	Downhearted, sad 5=all of the time 0=none of the time	Low in spirits, sad 5=all of the time 0=at no time
	Hopeless, nothing worthwhile 5=extremely so 0=not at all	Lack of interests 5=all the time 0=at no time
Restless (anxious)	Tense 5=extremely tense 0=not at all	Very restless 5=all of the time 0=at no time
Passive (apathetic)	Tired, worn out 5=all of the time 0=none of the time	Lacking in energy 5=all the time 0=at no time
	Losing control over talking or thinking 5=very much 0=not at all	Difficulty in concentration 5=all the time 0=at no time

Note.   PGWB = Psychological General Well-Being Index.

In measurement-based care, general population reference values for well-being scales such as the WHO-5 are essential for defining the goal of treatment (Bech 2012). Figure 7–1 shows the standardization of the WHO-5, where a score of 70 indicates the mean score in the general population (national norm).

Clinical Content in Personality Scales

The preexisting vulnerability (diathesis) to acute or chronic stressors is found in the personality traits, as illustrated in Figure 7–1. A mental reaction to a stressor does not just happen; it often has a history. Much research has been carried out on posttraumatic stress disorder, in which the ultimate mental reaction includes symptoms of anxiety, interpersonal sensitivity, and depression. As discussed by Breslau (2011), neuroticism as a personality trait accounts for the way these symptoms of anxiety, interpersonal sensitivity, and depression develop. A high negative correlation between neuroticism and well-being has been found in several studies.

A positive coping style in relation to a person's persistent disposition to deal with stressors has been called *fighting spirit* (Pettingale et al. 1985). Garnefski et al. (2008) used a questionnaire including positive coping style to measure post-

Trait disposition (diathesis): coping strategies	Mental reaction: WHO-5	
PTSG: Active coping (fighting spirit)	WHO-5	
• Thinking how to best cope with the situation		100
• Looking at the positive sides of the matter		
• Having a positive plan		
• Thinking how to change the situation		70 Norm (national mean)
• Considering yourself as a stronger person		
PTSD: Passive coping (neuroticism)		50
• Feelings easily hurt		40 Mild depression
• Often feeling lonely		30 Moderate depression
• Troubled by feelings of guilt		20 Severe depression
• Feeling tense or distressed		
• Considering yourself as a nervous person		0

FIGURE 7–1. Measuring coping strategies using questionnaires.

The scale is a standardization of the World Health Organization–Five Well-Being Index (WHO-5) to measure diathesis in relation to coping strategies for posttraumatic stress growth (PTSG) and posttraumatic stress disorder (PTSD).

traumatic stress growth in patients following a myocardial infarction. Garnefski et al. demonstrated a correlation coefficient of -0.81 between depression and the WHO-5.

Figure 7–1 shows a selection of the items from the studies by Pettingale et al. (1985) and Garnefski et al. (2008) measuring active coping, or fighting spirit. These personal growth items for active coping are also referred to by the term *eudaimonia*, that is, the diathesis aspect of well-being. The selection of items measuring passive coping, or neuroticism, in Figure 7–1 is derived from the Eysenck Personality Questionnaire (Eysenck and Eysenck 1976).

Simple global scales for these personality traits have been considered. For neuroticism, Rammstedt and John (2007) found that the items "considering yourself a nervous person" and "getting nervous easily" are sufficient. For fighting spirit, the item "considering yourself a strong person" seems to be sufficient.

Construct Validity or Scalability

The content validity of well-being scales is a test of their clinical plausibility or clinical validity. Content validity is a condition sine qua non. In a similar fashion, construct validity is an important psychometric property used to test the scalability of the questionnaire. From a measurement point of view, this scalability indicates to what extent the questionnaire under examination refers to one single construct, implying that the total score is a sufficient statistic, or more than one construct, implying that profile scores of the different constructs are more appropriate.

In their discussion of the term *construct validity*, Cronbach and Meehl (1955) refer to factor analysis as the psychometric method to use for to test construct validity. If more than one general factor is identified, the profile score or factor score will be the most valid expression for the outcome of the scale.

Among the well-being scales selected by the expert panel (Hall et al. 2011), the World Health Organization Quality of Life Assessment Instrument (WHO-QOL) was assessed as having 57% content validity. The WHOQOL originally contained 100 items covering several constructs. A brief version (WHOQOL-BREF) with 26 items was psychometrically analyzed by Power (2003), who used both factor analysis and an item response theory analysis (Rasch analysis) (Bech 2012). Factor analysis identified more than one general factor (Power 2003), and Rasch analysis showed that an eight-item subscale (WHOQOL-8) had acceptable construct validity. However, only one of these eight items (active [vital] component) is reflected in Table 7–2, namely, "Do you have enough energy for everyday life?"

Most of the WHOQOL-8 items are measured in terms of satisfaction, a result Power (2003) found disappointing. The problem with this mixed factor analysis and Rasch analysis is that Power (2003) did not a priori look at the content validity or the clinical validity of the WHOQOL, which is, as mentioned above, a condition sine qua non in the Rasch analysis (Bech 2012). Rasch analysis is a test of a hypothesis (scalability), not an explorative method for the creation of hypotheses.

Scalability of the WHO-5

This analysis places each of the five items (Table 7–2) on the latent dimension of well-being according to its prevalence (item location). Items located with high prevalence imply that they are present even in mild degrees of well-being, whereas items with low prevalence are only present at the more intense degrees of well-being. The two items at the top of the list in Table 7–2 ("Cheerful" and "Interested in things") were found to have high prevalence, and thus located at the milder degrees of well-being. The two items listed at the bottom of Table 7-2 ("Active" and "Fresh and rested") were found to have low prevalence, and thus located at the more intense degrees of well-being. The item "Relaxed" was located in between, thus indicating a moderate degree of well-being. According to the Rasch model, items with low prevalence must be preceded by items with a higher prevalence. A major advantage of the Rasch model over factor analysis is that item prevalence is a parameter in the model. Identifying item bias—that is, identifying to what extent any specific gender (male vs. female) or age-related (young vs. elderly) items are included—is also an important element in the Rasch analysis (Lucas-Carrasco et al. 2012).

As shown in Table 7–2, each of the WHO-5 items is scored from 0 to 5. The theoretical score range of the WHO-5 is therefore from 0 to 25. Conventionally, well-being scales should measure from 0 (worst thinkable state of well-being) to 100 (best thinkable state of well-being). Multiplying the raw score of the WHO-5 by 4 is therefore recommended. Figure 7–1 shows the standardization of the WHO-5 on this 0–100 scale with the general population norm of 70 (Bech et al. 2003).

Scalability of the PGWB

The PGWB was originally based on the factor structure of the 22 items included in this scale (Veit and Ware 1983). The factor analysis identified six underlying factors: anxiety, depression, general health, general positive well-being, loss of control, and vitality. Four of the items in the five-item PGWB shown in Table 7–2 were identified in the factor of general positive well-being. The remaining item (active and energetic) was included in the vitality factor. However, according to Veit and Ware (1983), using all 22 PGWB items as if they belonged to one single well-being factor by reversing the negatively phrased well-being items is not recommended; rather, they recommended a two-factor specification measuring psychological well-being versus psychological distress or ill-being.

The Wundt approach as recommended by Veit and Ware (1983) is shown in Tables 7–2 and 7–3. The items in the psychological well-being factor of the PGWB correspond to the WHO-5 items (Table 7–2).

The five PGWB ill-being items are listed in Table 7–3 together with items from the Major Depression Inventory (MDI). The MDI contains the items related to major depression according to DSM-IV and DSM-5 as well as depressive illness according to ICD-10 (World Health Organization 1993). The core items for an ICD-10 diagnosis are depressed mood, lack of interests, and lack of energy. The depression items in the PGWB do not include lack of interests because the PGWB has the positively formulated item "interested in things" (Table 7–3). To score the PGWB with all 22 items, 10 of the items must be reversed because the total score of the whole PGWB-22 is the sum of all the items. The PGWB items included in Table 7–3 are among the 10 items that need to be reversed.

A major issue in the Rasch analysis of the construct validity of a scale is local independence among the items. Local dependence refers to the extent to which the score of one item can automatically predict the score of another item. Local dependence implies a high intercorrelation between some pairs of items (Bech 2012). An examination of the 22 items in the PGWB shows that local dependence affects three depression items, namely, "feeling depressed," "feeling hopeless," and "feeling downhearted and sad." In other words, the PGWB has not controlled for local independence in the ill-being items (Table 7–3). However, local independence is in operation for all the items in Table 7–2.

Because a large number of intercorrelated items may be "rewarded" by increasing values of Cronbach reliability coefficient α, Feinstein (1987) noticed and criticized a tendency among psychosocial scientists working in academic institutions to increase the number of items in a scale, typically to approximately 20, to improve the Cronbach coefficient. However, as further stated by Feinstein (1987), the clinical investigator working outside the laboratory may want to shorten the number of items in a scale, particularly by eliminating the redundant items. Mixing positively and negatively formulated items also poses difficulties for the clinical investigator but again results from the fact that psychosocial laboratory workers are encouraged to mix the items to enlarge the standard deviations of their scales. Whereas the WHO-5 still exists in its original version from 1998, the PGWB has been modified in terms of both the time frame covered by the scale, for which the recommendation is the past 2 weeks, and the item quantifier, for which the frequency of the individual items has been revised (Bech 2004).

Scalability of Reversed Well-Being Scales

Among the 85 generic scales selected by the expert panel (Hall et al. 2011) as candidates to measure well-being, many scales primarily focusing on the ill-being dimensions, such as the Zung Anxiety Scale and the depression-oriented General Health Questionnaire, and the SF-36 include both positively and negatively formulated items. The content validity of these scales was found to be below 70% (Hall et al. 2011). For these scales to become well-being scales, the negatively formulated items must be reversed, similar to the process described for the PGWB. It is not clear why the panel group (Hall et al. 2011) did not consider the Center for Epidemiologic Studies Depression Scale or the Hospital Anxiety and Depression Scale (HADS). In the HADS, five of the seven items measuring depression are actually positively formulated and, to a large extent, correspond to the WHO-5 items (Bech 2012). However, from a clinical point of view, it is very problematic to measure depression severity with the HADS because it does not take the core items of depression into account (depressed mood, lack of interests, and lack of energy).

Scalability of Personality Scales

The time frame of WHO-5 is conventionally the past 2 weeks to ensure that the dynamic state of well-being covers an appropriate period, taking day-to-day variability into account. However, when relevant, this time frame can be reduced. For example, when monitoring treatment response in psychiatric care, Newnham et al. (2010) found it relevant to use the past 24 hours as the time frame (window) of the WHO-5. Originally, Dupuy (1984) had two windows for the PGWB, an acute version for the past week and a "chronic" version for the past 4 weeks.

When a personality trait such as the Eysenck neuroticism dimension is being measured, the respondent's lifelong, habitual trait is the focus of the examination. In the Eysenck neuroticism dimension, each item is negatively phrased. In a clinical validity study using many different personality scales, only Eysenck's neuroticism scale was associated with an experienced psychiatrist's assessment of neurotic severity (Bech et al. 1986).

The five passive coping items in Figure 7–1 were selected from Eysenck's neuroticism scale. These five items have no local dependence when they are used to measure passive coping or neuroticism. They can be considered subclinical levels of depression, including distress, interpersonal sensitivity, and guilt feelings.

The five items selected in Figure 7–1 to measure active coping, or fighting spirit, were derived from the scales made by Pettingale et al. (1985) and Garnefski et al. (2008). No local dependency seems to be in operation. When performing a clinical validity analysis of the fighting spirit dimension, clinicians need take into account to what extent this dimension overlaps with hidden bipolarity (Bech et al. 2013). Among the most valid items for hypomania in the Hypomanic Personality Scale are statements such as "I often feel excited and happy for no reason" and "I am considered to be a kind of a 'hyper' person"; these statements certainly have no overlap with active coping or fighting spirit.

Predictive Validity

A scale may be said to have predictive validity if it can predict some criterion obtained at a time after completion of the scale (Cronbach and Meehl 1955). Feinstein (1987) stipulates that the strictest form of predictive validity has three elements: a cutoff score on the scale at the baseline indicating the predictor, an outcome index describing the subsequent event whose likelihood is being predicted, and an expression for the relationship between the two. For example, the survival rate at 1 year (event) is 30% (the relationship) for certain cancer patients with decreased well-being (the baseline state) (Feinstein 1987).

Predictive Validity of Well-Being Scales

Predictive validity in Feinstein's sense has been evaluated by Birket-Smith et al. (2009) in patients with cardiovascular disorder. Using a baseline cutoff of >50 on the WHO-5, they found that 6 years later, patients with a score higher than the baseline cutoff had a survival rate of 80%, whereas patients with a score lower than the baseline cutoff had a survival rate of 20%.

Pilot studies using the PGWB have been collected, showing its validity to predict dropouts in a clinical study of antidepressants or to predict relapse in depressive episodes (Hunt and McKenna 1993). In this respect, the PGWB was superior to depression rating scales such as the Hamilton Depression Rating Scale. The PGWB confirmed the observation that stressful life events might not necessarily increase a patient's ill-being but could take some of the wind out of his or her sails.

Predictive Validity of Personality Scales

In the study by Pettingale et al. (1985), patients with breast cancer who had a fighting spirit score at baseline had a survival rate of 80% 5 years later. The high predictive validity of neuroticism in relation to physical illness events (diabetes, cardiovascular disease, cancer) has been reviewed by Lahey (2009).

Pharmacopsychometric Triangle

The pharmacopsychometric triangle (Figure 7–2) was developed to illustrate the validity of measuring positive well-being in clinical trials of antidepressants (Bech 2012). The upper left vertex (corner) of the triangle (A) lists the illness for which antidepressant medication is prescribed, namely, major depression. The upper right vertex (B) lists a scale measuring undesired effects of the medication (side effects). Finally, the lower vertex (C) lists patient-reported well-being (WHO-5) to indicate the treatment effect when taking into consideration both the desired (A) and the undesired (B) effects of the drug as indicated by the patients themselves.

Antidepressant medication is not produced to help persons with decreased well-being as such. Antidepressant medication is produced to treat major depression (A) with as few side effects as possible (B). By completing the WHO-5 (C), the patients themselves are reporting the final outcome of the treatment. The goal is to move patients' WHO-5 score from, for example, 30 (Figure 7–1) to the mean score in the general population, which is approximately 70.

The pharmacopsychometric triangle is actually an attempt to consider antidepressants as helpful practical adjuncts in more severely depressed patients. The WHO-5 assessment made by the patient as feedback about his or her benefit from the treatment should stimulate the dialogue between therapist and patient. As noted by Lehmann (1996), young psychiatrists unfortunately use DSM-IV as a kind of laundry list and psychopharmacology as a cookbook. However, measurement-based care of a depressed patient should include both assessments of side ef-

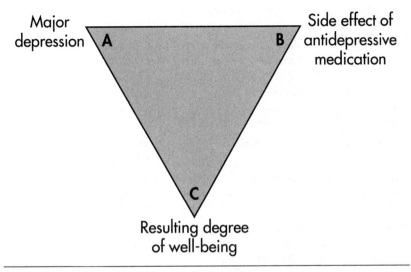

FIGURE 7–2. The pharmacopsychometric triangle.

fects and assessments of the patient's own subjective state of well-being. Clinical psychiatry is not psychopharmacology and should include empathy in the clinical dialogue between the therapist and his or her patient, often with reference to subjective well-being on the part of the patients and their relatives.

Comprehensive Overview of Assessment Tools

Table 7–1 gives an overview of the generic (i.e., illness-independent) scales, and Table 7–4 gives an overview of illness-specific quality-of-life scales. These tables are described in terms of construct, format for administration (self-, informant, or clinician administered), and psychometric properties with reference to the suggested review readings (McDowell 2010; Rush et al. 2008). The Mapi Research Trust PROQOLID database (Mapi Research Trust 2014) gives further details about which languages the scales have been translated into as well as other pertinent information.

Summary

Pure psychological well-being scales have to be written in clear language without overlap with symptoms of medical disorders or side effects of medication. To use a questionnaire in measurement-based care, the scalability has to be evaluated to ensure that the total scale score is a sufficient measure of the degree

Table 7–4.   Illness-specific quality-of-life scales

Scale	Illness assessed	Number of items	Administration	PROQOLID[a]
Spitzer's Quality of Life Index (QL-Index)	Chronic medical disorder	5	Interview (clinician)	+
Quality of Life Scale (QLS)	Schizophrenia	21	Interview (clinician)	+
Wisconsin Quality of Life Index (W-QLI)	Severe mental disorder	57	Interview (family members)	+
Lehman's Quality of Life Interview (QOLI)	Severe mental disorder	78	Interview (clinician)	–

Note.   See Rush et al. 2008 for more information on these scales. "+" indicates that the scale in question is included in the PROQOLID database; "–" indicates that it is not included.
[a]PROQOLID database (Mapi Research Trust 2014).

of well-being. It has been found that 5–10 questions in a scale are often suffi-cient. This holds true both for scales measuring the dynamic state of well-being and for scales measuring a preexisting dispositional factor or personality trait.

Scales that measure the dynamic state of well-being are especially used as outcome scales in measurement-based care, whereas scales that measure a per-sonality factor are especially used to predict outcome. A pharmacopsychomet-ric triangle illustrates how a measure of well-being is used to evaluate the benefit of treatment, taking into account the desired clinical effects and the unwanted side effects, thereby increasing the empathy in the dialogue between the thera-pist and his or her patient. Finally, the available scales are listed with reference to where much more detailed information about them can be obtained.

Clinical Key Points

- Although the dynamic state of mental well-being is a very subjective dimension, brief scales covering elements such as happiness, relaxation, and mental activity have been found to possess both clinical and psy-chometric validity.

- Most well-being scales actually contain the contrast ill-being, thereby also covering the elements of unhappiness, restlessness, and mental passivity. In some scales, a positive versus negative balance score is recommended; in other scales, the negatively formulated questions are reversed to give a summed score of well-being. Using a specific scale for well-being and another specific scale for ill-being is recommended.

- A mental reaction to stress does not just happen. It often has a history showing a preexisting factor or personality trait. Brief scales covering fighting spirit versus neuroticism have also been found to possess both clinical and psychometric validity.

- The predictive validity of well-being scales has especially been evaluated in patients with cardiovascular disorders. Patients with well-being scores above the median had a better survival outcome after 6 years than those scoring below the median.

- The predictive validity of personality scales has shown that patients with fighting spirit who consider themselves to be strong persons demonstrate posttraumatic growth rather than posttraumatic stress.

- Using well-being scales in measurement-based care to evaluate the balance between the desired clinical effects and the undesired side effects of an intervention might increase the empathy in the dialogue between the therapist and his or her patient.

References

American Psychiatric Association: Diagnostic and Statistical Manual of Mental Disorders, 3rd Edition. Washington, DC, American Psychiatric Association, 1980

American Psychiatric Association: Diagnostic and Statistical Manual of Mental Disorders, 4th Edition. Washington, DC, American Psychiatric Association, 1994

American Psychiatric Association: Diagnostic and Statistical Manual of Mental Disorders, 5th Edition. Arlington, VA, American Psychiatric Association, 2013

Bech P: Quality of life and rating scales for depression, in Antidepressants: Past, Present and Future. Edited by Preskorn SH, Feighner JP, Stranga CY, et al. New York, Springer, 2004, pp 148–170

Bech P: Clinical Psychometrics. Oxford, UK, Wiley Blackwell, 2012

Bech P, Jørgensen B, Jeppesen K, et al: Personality in depression: concordance between clinical assessment and questionnaires. Acta Psychiatr Scand 74(3):263–268, 1986 3788653

Bech P, Olsen LR, Kjoller M, et al: Measuring well-being rather than the absence of distress symptoms: a comparison of the SF-36 Mental Health subscale and the WHO-Five Well-Being Scale. Int J Methods Psychiatr Res 12(2):85–91, 2003 12830302

Bech P, Engell R, Bjerrum Møller S: Comparative validity of inventories and checklists for identifying depressed patients with hidden bipolarity. Neuropsychiatry 3:331–343, 2013

Birket-Smith M, Hansen BH, Hanash JA, et al: Mental disorders and general well-being in cardiology outpatients—6-year survival. J Psychosom Res 67(1):5–10, 2009 19539812

Blumental A: Language and Psychology. New York, Wiley, 1970

Bradburn NM: The Structure of Psychological Well-Being. Chicago, IL, Aldine, 1969

Breslau N: Causes of posttraumatic stress disorder, in Causality and Psychopathology. Edited by Shrout PE, Keyes KM, Ornstein K. Oxford, UK, Oxford University Press, 2011, pp 297–320

Cronbach LJ, Meehl PE: Construct validity in psychological tests. Psychol Bull 52(4):281–302, 1955 13245896

Croog SH, Levine S, Testa MA, et al: The effects of antihypertensive therapy on the quality of life. N Engl J Med 314(26):1657–1664, 1986 3520318

Dupuy HJ: The Psychological General Well-Being Index (PGWB), in Assessment of Quality of Life in Clinical Trials of Cardiovascular Therapy. Edited by Wenger NK, Mattson ME, Furberg CD, et al. New York, Le Jacq Publishing, 1984, pp 184–188

Eysenck HJ, Eysenck SBG: Psychoticism as a Dimension of Personality. London, Hodder & Stoughton, 1976

Feinstein AR: Clinimetrics. New Haven, CT, Yale University Press, 1987

Garnefski N, Kraaij V, Schroevers MJ, et al: Post-traumatic growth after a myocardial infarction: a matter of personality, psychological health, or cognitive coping? J Clin Psychol Med Settings 15(4):270–277, 2008 19104983

Hall T, Krahn GL, Horner-Johnson W, et al: Examining functional content in widely used Health-Related Quality of Life scales. Rehabil Psychol 56(2):94–99, 2011 21574727

Hunt S, McKenna S: Measuring quality of life in psychiatry, in Quality of Life Assessment Issues in the 1990s. Edited by Walker SR, Rosser RB. Dordrecht, Kluwer, 1993, pp 343–354

Jachuck SJ, Brierley H, Jachuck S, et al: The effect of hypotensive drugs on the quality of life. J R Coll Gen Pract 32(235):103–105, 1982 7097628

Lahey BB: Public health significance of neuroticism. Am Psychol 64(4):241–256, 2009 19449983

Lehmann HE: Psychopharmacotherapy, in The Psychopharmacologists. Edited by Healy D. London, Altman, 1996, pp 159–186

Lucas-Carrasco R, Allerup P, Bech P: The Validity of the WHO-5 as an early screening for apathy in an elderly population. Curr Gerontol Geriatr Res 2012:171857, 2012 22991511

Mapi Research Trust: PROQOLID. 2014. Available at: http://www.proqolid.org/about_proqolid. Accessed August 25, 2014.

McDowell I: Measures of self-perceived well-being. J Psychosom Res 69(1):69–79, 2010 20630265

Newnham EA, Hooke GR, Page AC: Monitoring treatment response and outcomes using the World Health Organization's Wellbeing Index in psychiatric care. J Affect Disord 122(1–2):133–138, 2010 19592116

Pettingale KW, Morris T, Greer S, et al: Mental attitudes to cancer: an additional prognostic factor. Lancet 1(8431):750, 1985 2858012

Power M: Development of a common instrument for quality of life, in EUROHIS: Developing Common Instruments for Health Surveys. Edited by Nosikov A, Gudex C. Amsterdam, The Netherlands, IOS Press, 2003, pp 145–164

Rammstedt B, John OP: Measuring personality in one minute or less: a 10-item short version of the Big Five Inventory in English and German. J Res Pers 41:203–212, 2007

Rush AJ, First MS, Blacker D: Handbook of Psychiatric Measures, 2nd Edition. Washington, DC, American Psychiatric Publishing, 2008

Selye H: Stress Without Distress. New York, JB Lippincott, 1974

Shimazu K, Shimodera S, Mino Y, et al: Family psychoeducation for major depression: randomised controlled trial. Br J Psychiatry 198(5):385–390, 2011 21343330

Vaillant GE: Positive mental health: is there a cross-cultural definition? World Psychiatry 11(2):93–99, 2012 22654934

Veit CT, Ware JE Jr: The structure of psychological distress and well-being in general populations. J Consult Clin Psychol 51(5):730–742, 1983 6630688

Ware JE, Gandek B; the IQoLA Project Group: The SF-36 health survey: development and use in mental health research and the IQoLA project. Int J Ment Health 23:49–73, 1994

World Health Organization: International Statistical Classification of Diseases and Related Health Problems, 10th Revision. Diagnostic Criteria for Research. Geneva, Switzerland, World Health Organization, 1993

Suggested Cross-References

Well-being is discussed in Chapter 6 ("What Is Well-Being?"), Chapter 13 ("Biology of Positive Psychiatry"), and Chapter 15 ("Positive Geriatric and Cultural Psychiatry").

Suggested Readings

McDowell I: Measures of self-perceived well-being. J Psychosom Res 69(1):69–79, 2010 20630265

Rush AJ, First MS, Blacker D (eds): Handbook of Psychiatric Measures, 2nd Edition. Washington, DC, American Psychiatric Publishing, 2008

Mapi Research Trust PROQOLID database. Available at: http://www.proqolid.org/. Accessed August 25, 2014.

Ware JE, Gandek B; the IQoLA Project Group: The SF-36 health survey: development and use in mental health research and the IQoLA project. Int J Ment Health 23:49–73, 1994

World Health Organization: International Statistical Classification of Diseases and Related Health Problems, 10th Revision. Diagnostic Criteria for Research. Geneva, Switzerland, World Health Organization, 1993

PART III

INTERVENTIONS IN POSITIVE PSYCHIATRY

8

Positive Psychotherapeutic and Behavioral Interventions

ACACIA C. PARKS, PH.D.

EVAN M. KLEIMAN, PH.D.

TODD B. KASHDAN, PH.D.

LESLIE R.M. HAUSMANN, PH.D.

PIPER S. MEYER, PH.D.

ANNE M. DAY, PH.D.

NICHEA S. SPILLANE, PH.D.

CHRISTOPHER W. KAHLER, PH.D.

Positive psychological interventions (PPIs), activities designed to promote positive outcomes via positive processes (Parks and Biswas-Diener 2013), have existed since the 1970s, starting with Fordyce's classic research teaching individuals to "act like a happy person." Consistent with Fordyce's original happiness studies (Fordyce 1977, 1983), as well as Martin Seligman's later call for research to improve the lives of individuals without disorder ("the other 80%") in his American Psychological Association presidential address (Seligman 1999), activities targeting happiness have primarily been developed and tested in nonclinical samples. However, PPIs have the potential to enrich the lives of individuals struggling with a range of physical and mental health conditions. In this chapter, we provide an overview of the growing body of research on the clinical applications of PPIs with an emphasis on showing by example how these activities can, with care and consideration, be tailored to specific populations.

Positive Psychological Interventions

Overview

PPIs include a broad range of activities such as savoring experiences, feeling and expressing gratitude, practicing kind acts, pursuing meaning, building hope, identifying and using one's strengths, and building compassion for oneself and others. Most studies examining the efficacy of PPIs have been conducted in experimental settings with nonclinical, healthy samples, in which single activities were assigned to individuals. Nevertheless, many PPI studies find small- to medium-sized reductions (Cohen's $d=0.31$ on average) in depressive symptoms, with more improvement overall occurring in samples with more baseline depressive symptoms (see Sin and Lyubomirsky 2009 for a meta-analysis).

Seligman et al. (2006) presented initial data on the impact of a "packaged" PPI program, one comprising multiple activities, which they called *positive psychotherapy* (PPT). Specifically, they evaluated PPT in samples with mild to moderate depressive symptoms (Study 1) and major depressive disorder (Study 2). PPT was administered either to groups (Study 1) or to individuals (Study 2). In both modalities, facilitators following a PPT manual introduced participants to a new activity each week. Participants were then asked to practice each activity as homework and report back the following week.

The group PPT program for mild to moderate depression consisted of activities delivered in a set sequence over a 6-week period (manualized by A.C. Parks and M.E.P. Seligman, "8-Week Group Positive Psychotherapy [PPT] Manual," unpublished manual, March 2007). Each week followed a similar format: an activity is introduced one week, and then participants use the activity between sessions and report back the following week. Any problems participants encountered with the activity for a given week are discussed and worked through at the start of the next session. Because the intervention used by Seligman et al. (2006) forms the basis for several of the programs discussed in this chapter, it is described in detail and is outlined in Table 8–1. The description of each activity is illustrated with clinical vignettes based on the first author's (A.C.P.) experience administering the activities in the manual to undergraduate and graduate students. Information on the empirical basis of each activity is given by Seligman et al. (2006).

Description of the Group PPT Program

Week 1: Using Your Strengths

Participants looked over a list of 24 character strengths from the VIA Institute on Character strengths classification system and spent time discussing which five strengths best characterized them. The groups then brainstormed ways to use those strengths more often in their lives over the next week and spent the week putting those ideas into practice. When they returned the following week, they reported their activities to their group and provided each other with troubleshooting in cases when the attempt did not go as planned. Participants reported a broad variety of experiences using their strengths. For example, one young woman resolved to use her curiosity more often by keeping abreast of local and global news; she set aside time each day to read articles online. A young man even found a way to make up for a weakness using one of his strengths; he was socially anxious and had mild Asperger's disorder, which made it difficult for him to interpret body language and facial expressions. One of his strengths was love of learning, so he made it a project to read everything he could about social signals and rules of social interaction. He then used that knowledge to help him observe social behavior and make sense of his previously incomprehensible social interactions.

Week 2: Three Good Things

Participants kept a nightly journal of three good things that happened at the end of each day. In this type of journal, the items can be big or small but should be specific (e.g., I had a great dinner with my three close friends vs. I have great friends), because previous research as well as clinical observation suggests that more general gratitude activities become stale and ultimately less effective if repeated too regularly (Lyubomirsky et al. 2005). The research on the *three good things* exercise suggests that although it leads to sustained increases in happiness, these increases occur at a delay, so it must be practiced consistently (Seligman et al. 2005). This empirical observation is consistent with clinical observation; participants generally reported finding this task very difficult, particularly in the first several days, and became proficient only with practice. Most participants described a process wherein they gradually became more observant of positive events throughout the day and worked harder to remember them, knowing they would need to record each event later. The end result was that participants gave greater attention to positive events than they would have otherwise and had little difficulty completing the task by the end of the first week.

Table 8–1.   Activities included in the original positive psychotherapy manual

Intervention	Description
Week 1: Using your strengths	Participants determine which 5 of 24 VIA character strengths represent them. Each day for a week, they use one of those strengths in a new way and record how they did it.
Week 2: Three good things	Each night for a week, participants write down three things that went well that day. Next to each positive event, they answer the question, "Why did this good thing happen?"
Week 3: Gratitude letter	Participants compose a letter detailing their gratitude to someone important in their life whom they have never properly thanked. They then read the letter to the person, preferably in person, and reflect on the experience.
Week 4: Savoring	Participants learn techniques for savoring sensory experiences. They are then asked to practice those techniques two to three times a day for a week.
Week 5: Active constructive responding	Participants are instructed to listen carefully for opportunities when people they care about share good news with them; they go out of their way to respond actively (i.e., visibly, enthusiastically) and constructively (i.e., positively).
Week 6: Life summary	Participants imagine how they hope a biographer might characterize them at the end of a long and fruitful life. They write a one- to two-page essay describing what traits and accomplishments they hope would define them, then reflect on whether they are pursuing those goals in everyday life.
Maintenance	Participants are asked to choose one or two activities to practice regularly for the next several months as a way of maintaining their gains. Activities can be modified as necessary to fit the individual's life.

Source.   A. C. Parks and M. E. P. Seligman, "8-Week Group Positive Psychotherapy (PPT) Manual," unpublished manual, March 2007.

Week 3: Gratitude Letter

Participants were asked to write a letter to a person in their lives to whom they felt very grateful but may never have thanked properly. They were then instructed to deliver the letter to the person, preferably by reading it to the recipient out loud in person or, if that was not possible, by reading it over the telephone. Although most participants noted that they expected the experience to be awkward, an overwhelming number of participants found the experience to be intensely positive. This experience matches up with experimental data by Seligman et al. (2005), which found the gratitude letter yielded a larger effect than any other PPI they tested at immediate posttest. However, it is worth discussing two instances in which the activity was not well received. One young woman chose to thank her parents, both of whom were Chinese; on receiving the letter thanking them for their dedication as parents, they took offense at the implication that they might have chosen to do otherwise. Because they considered parenting a duty rather than a choice— something the woman explained was typical in her parents' culture—their daughter's gratitude was both unnecessary and unwelcome. In another case, a middle-age woman expressed gratitude to her father; he regarded the display of affection with suspicion, certain that she was trying to manipulate him. These are the only two negative experiences that were observed with this activity over many years of teaching it. The majority of participants report a powerfully positive experience, often involving tears of joy, hugging, and sometimes even the other person responding by declaring their own gratitude.

Week 4: Savoring

Participants learned how to actively engage in everyday activities such as drinking coffee, enjoying a beautiful sunset, or appreciating a great conversation with a friend using skills for savoring those experiences. In the session, they were taught to savor a raisin, noticing all of the different aspects of the texture, smell, and taste. They were then asked to try to savor at least two activities a day for 2–3 minutes each. No participant struggled to learn or complete this activity; it seemed both accessible and pleasant for everyone. Although some claimed at the start of the introductory session to savoring that they already knew how to savor and did it on a regular basis, most acknowledged after completing the raisin activity that they could sharpen their skills further and went into the week of practice eager to try savoring in new contexts. Some participants did observe that it was more difficult to savor something that was an old habit, such as a daily shower or the same breakfast they ate every day, and instead chose to try new things (e.g., ordering a new dish in a restaurant or visiting a garden they had never been to) to try savoring them. Variation is important because research on hedonic adaptation finds that the same activity can become less interesting over time; thus, it is good to encourage participants to savor a combination of activities that fall in their daily routine and new activities.

Week 5: Active Constructive Responding

Participants learned about active constructive responding, which involves responding to others' good news with genuine enthusiasm and helping others capitalize on their good news by prolonging discussion of details of their experience. For example, when told that a friend had been offered a promotion, participants were taught how to respond with questions such as "When did you hear?" and statements like "Let me take you out for dinner to celebrate!" instead of simply saying "Congratulations." Participants were assigned the task using active constructive responding as often as possible. During introductory sessions, a subset of participants expressed concerns that they might not be able to use this skill spontaneously; to accommodate that concern, participants who struggled to use the skill were asked to instead record cases where they *could have* responded in an actively constructive way but did not. They could then brainstorm ways that they could improve their response in the future if they encountered a similar situation. Presumably, with more long-term practice of the activity via role-playing and brainstorming, individuals who are initially uncomfortable using it might eventually apply the skill in everyday life. A number of participants who did use the activity in their own lives during the week they were assigned to try it reported that it felt cheesy or disingenuous; however, those same participants reported that the responses they received were very positive. In other words, it seemed that what participants thought would be an over-the-top response to another person's good news appeared to be exactly what the other person was looking for.

Week 6: Life Summary

Participants wrote a one- to two-page essay detailing their legacy as it might be characterized by a biographer at the end of their long, fruitful life. Participants were asked to consider traits, accomplishments, and behaviors for which they hoped to be remembered. After completing the essay, participants were asked to consider how they spent their average day and to what extent the activities they chose aligned with the priorities they outlined in the essay. Most participants reported a substantial gap; for example, one college student noted that although he hoped to be remembered as a brilliant medical researcher, he spent most of his spare time playing video games, not studying or pursuing research experience. Another participant, a graduate student, noted that she hoped to be remembered as a dedicated and available parent yet often chose work over family. Both of these participants observed that they would like to readjust their behaviors to be more closely aligned with their long-term goals. Although most participants found the activity uplifting, two participants had an adverse reaction. One young man, who was very anxious, found that writing a life summary worsened his anxiety. Thinking about his hopes for the future made him worry that he would fail to achieve those hopes, and he felt too paralyzed by that fear to make any plans for pursuing his goals. Similarly, a young woman who was prone to more severe depression than the rest of the group noted that it made her feel hopeless for similar reasons. Her response was not as intensely negative as the young man's, but it, nevertheless, highlights that this activity is not for everybody.

The individual PPT program also consisted of working through a series of PPIs, but it was less rigidly structured. The facilitator worked from a predefined selection of PPIs described in a manual but chose each week's activity depending on what was going on in the individual's life at that time. Individual PPT, as tested by Seligman et al. (2006), went on for 12 weeks, twice as long as group PPT.

Both programs demonstrated initial efficacy compared with a control condition (Seligman et al. 2006). This set of studies, combined with a growing body of literature on the benefits of PPIs for reducing depressive symptoms in nonclinical populations (Sin and Lyubomirsky 2009), creates mounting evidence that PPIs can be used effectively to treat clinical depression. In recent years, other research groups have begun to craft and test PPIs for specific clinical populations. We provide an overview of four adaptations of PPT: schizophrenia, suicidality, smoking cessation, and chronic pain. Other PPIs in clinical populations exist. However, our goal was not to be exhaustive, but rather to provide clinical vignettes where PPIs have been successfully tailored to a new population; these vignettes can serve as a model for future efforts to use PPIs in new settings.

PPIs Adapted for Specific Clinical Populations

Schizophrenia

Individuals with schizophrenia struggle with a wide array of severe symptoms, including hallucinations and delusions, blunted affect, anhedonia, and avolition. Accordingly, treatments for schizophrenia are typically designed to target the deficits surrounding positive and negative symptoms, cognitive impairments, and relapse (Dixon et al. 2010). Over the last 15 years, individuals with a serious psychiatric disorder, along with researchers and practitioners, have advocated to expand the focus of treatment to include psychological recovery in order to experience a full and rewarding life (Andresen et al. 2003). The recent advent of positive psychology-based programs for clinical populations aligns perfectly with this call for new therapeutic approaches in schizophrenia.

PPIs have three elements that could help individuals with schizophrenia make progress toward an expanded psychological recovery. First, previous work shows that those with schizophrenia benefit most from concrete, skill-based strategies (Bellack et al. 2004). Because PPIs are both concrete and skill-based, they represent a good fit for this population. Second, PPIs directly target variables such as meaning and purpose, which are rarely addressed by existing psychosocial interventions. Meaning and purpose are not only valuable in their own right but also potentially helpful in reducing relapse by helping clients establish meaningful connections with people and activities. Third, using PPIs in conjunction with traditional psychosocial interventions for schizophrenia that are not directly designed to enhance well-being may lead to improvements in traditional symptoms and functional deficits through the development of meaningful coping strategies that build positive emotion. As a result of the enhancements offered by PPIs, individuals may also experience better symptom management, reductions in residual symptoms, fewer relapses, and a stronger repertoire of coping skills.

In a recent paper, PPIs were incorporated into an intervention called *positive living*, which specifically targeted improvements in psychological recovery for individuals with schizophrenia (Meyer et al. 2012). Overall, the program closely resembled that used by Seligman et al. (2006). Three elements were added to the procedure of the original group PPT manual to address common cognitive impairments associated with schizophrenia. These procedural modifications included asking participants to report on an ongoing positive goal each session; beginning and ending each session with a brief mindfulness exercise ("mindfulness minute"), because mindfulness has been useful in previous work on managing psychotic symptoms during therapy sessions; and creating worksheets for each positive psychology exercise.

Results from the positive living group suggest that this intervention is both feasible for and well tolerated by participants with schizophrenia. Meyer et al. (2012) conducted a pilot study on 16 participants in outpatient treatment for schizophrenia. They found that fewer than 20% of the participants dropped out of the program, and the attendance rate was 77%. During the group sessions, participants rarely discussed their symptoms or diagnosis but reported gains in both the broad area of well-being and clinical functioning. Specifically, participants in the program reported significant improvements in overall well-being, hope, savoring, and self-reported psychological symptoms immediately after intervention and 3 months later. Additional exploratory analyses suggested that participants experienced significant improvements in recovery related to hope, confidence, and goal orientation and reported a significant decrease in psychotic and paranoid symptoms that was maintained through the 3-month follow-up (Meyer et al. 2012).

The positive living pilot study demonstrated that an adapted version of PPT can be successfully implemented for individuals with schizophrenia and that the intervention may be associated with improvements in recovery and well-being. The value of an intervention aimed at improving well-being and psychological recovery could have a great impact on the design and development of future psychosocial interventions for schizophrenia. Using PPIs in conjunction with traditional psychosocial intervention treatments such as cognitive-behavioral therapy, social skills training, or psychoeducation may be a new route to enhance an individual's progress toward recovery. Studies that include PPIs as part of broader individual therapy interventions are now under way (Penn et al. 2014). Results from such studies will help us determine how best to use PPIs to promote psychological recovery and well-being in individuals with schizophrenia and other clinical populations.

Suicidality

Nearly 39,000 people die by suicide every year, and more than 20 times that number attempt or seriously consider suicide (Centers for Disease Control and Prevention 2012). Basic research suggests that positive psychological dimensions—specifically, gratitude, grit, and meaning in life—are relevant to reducing suicidality, which refers to both suicidal ideation and behavior. Although interventions that specifically target gratitude, grit, and meaning in life within the context of suicide have not been published, PPIs have been shown to reduce depressive symptomatology (Sin and Lyubomirsky 2009). Given that suicidality is a symptom often accompanying depression (Dumais et al. 2005), the effectiveness of PPIs among individuals with these common psychological conditions suggests that PPIs also hold promise for reducing suicidality.

Studies have found that adolescents (Li et al. 2012) and young adults (Kleiman et al. 2013a) who are grateful are less likely to be suicidal. Moreover, high levels of gratitude reduce the risk for suicidal ideation among individuals with high levels of hopelessness or depressive symptoms (both factors that confer high risk for suicidal ideation) (Kleiman et al. 2013a). These findings reinforce the idea that using PPIs to increase gratitude in individuals who are at risk for suicide can be beneficial.

Gratitude also works in tandem with grit to reduce suicidal ideation. Grit is a personality trait characterized by pursuing deeply valued goals with perseverance and passion (Duckworth et al. 2007). Researchers found that individuals who are both grateful and gritty showed the greatest decline in suicidal ideation over a 6-week period compared with individuals with any other combination of gratitude and grit (Kleiman et al. 2013b). These findings highlight the importance of addressing specific combinations of strengths simultaneously in individuals at risk for suicide.

Finally, the presence of purpose and meaning in life is associated with decreased risk for suicide (Heisel and Flett 2004; Kleiman and Beaver 2013). Thus, hypothetically, PPIs that increase meaning in life might serve to decrease suicidality. Several PPIs exist to increase meaning in life. For example encouraging individuals to engage in enjoyable, meaningful activities and having them reflect on the meaning gained from those activities might increase meaning in life. Recently, researchers found that creating a photographic journal of how life is personally meaningful can increase a sense of meaning in life (Steger et al. 2013).

One group of researchers examined the impact of nine different PPIs (Table 8–2) on the outcomes of hopelessness and optimism in suicidal inpatients (Huffman et al. 2014). Although these researchers did not directly assess changes in suicidality, they assessed factors that are strongly related to suicidality (i.e., hopelessness and optimism). The nine PPIs included writing a forgiveness letter; writing a gratitude letter; counting blessings; using personal strengths; performing acts of kindness; engaging in important, enjoyable, and meaningful activities; clarifying the best possible self in social relationships; clarifying the best possible self for accomplishments; and making a behavioral commitment to values-based activities (Table 8–2).

Eight of the nine PPIs led to at least a 50% increase in optimism and 50% decrease in hopelessness. The most effective PPI was the gratitude letter, which increased optimism by 94% and decreased hopelessness by 88%. The exception to these promising findings was the forgiveness letter, which failed to alter optimism and only reduced hopelessness by 27%. In addition to showing how effective PPIs can be in improving the lives of acutely suicidal individuals, this study can illuminate other lessons. First, the gratitude letter was not only the most effective PPI; it was also rated as the easiest to complete by the participants. Second, the study staff consisted of bachelor- and master-level clinicians who were supervised by licensed doctoral-level clinicians. This suggests that PPIs for suicide are effective when facilitated by individuals with small amounts of formal training. It is important to acknowledge, however, that training is essential when working with suicidal clients. Some of the PPIs, if not conducted by a trained individual, could potentially *increase* suicidal risk. For example, clients who do not believe they have anything to be grateful for during a gratitude exercise might be inclined to feel more hopeless, burdensome, and worthless. Nevertheless, the preliminary work in this population suggests that under the right conditions, PPIs could be a simple, effective, and low-cost way to reduce suicidal ideation.

Smoking Cessation

Negative affect during and after a smoking cessation attempt adversely affects treatment outcome (Kinnunen et al. 1996). To address this, several efforts have been made to incorporate a mood management component into smoking cessation treatment, most of which have focused on reducing negative affect or depressive symptoms. However, for individuals without a history of depression, focusing on the management of depressive symptoms actually increases self-reported negative affect (Kahler et al. 2002). Focusing instead on positive emotions through the use of PPIs, however, may increase the success of quitting smoking (Leventhal et al. 2008).

Table 8–2. Positive psychology interventions with theoretical or empirical support for reducing suicide risk

Intervention	Description
Acts of kindness	Clients perform three acts of kindness for others during the day and write about them.
Behavioral commitment to values-based activates	Clients select a life principle (e.g., being healthy) and make a small behavioral step toward this principle (e.g., going for a 10-minute walk).
Best possible self, accomplishments	Clients imagine their future accomplishments and write them down.
Best possible self, social relationships	Clients imagine their most optimal future relationships with others and write them down.
Counting blessings	Clients recall the events for which they are grateful and record them in detail.
Forgiveness letter	Clients recall a hurtful event from the past and write a letter forgiving the individual responsible. This letter is not sent.
Gratitude letter	Clients write a letter to express gratitude to someone who did a kind act for them. Participants decide whether to send the letter.
Gratitude visit	Clients write a letter of gratitude to someone to whom they are grateful and then hand deliver the letter to discuss it with that person.
Important, enjoyable, and meaningful activities	Clients complete an important act (e.g., something for their health) as well as enjoyable meaningful activities alone and with others.
Personal strength	Clients identify their signature strengths, deliberately use them over the next day, and then write about this experience.[a]
Three good things	Clients make a list of three things they are grateful for at the end of every day (or week).

Note. See Huffman et al. 2014 and Seligman et al. 2005 for more information on these positive psychology interventions.
[a]See VIA Survey of Character Strengths (VIA Institute on Character 2014) on signature strengths.

Positive psychotherapy for smoking cessation (PPT-S) has been designed to enhance positive affect among smokers before and during a quit attempt. To date, only one study has examined the feasibility of PPT-S (Kahler et al. 2014). In a six-session program, participants were guided through five different PPIs aimed at enhancing positive affect (derived from the original PPT protocol in A.C. Parks and M.E.P. Seligman, "8-Week Group Positive Psychotherapy [PPT] Manual," 2007) with the intention of bolstering participants' moods prior to quit day and during the quit attempt. PPT-S was administered individually in conjunction with rec-ommended smoking cessation strategies that included addressing high-risk smoking situations, emphasizing the importance of enlisting social support, and use of a transdermal nicotine patch for 8 weeks (Fiore et al. 2008).

Four PPIs from the original PPT manual were used (Table 8–1): the three good things exercise, the gratitude letter, savoring, and active constructive responding. Additionally, the study included a new activity, savoring kindness, which involved counting and savoring the acts of kindness that one engaged in on a daily basis. Like the three good things exercise, the examples could be big or small but had to be specific. Participants began PPT-S 2 weeks prior to attempting to quit smok-ing to give the three good things exercise, which has been observed to work only after a period of continuous use, a chance to enhance the participants' positive af-fect. The gratitude letter was scheduled to occur immediately prior to the partic-ipants' quit date because it has the most empirical support for providing the greatest boost in positive affect. Participants then completed the remaining ac-tivities at the rate of one per week. At the end of the sixth session, participants en-gaged in a memory-building exercise in which they reflected on their quit at-tempt and chose one of the five activities to continue doing in their lives.

In a pilot study, PPT-S was well liked by participants and was associated with a 31.6% quit rate 26 weeks after the initiation of treatment (Kahler et al. 2014), which is a relatively high rate considering that other research reported 23% of the participants were still abstinent at 26 weeks (Fiore et al. 2008). The fact that al-most one-third of the smokers remaining in the study quit is noteworthy because smokers in this study were chosen for having high levels of negative affect, which is a predictor of poorer outcome in smoking cessation (Leventhal et al. 2008).

The purpose of this pilot study was to adapt and refine the PPT manual to use in a smoking cessation study and to obtain initial effect sizes, but these pre-liminary results provide promising evidence of the efficacy of PPT-S. However, because of the lack of a control group, causal statements cannot be made about the role of PPT-S in affecting participants' moods. Participants self-reported in-creases in depressive symptoms prior to the quit date, but mood remained rel-atively stable after that point. In addition, an increase in negative mood occurred after the end of treatment, which may have been the result of treatment ending; by the 16- and 26-week follow-up appointments, negative mood had again sta-bilized (Kahler et al. 2014).

In summary, PPT-S shows promise. It is a feasible protocol that is relatively easy to implement and requires very little other than pen and paper, and participants reported both liking and attempting to implement each of the assigned activities (Day et al. 2014; Kahler et al. 2014).

Chronic Pain

According to the biopsychosocial model of pain, pain is determined not only by underlying biological manifestations of disease but also by the psychological and social circumstances in which the disease is experienced (Somers et al. 2009). In patients with arthritis, for example, depression is associated with worse pain and functioning (Marks 2009; Patten et al. 2006). Pain-related cognitions, including self-efficacy with managing pain, pain coping strategies, and pain catastrophizing (i.e., magnifying pain symptoms), are also associated with arthritis pain and functional impairment (Somers et al. 2009). Because psychosocial factors can cause pain to be more or less extreme than one would expect on the basis of biological indicators alone, targeting psychosocial factors using PPIs may help reduce pain.

Hausmann et al. (2014) showed that PPIs disseminated online resulted in a long-term reduction in self-reported bodily pain. Given that the online study targeted a general population rather than individuals with chronic pain, Hausmann and colleagues have since developed a PPI program for use in a very specific clinical population: patients seeking treatment for pain due to knee or hip arthritis in U.S. Department of Veterans Affairs (VA) medical facilities. They set out to develop a 6-week Staying Positive With Arthritis Program that would feature one PPI each week for 6 weeks. Patients referred to instructions for each PPI provided in a Staying Positive With Arthritis workbook and received additional clarification and support during weekly calls with a trained interventionist.

To develop the workbook, Hausmann and colleagues selected PPIs that had been shown to have positive effects on well-being for 1 month or more, were simple to complete, did not require extensive training or follow-up, worked well when self-administered, and could be adapted for use by those with low literacy. The set of PPIs included three that were adapted from the original PPT program (A.C. Parks and M.E.P. Seligman, "8-Week Group Positive Psychotherapy [PPT] Manual," 2007) (i.e., three good things, gratitude letter, and savoring) and two that were drawn from other sources. An acts of kindness PPI was added given that practicing kindness is associated with increased subjective well-being (Lyubomirsky et al. 2005). On the basis of evidence that completing five acts of kindness in a single day produces larger improvements in well-being than distributing five kind acts over a week, the acts of kindness PPI involved completing five kind acts in one day. An increasing pleasant activity PPI was also added; it involved

1) identifying from a list of pleasant activities those that provide the participant with a sense of enjoyment and achievement or bring the participant closer to others, 2) engaging in at least four pleasant activities per day for a week, and 3) recording them in an activity diary. Increasing pleasant activities is one of the most well-researched strategies for improving psychological well-being (Mazzucchelli et al. 2010). Hausmann and colleagues included it in the Staying Positive With Arthritis Program because of its effectiveness across different populations and its ease of administration.

Hausmann and colleagues compiled instructions for each PPI into a Staying Positive With Arthritis workbook. Page 1 included an overview of the program and a rationale for why being positive is good for individuals with arthritis. The rationale acknowledged that it can be hard to notice the good things in life when you have pain. It also explained that the program was designed to teach individuals habits that would help them learn to notice and enjoy good things, which would help them cope with the challenges of arthritis. Subsequent pages included instructions for each PPI along with PPI-specific worksheets.

Hausmann's research group gathered feedback on the initial draft of the workbook from 10 veterans with arthritis. After allowing veterans to read and review the workbook on their own, they asked if the veterans would be willing to complete each PPI (why or why not) and how each PPI could be improved. Responses were overwhelmingly positive, with veterans indicating that they would be willing to try all of the PPIs. Veterans also expressed that they thought doing the PPIs would benefit them by providing motivation and enjoyment and would help them feel good about themselves in general.

All veterans were able to read and comprehend the original instructions, which were written at a sixth-grade reading level to accommodate a broad range of literacy levels. However, some veterans had difficulty with terms that are traditionally used to describe popular positive activities, such as gratitude and savoring. Hausmann and colleagues therefore revised the activity instructions to replace the problematic terms with language that was understood more easily in the target population. This change resulted in recasting the gratitude letter as expressing thanks and savoring pleasures as making good moments last. Using the overall feedback they received, they also revised the introduction and all instructions to present everything as simply as possible, which resulted in the final workbook being written at a fourth-grade reading level.

Hausmann and colleagues are now in the process of pilot testing the full 6-week program in a small sample of veterans with arthritis. The program is being delivered via the refined activity workbooks and oral instructions provided during weekly telephone calls from trained interventionists. The interventionists have a bachelor's or master's degree in a health-related field but are not required to have any additional clinical certification. An interventionist meets individually with each participant in person at the VA medical facility where the veteran receives his or her health care to explain the program and review the first activity in the workbook. Although the workbook contains all instructions needed to complete the full program, the interventionist conducts weekly telephone calls that last 10–15 minutes to provide any additional support that is needed. During these calls, the interventionist asks about the previous week's activity, reviews instructions for the next week's activity, and helps troubleshoot anticipated barriers to completing it. For the first 5 weeks, one new activity is completed each week in a set order. In week 6, participants select an activity from previous weeks to complete again. Repeating an activity serves to engage veterans in identifying positive activities that appeal to them and to give them additional practice building positive activities into their daily lives. At the conclusion of week 6, the interventionist encourages veterans to continue using activities from the program.

Evidence from prior work suggests that PPIs reduce pain (see Hausmann et al. 2014), although little systematic effort has been made to incorporate PPIs into the clinical care of patients with a chronic pain condition. Hausmann and colleagues have attempted to fill this gap by designing a Staying Positive With Arthritis Program for veterans who have chronic arthritis pain. They have taken several steps to maximize the potential impact of the program, including selecting activities that have shown benefits for overall well-being, tailoring the activities on the basis of feedback from patients in the target population, and structuring the program so that it incorporates features of the most efficacious PPIs. Although it is premature to draw conclusions about the impact of the Staying Positive with Arthritis Program, Hausmann's research group is optimistic that it will help veterans overcome the challenges of living with arthritis.

Future Directions

In this chapter, we have provided an overview of four innovative adaptations of PPIs for new clinical populations. A few general recommendations can be gleaned from these vignettes to assist anyone interested in PPI adaptations.

Evaluate Whether There Is a Sound Rationale for Using PPIs in a Given Population

We advise researchers and clinicians seeking to try PPIs in new populations to follow Parks and Biswas-Diener's (2013) recommendation that PPIs must have a foundation in research and, ideally, in theory. Each of the PPI programs presented in this chapter was created because a rationale existed for why increasing positive emotion would benefit the population being targeted. In smoking cessation, the presence of negative affect predicts failure to quit. In chronic pain, negative affect amplifies pain symptoms.

Consider Each PPI's Relevance for the Target Audience

Each PPI program described in this chapter contains its own variation on the individual PPIs that are included. This variation makes sense because some PPIs are more appropriate than others for a given audience. For example, the schizophrenia-focused PPI program contained a mindfulness minute, which is not a traditional PPI, because mindfulness seemed to help clients focus on the present moment when the group was meeting. Similarly, the smoking cessation PPI program originally contained the six PPIs from the group PPT (A.C. Parks and M.E.P. Seligman, "8-Week Group Positive Psychotherapy [PPT] Manual," 2007). Following feedback on the program, however, two PPIs were removed, and one new PPI was added. The suicidality-focused program was not explicitly based on Parks and Seligman's PPT program but, instead, integrated PPIs from throughout the literature. The chronic pain program had a mixture of all the sources—half the activities were from Parks and Seligman's original manual, and the other half were drawn from the broader literature.

Adjust the Intervention to an Appropriate Reading Level

The original PPT programs reported by Seligman et al. (2006) were designed for college students; therefore, the manuals were geared toward individuals with a college reading level. When adapting an intervention for use in a new audience, one must always consider the appropriate reading level and, ideally, pilot test the intervention to make sure the target population can understand its content. PPIs for veterans, for example, were initially revamped to be accessible at a sixth-grade reading level and then further adjusted to a fourth grade reading level after pilot testing the materials in a small group of veterans.

Select the Best Possible Format for Administering PPIs

In some populations, it may be more or less appropriate to ask participants to do an intervention in a self-guided format (as in chronic pain), in individual sessions (as in smoking cessation), or even as part of inpatient care (as in suicidality). Although Web- and smartphone-based PPIs were not used in the populations described here, a large body of research has found technology-based interventions to be effective treatments for various mental disorders (Andersson and Cuijpers 2009). Therefore, technology-based delivery should definitely be considered when adapting PPIs for new clinical populations.

Summary

Positive psychological interventions are becoming more widely used in clinical populations. Evidence suggests that fostering positive emotion, as PPIs do, can lead to global improvements in quality of life and reduce symptoms associated with a variety of clinical conditions. We intend this chapter to serve as an initial guide for practitioners hoping to incorporate PPIs into clinical care delivered across diverse populations. By illustrating how PPI programs have been successfully adapted to help individuals with schizophrenia, suicidal thoughts, smoking cessation, and chronic pain, we hope that this chapter will inspire and guide future adaptations of PPI for additional populations.

Clinical Key Points

- Positive psychological interventions (PPIs) have demonstrated both feasibility and utility in treating depression.

- PPIs have been successfully adapted to and tested in new clinical populations, including individuals with schizophrenia, suicidality, nicotine dependence, and chronic pain.

- Clinicians and researchers hoping to develop their own adaptations can use this chapter, as well as the suggested readings, as a guide.

References

Andersson G, Cuijpers P: Internet-based and other computerized psychological treatments for adult depression: a meta-analysis. Cogn Behav Ther 38(4):196–205, 2009 20183695

Andresen R, Oades L, Caputi P: The experience of recovery from schizophrenia: towards an empirically validated stage model. Aust N Z J Psychiatry 37(5):586–594, 2003 14511087

Bellack AS, Mueser KT, Gingerich S, Agresta J: Social Skills Training for Schizophrenia: A Step-By-Step Guide. New York, Guilford, 2004

Centers for Disease Control and Prevention: WISQARS Injury Mortality Report: Web-Based Injury Statistics Query and Reporting System (WISQARS). 2012. Available at: http://webappa.cdc.gov/cgi-bin/broker.exe. Accessed August 26, 2014.

Day AM, Clerkin EM, Spillane NS, et al: Adapting positive psychotherapy for smoking cessation, in Wiley-Blackwell Handbook of Positive Psychological Interventions. Edited by Parks AC. Oxford, UK, Wiley-Blackwell, 2014, pp 358–370

Dixon LB, Dickerson F, Bellack AS, et al; Schizophrenia Patient Outcomes Research Team (PORT): The 2009 schizophrenia PORT psychosocial treatment recommendations and summary statements. Schizophr Bull 36(1):48–70, 2010 19955389

Duckworth AL, Peterson C, Matthews MD, et al: Grit: perseverance and passion for long-term goals. J Pers Soc Psychol 92(6):1087–1101, 2007 17547490

Dumais A, Lesage AD, Alda M, et al: Risk factors for suicide completion in major depression: a case-control study of impulsive and aggressive behaviors in men. Am J Psychiatry 162(11):2116–2124, 2005 16263852

Fiore MC, Jaen CR, Baker TB, et al: Treating Tobacco Use and Dependence: 2008 Update: Clinical Practice Guideline. Rockville, MD, U.S. Department of Health and Human Services, Public Health Service, 2008

Fordyce MW: Development of a program to increase personal happiness. Journal of Counseling Psychology 24:511–521, 1977

Fordyce MW: A program to increase happiness: further studies. Journal of Counseling Psychology 30:483–498, 1983

Hausmann LR, Parks A, Youk AO, et al: Reduction of bodily pain in response to an online positive activities intervention. J Pain 15(5):560–567, 2014 24568751

Heisel MJ, Flett GL: Purpose in life, satisfaction with life, and suicide ideation in a clinical sample. J Psychopathol Behav Assess 26:127–135, 2004

Huffman JC, DuBois CM, Healy BC, et al: Feasibility and utility of positive psychology exercises for suicidal inpatients. Gen Hosp Psychiatry 36(1):88–94, 2014 24230461

Kahler CW, Brown RA, Ramsey SE, et al: Negative mood, depressive symptoms, and major depression after smoking cessation treatment in smokers with a history of major depressive disorder. J Abnorm Psychol 111(4):670–675, 2002 12428781

Kahler CW, Spillane NS, Day A, et al: Positive psychotherapy for smoking cessation: treatment development, feasibility and preliminary results. J Posit Psychol 9(1):19–29, 2014 24683417

Kinnunen T, Doherty K, Militello FS, et al: Depression and smoking cessation: characteristics of depressed smokers and effects of nicotine replacement. J Consult Clin Psychol 64(4):791–798, 1996 8803370

Kleiman EM, Beaver JK: A meaningful life is worth living: meaning in life as a suicide resiliency factor. Psychiatry Res 210(3):934–939, 2013 23978733

Kleiman EM, Adams LM, Kashdan TB, et al: Grateful individuals are not suicidal: buffering risks associated with hopelessness and depressive symptoms. Pers Individ Dif 555:595–599, 2013a

Kleiman EM, Adams LM, Kashdan TB, et al: Gratitude and grit indirectly reduce risk of suicidal ideations by enhancing meaning in life: evidence for a mediated moderation model. J Res Pers 47:539–546, 2013b

Leventhal AM, Ramsey SE, Brown RA, et al: Dimensions of depressive symptoms and smoking cessation. Nicotine Tob Res 10(3):507–517, 2008 18324570

Li D, Zhang W, Li X, et al: Gratitude and suicidal ideation and suicide attempts among Chinese adolescents: direct, mediated, and moderated effects. J Adolesc 35(1):55–66, 2012 21774977

Lyubomirsky S, Sheldon KM, Schkade D: Pursuing happiness: the architecture of sustainable change. Rev Gen Psychol 9:111–131, 2005

Marks R: Comorbid depression and anxiety impact hip osteoarthritis disability. Disabil Health J 2(1):27–35, 2009 21122740

Mazzucchelli TG, Kane RT, Rees CS: Behavioral activation interventions for well-being: a meta-analysis. J Posit Psychol 5(2):105–121, 2010 20539837

Meyer PS, Johnson DP, Parks A, et al: Positive Living: a pilot study of group positive psychotherapy for people with schizophrenia. J Posit Psychol 7:239–248, 2012

Parks AC, Biswas-Diener R: Positive interventions: past, present and future, in Mindfulness, Acceptance, and Positive Psychology: The Seven Foundations of Well-Being. Edited by Kashdan T, Ciarrochi J. Oakland, CA, Context Press, 2013, pp 140–165

Patten SB, Williams JV, Wang J: Mental disorders in a population sample with musculo-skeletal disorders. BMC Musculoskelet Disord 7:37, 2006 16638139

Penn D, Meyer P, Gottlieb J, et al: Individual Resiliency Training (IRT) Manual. 2014. Available at: https://raiseetp.org/studymanuals/IRT%20Complete%20Manual.pdf. Accessed August 26, 2014.

Seligman MEP: The president's address. Am Psychol 54:559–562, 1999

Seligman ME, Steen TA, Park N, et al: Positive psychology progress: empirical validation of interventions. Am Psychol 60(5):410–421, 2005 16045394

Seligman ME, Rashid T, Parks AC: Positive psychotherapy. Am Psychol 61(8):774–788, 2006 17115810

Sin NL, Lyubomirsky S: Enhancing well-being and alleviating depressive symptoms with positive psychology interventions: a practice-friendly meta-analysis. J Clin Psychol 65(5):467–487, 2009 19301241

Somers TJ, Keefe FJ, Godiwala N, et al: Psychosocial factors and the pain experience of osteoarthritis patients: new findings and new directions. Curr Opin Rheumatol 21(5):501–506, 2009 19617836

Steger MF, Sheline K, Merriman L, et al: Using the science of meaning to invigorate values-congruent, purpose driven action, in Mindfulness, Acceptance, and Positive Psychology: The Seven Foundations of Well-Being. Edited by Kashdan TB, Ciarrochi J. Oakland, CA, Context Press, 2013, pp 240–266

VIA Institute on Character: VIA Survey. 2014. Available at: http://www.viacharacter.org/www/. Accessed August 26, 2014.

Suggested Cross-References

Psychotherapy is discussed in Chapter 5 ("Recovery in Mental Illnesses") and Chapter 9 ("Positivity in Supportive and Psychodynamic Therapy").

Suggested Readings

Huffman JC, DuBois CM, Healy BC, et al: Feasibility and utility of positive psychology exercises for suicidal inpatients. Gen Hosp Psychiatry 36(1):88–94, 2014 24230461

Meyer PS, Johnson DP, Parks A, et al: Positive Living: a pilot study of group positive psychotherapy for people with schizophrenia. J Posit Psychol 7:239–248, 2012

Parks AC, Seligman MEP: 8-Week Group Positive Psychotherapy (PPT) Manual. Unpublished manual, available by request, 2007

Seligman ME, Rashid T, Parks AC: Positive psychotherapy. Am Psychol 61(8):774–788, 2006 17115810

Sin NL, Lyubomirsky S: Enhancing well-being and alleviating depressive symptoms with positive psychology interventions: a practice-friendly meta-analysis. J Clin Psychol 65(5):467–487, 2009 19301241

Positivity in Supportive and Psychodynamic Therapy

RICHARD F. SUMMERS, M.D.

JULIE A. LORD, M.D.

In this chapter we explore the contribution of positive psychology to the theory and practice of supportive and psychodynamic therapy and make three major points: 1) Positive emotion and negative emotion coexist in our patients, and this requires that we conceptualize how a psychotherapy impacts positive experiences as well as suffering, and strengths along with limitations. 2) Supportive psychotherapy is better characterized as the application of positive psychology principles directed toward enhancing positive emotions and experiences than it is by its traditional defining elements, the bolstering of defenses and avoidance of exploratory interventions. 3) The traditional psychodynamic and psychoanalytic notions of therapeutic alliance, working through, and termination can be deepened and expanded by insights from positive psychology. We conclude the chapter by discussing the role of positive psychology on medical education. Our ideas are reflective and theoretical and suggest new avenues for empirical study.

Coexistence of Positive and Negative Emotions

The practicing clinician, as well as the research evaluator, assesses symptoms on continua from mild to severe. More or less depressed, more or less anxious, more or less psychotic—each symptom domain has a continuum. When clinicians ask how ill the patient is, they are implying a single dimension of symptom severity. Typical clinical assessment scales reflect a range from normality to mild to severe symptomatology.

However, evidence supports a dual-continuum model of positive and negative affectivity; that is, these affective experiences may coexist and manifest independently of one another. The Positive and Negative Affect Schedule (Watson et al. 1988) assesses the presence of both positive and negative emotions. Using this measure, Costa et al. (1992) suggested that positive and negative emotional expression are stable traits over time and that the degree of lability in positive and negative affectivity is also stable over time. Surprisingly, positive and negative emotions show little correlation (Watson et al. 1988). If they were simply the opposite ends of a single continuum, they should be strongly negatively correlated.

Positive emotion may reflect the activity of specific brain systems. For example, love, hope, and enthusiasm involve the hippocampus, which allows people to remember and picture those they love. The anterior cingulate gyrus seems to mediate attachment, and the prefrontal cortex is involved in reward, punishment, and moral decision making. Activity in the left lateral prefrontal cortex is associated with positive emotion, whereas the contralateral area is associated with negative emotion, and the intensive meditation practice of Buddhist monks generates powerful positive emotion and deep relaxation and increases left lateral prefrontal cortical activity (Davidson and Harrington 2002). All of these areas, along with mirror neurons in the insular cortex and the spindle cells, seem to be involved in promoting attachment, engagement, and positive emotion. Although there is certainly overlap between these brain systems and those involved in psychiatric symptoms such as depression and anxiety, the dual-continuum model suggests that important differences may also exist.

Positive emotion itself seems to be an important predictor of beneficial outcomes. The Rush Nun Study (Danner et al. 2001) followed 180 nuns over their adult life spans and found positive emotion to be significantly correlated with longevity. Similarly, observers rated the degree and genuineness of Mills College graduates' smiles in their yearbook photographs and concluded that early positive affect was strongly correlated with marital satisfaction many years later (Harker and Keltner 2001).

Peterson's (2006) compilation of correlates of happiness and life satisfaction suggests that age, gender, education, social class, income, having children, ethnicity, intelligence, and physical attractiveness have very little to no correlation. Large correlations were reserved for the relationship of happiness and life satisfaction with self-reports of gratitude and optimism, being employed, frequency of sexual intercourse, percentage of time experiencing positive affect, happiness of an identical twin, and self-reports about self-esteem.

As interesting conceptually as the dual-continuum model might be, it has rather important implications for clinical work and for psychotherapy in particular. Traditional clinical assessment relies primarily on the single-continuum model. Although lip service is typically paid to assessing strengths, clinicians do little systematic thinking about this domain and give it little attention, and they do not typically do much with these assessments.

We suggest that although a comprehensive assessment certainly includes the review of symptoms and systems that make up a traditional psychiatric interview, an inventory of strengths is equally important. From the perspective of the dual-continuum model, each patient has a particular combination of strengths and symptoms and positive and negative affects.

Indeed, a simple 2×2 matrix (Table 9–1) may help distinguish among patients with different combinations of affectivity. Some have high positive affect and high negative affect (satisfied and fulfilled, but with ongoing distress and suffering), whereas others have high positive affect and low negative affect (much enjoyment of life with relatively few symptoms), low positive affect and high negative affect (much suffering with little satisfaction, buffering, and resilience), and low positive affect and low negative affect ("flatline" life).

This simple heuristic for assessing and categorizing patient symptoms and strengths might allow clinicians to think more clearly about typical clinical dilemmas that are otherwise harder to conceptualize and articulate. People with high positive and low negative affect are unlikely to come for treatment. Those with high positive and high negative affect, we would suggest, are some of the most satisfying patients to work with. They have significant suffering but also the strengths and capacity for positive experience that allows them to make the most of therapy. If a reduction in negative affect takes place, they may be able to capitalize on this and make positive changes in their lives. Those with low positive and low negative affect may not have as fulfilling lives as they might hope, but they are less likely to come for treatment, and when they do, the typical clinician will struggle to find target symptoms to work on. Finally, the patients with low positive and high negative affect may be those with the most concerning prognosis. They have significant suffering but fewer strengths to employ, less of an ability to tolerate the rigors of making changes, and little to fall back on when their symptoms exacerbate.

The myth that positive and negative emotions are at opposite ends of a single continuum is part of the incorrect therapeutic notion that removal of symptoms results in wellness. Awareness that positive and negative emotions are two dis-

Table 9–1. Clinical assessment of positive and negative affects

	High positive affect	Low positive affect
Low negative affect	Satisfied, many strengths, little suffering	"Flatline," stable low affect, no significant symptoms, limited positive experiences and strengths
High negative affect	Significant strengths and positive affects with concurrent significant suffering from negative experiences and symptoms	Difficult-to-treat patients with much suffering and fewer strengths to build up

tinct dimensions of affective life, rather than opposite sides of the same coin, may help to expand patients' awareness, allow for a more accurate and nuanced narrative understanding of self, open the door to targeting positive emotions for psychotherapeutic intervention, and make attainment of the good life a goal to consider in psychotherapy. The clinical vignette later in this chapter helps to illustrate these ideas.

Proposed New Conceptualization: Supportive Psychotherapy Is Applied Positive Psychology

The dual-continuum model opens up new possibilities for understanding how established treatments work, that is, their mechanisms of action. We believe that supportive psychotherapy may promote change through increased positive affect, increased engagement, and more effective utilization of strengths rather than by reducing symptomatology and dysfunction.

Each type of psychotherapy can be characterized by its basic assumptions, proposed mechanism of action, focus in sessions, typical goals, and characteristic interventions or techniques. We describe the traditionally understood mechanism of action, goals, and interventions of supportive psychotherapy and contrast these notions with our proposed new conceptualization of this therapy based on the dual-continuum model and the principles of positive psychology. The main points of this discussion are summarized in Table 9–2.

Traditional Model of Supportive Psychotherapy

Supportive psychotherapy is typically defined more by what it is not than by what it actually is. Traditionally, supportive psychotherapy is based on the *assumption* that underlying conscious and unconscious conflict results in maladaptive cop-

Table 9–2. Comparison of traditional and positive supportive psychotherapy models

	Traditional conceptualization	Positive conceptualization
Assumptions	• Conscious and unconscious feelings influence our thoughts, feelings, and behavior • Psychological defenses are employed to manage conflicts and intolerable feelings • Use of immature or maladaptive defenses causes symptoms and problematic behaviors, leading to psychopathology	• Positive and negative emotions exist on independent continua • Well-being is influenced by both positive and negative emotions • Positive emotions and character strengths can buffer against stress and loss
Mechanism of action	• Use of more adaptive defenses and functional behaviors, resulting in symptom reduction and increased self-esteem • Corrective emotional experience	• Enhancement of positive emotions, engagement, and more effective utilization of strengths • Improvement of well-being through enhancement of positive affective dimension
Focus in session	• Here and now • Current problematic relationships, maladaptive patterns of conscious behavior, and emotional responses • Earlier experiences discussed as needed to understand origin of current behaviors	• Here and now • Positive and negative aspects of patient's conscious life, including relationships, periods of optimal functioning, and personal strengths and values
Therapeutic goals	• Improve self-esteem, psychological functioning, and adaptive skills • Improvement in one domain to promote improvement in the other two • Bolster existing strengths	• Same as traditional model • Minimize interference with pursuit of positive experiences

Table 9–2. Comparison of traditional and positive supportive psychotherapy models *(continued)*

	Traditional conceptualization	Positive conceptualization
Techniques		
General	• Conversational tone • Keep emotions at manageable level	• Conversational tone • Balance attention to positive and negative
Therapeutic relationship	• Use positive transference to promote hope and engagement in therapy • Address and diffuse negative transference promptly	• Express positive emotion when genuine • Emphasize empathy with both negative and positive experiences • Use positive transference to promote hope and engagement in therapy • Address and diffuse negative transference promptly
Interventions	• Foster and protect the therapeutic alliance • Manage the transference • Hold and contain the patient • Lend psychic structure • Maximize adaptive coping strategies • Provide a role model for identification • Decrease alexithymia • Make connections between patient's behavior, others' reactions, and outcomes or events	• Mirroring positive experiences • "Positive space" • Capitalization • Savoring techniques • Gratitude interventions • Forgiveness interventions • Counting kindnesses • Reminiscing

ing strategies that account for the symptoms and suffering. Supportive therapy is seen as lying on one end of a supportive-expressive spectrum, with psychodynamic therapy lying at the other (Gabbard 2009). The difference between the two is the degree to which exploratory, uncovering, or anxiety-increasing interventions are employed. Supportive psychotherapy refers to treatments that largely eschew these interventions (Winston et al. 2004). Furthermore, supportive psychotherapy draws on cognitive-behavioral therapy, behavioral activation, problem-solving therapy, and interpersonal therapy (Gabbard 2009).

The *mechanism of action* of supportive psychotherapy has been variously described as improvement of reality testing, enhanced self-esteem, and decrease in dysfunctional behaviors (Winston et al. 2004). These terms are really descriptions of the aims of the treatment and do not specifically describe mechanisms, such as increased awareness leading to new behavior or a new relationship leading to changed self-esteem. The corrective emotional experience, facilitated by an empathic "holding environment" (Gabbard 2009), is also considered to be important. All of these mechanisms involve the idea that patients get better because they use their strengths better and minimize their dysfunctional patterns. Just as supportive therapy interventions are often described by what they are not, the mechanism of action of supportive psychotherapy is noticeably not well articulated in the literature.

The *focus* in supportive psychotherapy is on the here and now, instances of relationship difficulty, and dysfunctional coping. Past patterns of adaption are useful only insofar as they help the patient work on the present difficulties. Possible historical causes of the current difficulties are not considered to be important.

The traditional *goals* of supportive psychotherapy are well elaborated. They include improvement of self-esteem, psychological functioning, and adaptive skills (Misch 2000; Winston et al. 2004). Definitions of these terms are as follows:

- *Self-esteem* is a person's self-regard, self-efficacy, confidence, and hope. Self-esteem is influenced by a person's attributional or explanatory models for life events. Does the person perceive that he or she can influence outcomes in his or her life with his or her actions? Or does he or she believe that his or her fate is controlled by external factors or simple luck?
- *Psychological functioning* is the way a person makes sense of himself or herself and his or her world. It includes the capability for reality testing, cognitive abilities, the capacity to organize thoughts and behavior, affect regulation, the capacity to relate to others, and morals.
- *Adaptive skills* are behaviors, that is, what a person does in response to his or her assessment of events and relationships.

Supportive therapy is seen as focusing on the person's current life and conscious thoughts, rather than unconscious feelings or conflicts. It is called *support-*

ive psychotherapy because the primary *interventions* involve supporting what is already working for the person rather than helping him or her explore and change his or her defensive structure. Existing strengths and adaptive psychological defenses are bolstered to help the patient recover. At the same time, maladaptive defenses and behaviors are minimized to reduce symptoms and promote better functioning. In contrast, psychodynamic therapy aims to help the patient by increasing awareness of unconscious feelings and conflicts, opening the door to more fundamentally improved self-awareness, more accurate perceptions, and more effective behavioral responses (Summers and Barber 2010).

Supportive psychotherapy focuses on the here and now—current symptoms, problematic relationships, and maladaptive behavioral and emotional patterns (Gabbard 2009). Many patients seeking therapy are demoralized and feel as if they have little control over what is happening in their lives. An important technique of supportive therapy is to help patients make connections between their actions and resulting events and others' reactions to them (Misch 2000; Winston et al. 2004). Recognizing these connections helps to increase self-efficacy and shift the locus of control back to the patient. This awareness can have a remoralizing effect and can promote self-understanding. It also sets the stage for patients to try out more adaptive behaviors and to experience feelings of success and mastery. Although the focus is on the present, earlier experiences may be discussed to help the patient understand the source of the current maladaptive patterns (Gabbard 2009; Winston et al. 2004).

In summary, the traditional conceptualization of supportive psychotherapy has a relatively less well described mechanism of action, but clear goals and techniques emphasize supporting existing strengths and capacities to improve function and decrease symptoms.

Traditional Clinical Approach

The first steps in supportive therapy are assessing the patient and making a case formulation. The supportive therapist evaluates the patient's level of functioning, self-esteem, psychological functioning, and adaptive skills (Winston et al. 2004). He or she inquires about the patient's current life circumstances, prior experiences, relationships, and ability to cope with stress and asks about treatment goals. A key purpose is to understand the patient's usual baseline functioning, existing resources and strengths, and maladaptive patterns. The assessment helps define targets for the therapist's interventions. In other words, what can the therapist bolster, and what must the therapist try to minimize?

In supportive therapy, interventions are aimed toward improving self-esteem, psychological functioning, and adaptive skills (Gabbard 2009; Misch 2000; Winston et al. 2004). Interventions to improve self-esteem include praise, reassurance and normalizing, and encouragement. Interventions that improve psychological functioning, such as structuring the patient's environment or experiences, naming the problem, rationalizing, reframing, minimization, clarification, confrontation, and interpretation, often also decrease anxiety or increase awareness. Interventions intended to increase adaptive skills often impart knowledge. Examples include advice, teaching, anticipatory guidance, and modeling. Improvement in one domain often promotes improvement in the others.

Supportive Therapy as Applied Positive Psychology

Supportive psychotherapy does work, and we are not suggesting otherwise (Cuijpers et al. 2008). Rather, we offer an alternative conceptualization of *how* it works, that is, its mechanism of action. Using the *assumptions* outlined in the earlier section "Coexistence of Positive and Negative Emotions," we suggest that the *mechanism of action* of supportive psychotherapy is new positive experiences—increased positive affect, increased engagement, and more effective utilization of strengths. We suggest that this mechanism is more clear and parsimonious than the traditional mechanism of action.

This proposed mechanism supports a different explanatory framework for supportive therapy. The basic assumption is that the primary therapeutic action takes place on the positive continuum rather than on the negative continuum. That is, supportive psychotherapy does more to make people feel better than it does to make them feel less bad. Thus, our conceptualization of supportive therapy fundamentally shifts the emphasis away from intervening on the negative continuum. We flesh this idea out using the same framework for describing psychotherapy used in the "Traditional Clinical Approach" subsection.

The *focus* in sessions using the positive model is on experiences that have been meaningful, positive, and fulfilling. The therapist certainly empathizes with and inquires about losses, frustration, resentment, fear, and depression. However, special attention is paid to those areas of the patient's life and experience that involve pleasure, satisfaction, joy, fulfillment, poignancy, success, and meaning. The therapist tries to create a "positive space" in the therapeutic relationship for these present and past experiences to be described and experienced in unhurried depth. The positive space is analogous to the Winnicottian notion of the therapeutic relationship as a holding environment for intolerable negative affects (Winnicott 1960). The therapeutic *goals* are essentially the same as those in the traditional model, but an additional goal is to minimize those patterns that interfere with the ability to experience positive emotion.

Seeing supportive psychotherapy as a venture focused on enhancement of positive experiences opens up the possibility of reframing typical supportive *interventions*. Indeed, striking parallels exist between common supportive psychotherapy strategies and the positive interventions that are a focus of positive psychology research.

Several strategies have been identified to promote positive experiences. These strategies include techniques to promote gratitude, increase awareness and frequency of positive emotions, and encourage the use of personal strengths (Bryant et al. 2005; Garland et al. 2010; Johnson et al. 2013; Otake et al. 2006; Seligman et al. 2005; Sin and Lyubomirsky 2009; Wood et al. 2011). Although these techniques are often offered as approaches to enhance life satisfaction for nonclinical populations, they are also used in clinical settings. Various forms of positive psychotherapy have been described and studied. For example, Seligman et al. (2006) studied group and individual versions of manualized positive psychotherapy in depressed university students. The group treatment protocol contained the following exercises: using signature strengths, thinking of three good things, writing a positive obituary, going on a gratitude visit, active constructive responding, and savoring. The treatment took place over 6 weeks for 2 hours per week. The group treatment intervention produced reduced levels of depression over 1 year of follow-up. The individual treatment protocol was based on 12 positive exercises and took place in 14 sessions over no more than 12 weeks. The individual treatment intervention produced higher remission rates compared with treatment as usual or treatment as usual plus medication.

We are not suggesting that supportive psychotherapy be scrapped to make way for a newly branded positive therapy. Rather, we suggest that clinicians can learn to improve the specificity and, hopefully, the efficacy of supportive psychotherapy by being more clear about its previously unacknowledged use of positive techniques. This understanding may help clinicians clarify their approach to patients they are treating supportively.

To further develop this point, in Table 9–3 we list the traditional supportive psychotherapy interventions described by Misch (2000) and suggest how they might be reframed as positive interventions. We note the interventions that seem similar to known positive psychology interventions that have been studied.

Clinical Vignette

A clinical vignette of supportive psychotherapy serves to illustrate these points. After a brief history, we formulate the case using both the traditional model and the new positive model and then discuss the traditional and positive techniques suggested by our proposed model.

Annette is a 55-year-old woman with a lifelong history of recurrent depression. Her previous treatments included antidepressants and a lengthy psychodynamic treatment from which she gained significant insight, although she still experienced bouts of depression. She is in a long-term, supportive marriage. She has two adult daughters. She is intelligent, highly educated, well-traveled, and religious. She has had a long career in higher education and feels especially rewarded

Table 9–3. Comparison of traditional supportive psychotherapy interventions and positive psychology interventions

Typical supportive psychotherapy strategy	Reframed positive psychology strategy	Known positive psychology interventions[a]
Patient assessment and case formulation	Assess positive characteristics such as experience of positive emotions, gratitude, optimism, environmental mastery, self-worth, self-efficacy, and positive social relationships Explore periods of optimal functioning, character strengths, and use of strengths	Use standardized measurements such as PANAS, which assess for positive and negative affect elements Identify personal strengths (e.g., VIA Strengths Inventory) (Seligman et al. 2005) Broad-minded affective coping (Johnson et al. 2013) Reminiscing (Bryant et al. 2005)
Foster and protect the therapeutic alliance	Promote experience of a positive relationship through warmth, collaboration, trust, and emotional safety Respond actively and productively to positive events in the patient's life	Capitalization (Gable et al. 2004)
Manage the transference	Address negative responses and use genuine warmth and interest to promote positive affective response to therapist	—[a]
Hold and contain the patient	Promote self-experience of consistency, self-respect, and predictability	—[a]
Lend psychic structure	Role model to enhance character strengths	—[a]

Table 9–3. Comparison of traditional supportive psychotherapy interventions and positive psychology interventions (continued)

Typical supportive psychotherapy strategy	Reframed positive psychology strategy	Known positive psychology interventions[a]
Maximize adaptive coping strategies	Promote engagement and approach coping style rather than disengagement and avoidance of problems	Use of signature strengths in novel way (Seligman et al. 2005)
	Focus on success experiences in use of new attitudes and behaviors	
	Encourage appropriate use of support network and available resources	
Provide a role model for identification	Enhance character strengths through modeling	—[a]
Decrease alexithymia	Enhance self-awareness and mastery by naming affects	Gratitude exercises (Seligman et al. 2005)
	Attend to positive affects through explicit exploration of positive emotional states and experiences	Broad-minded affective coping (Johnson et al. 2013)
	Increase periods of positive emotion and improve ratio of positive to negative emotions	Interventions to raise positive affect (Garland et al. 2010)
Make connections between patient's behavior, others' reactions, and outcomes or events	Enhance self-awareness and social intelligence	Three good things exercise (Seligman et al 2005)
	Build self-efficacy and positive expectancy	Forgiveness interventions (Wade et al. 2014)
		Meaning-making activities and life narratives
Raise self-esteem	Promote positive self-experiences	Three good things exercise (Seligman et al. 2005)
	Create a "positive space"	Gratitude exercises (Seligman et al. 2005)

Table 9–3. Comparison of traditional supportive psychotherapy interventions and positive psychology interventions *(continued)*

Typical supportive psychotherapy strategy	Reframed positive psychology strategy	Known positive psychology interventions[a]
Ameliorate hopelessness	Promote positive expectancy about the future	—[a]
Focus on the here and now	Enhance positive affect through present centeredness Shift focus to induce positive emotions and events when appropriate	Mindfulness and meditation (Garland et al. 2010) Counting kindnesses (Otake et al. 2006) Gratitude exercises (Seligman et al. 2005) Three good things exercise (Seligman et al. 2005)
Encourage patient activity	Promote mastery experiences through realistic goal setting and coaching to "set patient up for success" Reinforce by talking explicitly about successful activities and resultant positive emotions in therapy sessions Guide patient toward activities likely to create more positive experiences	Identify and use strengths interventions (Seligman et al. 2005; Wood et al. 2011) Three good things exercise (Seligman et al. 2005) Counting kindnesses (Otake et al. 2006)
Educate the patient (and family)	Enhance capacity for strategic planning about positive experiences	—[a]
Manipulate the environment	Increase access to positive experiences such as opportunities for rewarding social contact, pleasant emotions, and mastery experiences	Group positive psychotherapy (Meyer et al. 2012; Seligman et al. 2006)

Note. PANAS = Positive and Negative Affect Schedule.
[a]No empirical support currently.
Source. Description of traditional supportive strategies adapted from Misch 2000.

by working with students. She enjoys literature and the arts. She has durable friendships, good relationships with her siblings, and a close relationship with her sister-in-law, Louise.

Annette's mother had major depressive disorder and alcohol use disorder and ultimately committed suicide. Her mother died while Annette was studying abroad on a prestigious academic fellowship. Annette worried about the possibility of her own early death by suicide. She recognized that staying busy and physically active previously helped her mood. However, she feared that, as she aged, she would not be able to stay active enough to keep the depression at bay. She feared that "deep down, [she was] broken," like her mother. Even when not depressed, Annette has a lingering feeling of disappointment in herself because she believes that she has not lived up to her potential.

Her presenting depressive symptoms include low mood, feelings of worthlessness, excessive guilt, passive suicidal ideation without planning or intent, impaired concentration, anergia, slowing, hypersomnia, overeating with sugar cravings, and rejection sensitivity. She has difficulty working and has curtailed her other activities. When she is with others, she feels disconnected and distant, as if she is "putting on a front."

Traditional Case Formulation

Annette has multiple strengths, including her insightfulness, engagement in meaningful activities, close relationships, and educational achievement. She has a fear that inactivity will lead to despair and suicide. The traditional supportive psychotherapist would foster a therapeutic alliance, help contain the negative affects of hopelessness and guilt, role model some healthy responses, and encourage behavioral activation and a reasonable and not overly ambitious return to the previous actively functional status. Annette would build on her strengths and activities, and the therapist would help her address her avoidance and get back to her regular life. Annette would be expected to feel an improvement in self-esteem, greater sense of self-efficacy, and, hopefully, a corresponding decrease in her neurovegetative symptoms of depression.

New Case Formulation

The positively oriented supportive psychotherapist would certainly agree with all of the above. However, although Annette may be suffering greatly and engaging in dysfunctional coping strategies—for example, negatively biased perceptions and self-experiences and avoidance—she has a great continuing capacity for positive experiences. From the perspective of the dual-continuum model, she is a person with high negative and high positive experiences. The positive supportive psychotherapist would work to develop the positive space in the therapeutic relationship to allow the patient to reflect on and feel her positive emotions and strengths. It would be important to help the patient identify her character strengths and to help her use these strengths in new ways.

Positive Supportive Psychotherapy Approach

In the clinical vignette presented in the previous section, Annette was treated using the positive model. In the initial assessment, the therapist actively inquired about positive aspects of Annette's life: examples of successful behavior, supportive relationships, and positive emotional states. As therapy progressed, positive techniques played a prominent role: strengths-based interventions, promoting positive experiences, savoring positive emotions, gratitude building, and capitalization.

Assessing Prior Successes and Positive Relationships

During the initial visit, Annette reported that she quit drinking 25 years ago. The therapist appreciatively inquired about how and why she got sober. Pregnancy and her unhappy childhood motivated her. Her sister-in-law, Louise, also grew up in an alcoholic family, and Annette and Louise made a pact to raise their children in stable, sober homes. Together, they had alcohol-free family holiday and birthday celebrations for years, and Louise remained a close confidant. "We wanted times like Christmas to be fun and focused on the kids, not everybody getting drunk and arguing. We'd both had enough of that." The therapist reflected the information back to the patient with liberal use of praise. "It sounds like you got sober because you really wanted your children to have a different family life from yours. Your love for them is a strong motivator for you. This shows commitment to your kids. It also sounds like Louise shares this value. You two worked together to make family times like Christmas special and happy—a completely different model from what you knew growing up. You changed the pattern. How do you feel about that?"

Next, the therapist probed for information about Louise. Annette usually saw Louise a couple of times per week to take walks together or have coffee. Louise was talkative, with a good sense of humor and a big heart. Annette usually liked being around her. A favorite activity was planning the annual multifamily vacation together. Recently, however, she had not called Louise as often. "After all, who wants to hear about it? There's nothing anybody can say to help me, so why bother? And I don't have the energy to fake it. Louise is so busy with her own life. I don't want to bug her." With further probing, Annette confirmed that Louise had been supportive during past depressive episodes, and the therapist encouraged her to try a little harder to connect and spend time together.

Identifying Sources of Positive Emotion
and Pleasant Activities

The therapist inquired about positive experiences. "You mentioned that you really like working with young people—this sounds like a bright spot in your life. Tell me more about it. What is the most enjoyable part? Can you share some details?" At work, Annette advised graduate students. She especially liked working with foreign students because she enjoyed learning about their cultures and serving as a "surrogate parent." Annette herself loved studying abroad in Spain during college. Two years ago, she returned to Spain to study Spanish art for 6 months. It was an inspiring experience because "the art and language are beautiful."

Strengths-Based Interventions

Annette has evident strengths of kindness and love of learning—good foundations for a strengths-based intervention. The therapist explicitly raised Annette's awareness of her strengths using reflection and realistic praise grounded in Annette's experiences and values. The therapist also asked Annette to complete the VIA Survey of Character Strengths (Seligman et al. 2005). Next, the therapist and Annette searched for new opportunities for strengths implementation, using anticipatory guidance to prepare for taking action. Annette began volunteering as an English tutor for immigrant church members, an experience that she found rewarding.

Encouraging Activities to Increase Pleasant Emotions

The therapist noted Annette's enjoyment of art and literature and encouraged activities that leveraged her appreciation of beauty. With a push from the therapist, Annette identified ways to increase her activity and boost pleasant emotions. Early in treatment, poor concentration made reading less enjoyable, so Annette went to the movies and listened to audiobooks as an alternative. She attended an art exhibit with a friend. When her concentration improved, Annette resumed attendance at her book club.

Increasing Positivity Through Capitalization,
Gratitude, and Savoring

Annette came into one session brimming with excitement. One of her former students was awarded a prestigious academic prize, and she had invited Annette to the award ceremony. All of the university dignitaries were there, and Annette received compliments for her outstanding mentoring. The student herself thanked Annette for acts of kindness, such as inviting her to celebrate holidays at her home and coaching her for her thesis defense. During the ceremony, Annette tried to "take a picture in [her] mind" by noticing every detail of the experience, including the sounds, the colors, and even the taste of the food. During the session, the therapist and Annette savored every detail together. Annette labeled her emotions and described how they made her body feel, including how she felt telling the therapist about it. "My heart felt warm and all in one piece. I didn't feel broken at all. I felt joy. And, now, it feels different to tell you about it, rather than just remembering it by myself. It's stronger, somehow. I couldn't wait to share it." She then described an enhanced sense of her own worth and gave specific examples of other people for whom she made an important difference.

After discussing Annette's new experience, the therapist asked Annette about sharing the good news with other people. Had she told anyone else? How did they react? The therapist followed up with psychoeducation: sharing good news with responsive, close people builds more positive emotions. Annette planned to call Louise so that she could tell her about it. She felt confident that Louise would be interested and encouraging.

Summary

Building on the dual-continuum model of emotional experience, in this section we have argued that supportive psychotherapy may be viewed as a series of interventions designed to enhance positive emotion, strengths, and engagement. Supportive psychotherapy involves a wide range of interventions, and this conceptualization may provide a simple and clear understanding of what these interventions have in common and may reflect an essential mechanism of action. Our clinical example illustrates this emphasis on enhancing positive experiences and sparing attention to minimizing dysfunctional patterns.

Positivity in Psychodynamic Therapy

Next, we consider the contribution of positive psychology to the theory and practice of psychodynamic therapy. The traditional psychodynamic model relies fundamentally on the exploration of old, painful experiences and the elucidation of their distorting effects on present experience. We believe that positive psychology suggests a number of interesting and valuable additions to this model and its application in therapy. The four following observations are necessarily speculative and are points of departure for future study rather than firm conclusions.

Therapeutic Alliance

Patients come for treatment because they are suffering, but we suggest that perhaps they become engaged in treatment and form a therapeutic alliance because of the juxtaposition of new positive experiences with the therapist along with the pain and suffering they bring to the relationship. Bordin (1979) sees the therapeutic alliance as being built on three components: shared goals for the treatment, mutual understanding of the tasks to be performed by patient and therapist, and the affective bond that develops between them. Just as Fredrickson (2001), in her research on broaden-and-build theory, found that a positive affective state enhances a patient's ability to perform anxiety-producing activities, positive affect in the patient may facilitate commitment to the necessary but difficult tasks of therapy: honesty, verbalization, and self-reflection. It is even more likely that the affective bond will be facilitated by positive affective experience. Thus, two of three components that Bordin describes deepen in the presence of positive emotion. Analogously, Tronick et al. (1978) found that negative affect diminishes relationship strength in observations of mothers and infants.

If positive affect in the patient is a crucial ingredient in the therapeutic alliance, what brings this about? Is it spontaneous in the patient or a reflection of positive affect in the therapist? A consideration of therapist emotion, especially positive emotion, can become bogged down in discussions of countertransference enactments and who is generating what affect in the interpersonal field. The observation we are making here is something simpler: positive feeling toward the patient, arising from the therapist and reflecting the therapist's own personal values and character, may facilitate the development of therapeutic alliance. Of course, this presumes that therapists find ways of reacting to patients with genuine positive affect and not false enthusiasm. Positive affect in early psychotherapy may also develop when the therapist encourages discussion of the patient's positive experiences. New approaches for enhancing early positive affective engagement could decrease the substantial early dropout rate in treatment and increase the effectiveness of the treatment by building a stronger therapeutic alliance.

Positive Experiences

Positive affect may play just as important a role in psychodynamic therapy as we have suggested it plays in supportive therapy. Hidden positive affects, along with the usual and expected hidden negative effects of anxiety, fear, and anger, should be observed and discussed. The traditional recommendation to put problems into words so that they can be solved, which is the basis for much psychotherapeutic activity, may have a companion prescription concept that indicates that patients ought to articulate positive affects because that begets more positive affect. This idea relates to the extended discussion of positive interventions and their centrality in supportive psychotherapy.

Clinicians have typically worried that excessive attention to supportive interventions could undermine exploratory psychodynamic therapy. However, when therapy is conceptualized as the exploration and expression of positive affect, less of a contradiction exists. After all, if positive affects and negative affects are not correlated, then discussion of and enhancement of positive emotions do not detract from articulation and experience of negative ones. It is a matter of tactics to determine how to combine attention to positive and negative emotions. Empathy dictates following the patient, and cheerily suggesting the positive in the midst of a discussion of pain and loss is surely insensitive and counterproductive. However, perhaps the strategy of psychodynamic psychotherapy should include asking more about positive experiences without fear of making pain less accessible. Psychodynamic therapy outcome might be enhanced if therapy is not solely the place to go to discuss negative feelings and problems.

Working Through

The laborious process of psychotherapeutic working through may be more effective in the context of positive affect. This is true for both the psychodynamic version of working through, which involves repeated comparison between old feelings and thoughts and current experiences, and the cognitive-behavioral correction of dysfunctional thoughts and evaluation of new behavioral responses. The better cognitive flexibility and problem-solving ability Fredrickson (2001) found in positively toned situations should speed and enhance the self-observation, motivation, and flexibility required to change. This is probably the explanation for why tactful irony and humor are so useful in therapy and why some difficult experiences are processed only after they are over and the patient can relax and reflect safely. Self-observation during moments of positive affect may allow patients to see themselves and others in new ways and may facilitate their tolerating difficult perceptions and finding creative responses.

Termination

The literature on psychotherapy termination is mainly focused on the resolution of symptoms, conflicts, and problems. Traditional psychodynamic psychotherapy regards the experience of, and insight about, ending the therapeutic relationship to be an important aspect of therapy. It allows for reexperiencing of old losses in a new light and grieving the loss of the valued therapeutic relationship. The patient is considered to be ready for termination when the problems he or she came with have been sufficiently ameliorated.

The positive perspective on termination brings out another aspect of this phase of therapy: to what extent has the patient achieved an ability to respond with resilience to future life stressors, and what is the nature and extent of the patient's character strengths? Inclusion of the positive perspective reframes termination as appropriate when the optimal balance of symptom amelioration and strength development has occurred. Perhaps some patients could leave therapy earlier than they do now because they have achieved enough resilience even though they still have some of the problems that brought them to treatment. Likewise, some patients may leave treatment feeling better but should stay longer because they need more help to develop the ability to buffer the storms of life.

Assessing resilience and character strengths is surely more difficult than assessing the degree of symptom resolution, but there is room for improvement in clinicians' abilities to do so. For example, perhaps a 3-month or 6-month follow-up appointment for the specific purpose of assessing a patient's capacity to deal with stressful and negative experiences during the interim could be a standard psychodynamic termination technique.

Positive Psychology Applications in Medical Education

In addition to its importance to psychotherapy, positive psychology has potential applications at multiple levels of academic medicine, and we see medical education as a fruitful area for further innovation. Positive psychology practices are emerging in organizational management of academic medical centers and in undergraduate medical education. In psychiatry training programs, psychiatric educators could also incorporate positive psychology in supervision and formal classroom teaching.

Organizational Culture in Academic Medicine

Positive psychology is emerging in medical education at the academic medical center level. Appreciative inquiry (AI) is a management methodology that spotlights an organization's positive functioning as a means to understand and change institutional culture, in contrast to the traditional deficit model approach of problem identification, cause analysis, and corrective action (Cottingham et al. 2008; Plews-Ogan et al. 2007). At its core, AI is based on inquiry into what is going well as a stimulus for discovery, aspiration, and transformation. Academic medical centers are applying positive methods to facilitate organizational change through AI.

Two example institutions are the Indiana University School of Medicine and the University of Virginia. In 2003, the Indiana University School of Medicine launched a longitudinal culture change project aimed at aligning their informal medical school curriculum with their formal competency-based curriculum (Cottingham et al. 2008). Their team started by conducting appreciative interviews to elicit stories of best performance at all levels of the organization (medical students, residents, hospital staff, and faculty physicians). From those interviews, four key themes emerged: the wonderment of medicine, the importance of connectedness, passion for one's work, and believing in everyone's capacity to learn and grow. Reflection on these themes stimulated new initiatives and changes in the relational culture. Sample outcomes included publication of a student-initiated handbook of high-point professional experiences distributed at their 2004 white coat ceremony, a redesign of the admissions processes to recruit students with a strong relational orientation, and new meeting formats that encourage sharing and collaboration.

Similarly, in 2006, the University of Virginia initiated an AI-based organizational change project to improve their graduate medical education programs (Plews-Ogan et al. 2007). Their team started with appreciative interviews to elicit stories of being at one's best and feeling connected to values and sense of calling. From those interviews, four themes emerged: working together as a community; self-awareness and reflection; human connection and empathy; and excitement, joy, and innovation. The ripple effects from their AI project included a pocket notebook of inspiring medical student experiences given to first-year students at their white coat ceremony, using appreciative check-ins to open meetings, spreading "appreciative gossip" about good news, and inclusion of AI in their Leadership in Academic Medicine course.

Undergraduate Medical Education

Positive practices also appear in undergraduate medical education. Garman (2007) conducted a study of the impact of positive formative feedback on third-year students' clinical skills during a longitudinal primary care clerkship at the University of California, San Diego School of Medicine. In this study, students were randomly assigned to coaching groups (four to five students per group) in which faculty provided AI-based formative feedback about students' video-recorded clinical performances with standardized patients. Coaching group sessions were audio-recorded and coded for positive and negative formative feedback comments. Garman found that student coaching groups who scored one standard deviation above the class mean on the clinical skills performance exam experienced an average of 3.8 positive formative feedback statements to every 1 negative statement. Student coaching groups who scored one standard deviation below the class mean experienced an average of 1.2 positive formative feedback statements for every 1 negative statement. On the basis of the results of this study, University of California, San Diego faculty members have continued to emphasize positive formative feedback in the clerkship program.

In another example, the University of South Florida Health Morsani College of Medicine recruited its first class of medical students into its Scholarly Excellence Leadership Experiences Collaborative Training (SELECT) track program in 2011 (Martin 2011). The SELECT track is a specialized program designed to cultivate positive personal leadership abilities, self-awareness, and emotional resilience. In addition to the usual admissions criteria, the SELECT admissions process includes "behavioral event interviews" designed to gauge emotional intelligence. Students are then recruited on the basis of their emotional intelligence as well as academic achievement. This track includes one-on-one coaching, small groups, and seminars intended to cultivate emotionally intelligent leaders in medicine.

Supervision

Positive psychology instruction can be embedded in psychiatry supervision. The intent is for residents learn to gauge their patients' positive potentialities (as well as their distress) and to use positive interventions to improve well-being. We recommend the following educational elements in supervision:

- Application of the dual continua to clinical cases
- Inclusion of patients' positive capacities in case conceptualization
- Coaching in use of positive interventions
- Modeling through supervisors' conduct and attitudes during supervision

Supervisors should introduce the dual-continuum model and provide suggestions for gathering the relevant information to make a clinical assessment. Because the traditional medical model predominates in medical education, residents may need prompting to inquire about patients' strengths, positive relationships, opportunities for pleasant emotions, and areas of life engagement. Next, regardless of therapeutic orientation, supervisors can help residents synthesize clinical information into a balanced case conceptualization. This conceptualization should include a description of the patient's unique combination of positive and negative affectivity, positive capacities, and strengths. On the basis of the case conceptualization, supervisors may point out opportunities to apply positive interventions and coach residents on their use.

In addition to learning from explicit instruction, residents learn from their supervisors' attitudes and behavior (Wear and Skillicorn 2009). By including a positive focus in supervision, supervisors can *show* the desired stance and techniques to residents, rather than just *telling* residents about them. This modeling starts with making supervision a place to talk about resident successes *and* struggles. As in psychotherapy, supervision should include discussion about what is going right in treatment, as well as residents' struggles and uncertainties. Residents learn by explicit discussion of their clinical reasoning and exactly what they did during successful treatments. Thinking aloud with a supervisor about what went well reinforces knowledge and promotes mastery, and it demonstrates the value of talking about positive as well as negative aspects. Perhaps more importantly, supervision is also a place to talk about the positive emotions that come from helping patients, not just negative countertransference.

Early in training, residents may be surprised by the intensity of their emotions for patients, including positive feelings such as mastery, excitement, gratitude, and warmth. They may feel close to their patients, invested in their outcomes, and excited about special moments in the treatment. Supervisors model valuing the positive by appreciatively inquiring about those aspects of the residents' experiences. Furthermore, by responding actively and constructively to residents' positive emotions and engaging experiences, supervisors model techniques such as capitalizing on positive events and gratefully savoring meaningful professional work. In this way, the supervisor's stance cultivates an orientation toward patients' positivity as well as suffering, a sense of engagement, and positive professional habits such as savoring positive emotions and engaging fully.

Classroom Curriculum

Positive psychology research has begun to define well-being and identify factors that contribute to a meaningful, flourishing existence. Despite the science behind positivity, these essential concepts are not emphasized in modern psychiatric education. The vast majority of training focuses on diseases, deficits, and alleviating suffering. Medical students and residents learn to classify symptoms, identify diseases, and apply treatments to reduce disease impact. At best, instructors do an incomplete job of teaching trainees to recognize patients' strengths, humanity, and resilience. Training in interventions to increase positivity is even sparser. We suggest that psychiatric education needs to add an explicit focus on positivity alongside the traditional medical model.

At the curricular level, instruction should include definitions of well-being, an introduction to the theory of positive psychology, and an overview of the research on factors that contribute to well-being. Training should also include clinical applications, such as empirically validated strengths and gratitude interventions.

Summary

Positive psychology has made a major contribution to psychiatry through new theory, practical applications, and valuable empirical research. We suggest a reconceptualization of supportive psychotherapy as applied positive psychology, provide several new perspectives on psychodynamic therapy, and describe new approaches to medical education based on these new ideas.

Clinical Key Points

- Positive and negative affects coexist and should be separately assessed in clinical evaluation.

- Enhancement of positive affect, experience, and engagement is the essential mechanism of action in supportive psychotherapy.

- Specific techniques for enhancing positivity have been studied empirically, and these approaches are the basis for effective supportive psychotherapy.

- Attention to positive affect in psychodynamic therapy may enhance therapeutic alliance formation, strengths development, and the working through process and may be an important consideration in termination.

- Attention to positive emotion may be a critical ingredient in effective medical education for the individual learner as well as the culture of the academic medical center.

References

Bordin ES: The generalizability of the psychoanalytic concept of the working alliance. Psychotherapy 16:252–260, 1979

Bryant FB, Smart CM, King SP: Using the past to enhance the present: boosting happiness through positive reminiscence. J Happiness Stud 6:227–260, 2005

Costa PTJr, Fagan PJ, Piedmont RL, et al: The five-factor model of personality and sexual functioning in outpatient men and women. Psychiatr Med 10(2):199–215, 1992 1615160

Cottingham AH, Suchman AL, Litzelman DK, et al: Enhancing the informal curriculum of a medical school: a case study in organizational culture change. J Gen Intern Med 23(6):715–722, 2008 18389324

Cuijpers P, van Straten A, Andersson G, et al: Psychotherapy for depression in adults: a meta-analysis of comparative outcome studies. J Consult Clin Psychol 76(6):909–922, 2008 19045960

Danner DD, Snowdon DA, Friesen WV: Positive emotions in early life and longevity: findings from the nun study. J Pers Soc Psychol 80(5):804–813, 2001 11374751

Davidson RJ, Harrington A: Visions of Compassion: Western Scientists and Tibetan Buddhists Examine Human Nature. New York, Oxford University Press, 2002

Fredrickson BL: The role of positive emotions in positive psychology: the broaden-and-build theory of positive emotions. Am Psychol 56(3):218–226, 2001 11315248

Gabbard GO: Textbook of Psychotherapeutic Treatments. Washington, DC, American Psychiatric Publishing, 2009

Gable SL, Reis HT, Impett EA, et al: What do you do when things go right? The intrapersonal and interpersonal benefits of sharing positive events. J Pers Soc Psychol 87(2):228–245, 2004 15301629

Garland EL, Fredrickson B, Kring AM, et al: Upward spirals of positive emotions counter downward spirals of negativity: insights from the broaden-and-build theory and affective neuroscience on the treatment of emotion dysfunctions and deficits in psychopathology. Clin Psychol Rev 30(7):849–864, 2010 20363063

Garman K: Broadening and Building Medical Students' Clinical Performance: An Action Research Study. Poster Presentation. Washington, DC, Gallup International Positive Psychology Summit, October 4–7, 2007

Harker L, Keltner D: Expressions of positive emotion in women's college yearbook pictures and their relationship to personality and life outcomes across adulthood. J Pers Soc Psychol 80(1):112–124, 2001 11195884

Johnson J, Gooding PA, Wood AM, et al: A therapeutic tool for boosting mood: the broadminded affective coping procedure (BMAC). Cognit Ther Res 37:61–70, 2013

Martin M: New medical education program selects students for "emotional intelligence." 2011. Available at: https://www.aamc.org/newsroom/reporter/december2011/268876/emotional-intelligence.html. Accessed August 26, 2014.

Meyer PS, Johnson DP, Parks A, et al: Positive Living: a pilot study of group positive psychotherapy for people with schizophrenia. J Posit Psychol 7:239–248, 2012

Misch DA: Basic strategies of dynamic supportive therapy. J Psychother Pract Res 9(4):173–189, 2000 11069130

Otake K, Shimai S, Tanaka-Matsumi J, et al: Happy people become happier through kindness: a counting kindness intervention. J Happiness Stud 7(3):361–375, 2006 17356687

Peterson C: A Primer in Positive Psychology (Oxford Positive Psychiatry Series). New York, Oxford University Press, 2006

Plews-Ogan M, May NB, Schorling JB, et al: Feeding the Good Wolf: Appreciative Inquiry and Graduate Medical Education. Chicago, IL, ACGME Bulletin, 2007

Seligman ME, Steen TA, Park N, et al: Positive psychology progress: empirical validation of interventions. Am Psychol 60(5):410–421, 2005 16045394

Seligman ME, Rashid T, Parks AC: Positive psychotherapy. Am Psychol 61(8):774–788, 2006 17115810

Sin NL, Lyubomirsky S: Enhancing well-being and alleviating depressive symptoms with positive psychology interventions: a practice-friendly meta-analysis. J Clin Psychol 65(5):467–487, 2009 19301241

Summers RF, Barber JP: Psychodynamic Therapy: A Guide to Evidence-Based Practice. New York, Guilford, 2010

Tronick E, Als H, Adamson L, et al: The infant's response to entrapment between contradictory messages in face-to-face interaction. J Am Acad Child Psychiatry 17(1):1–13, 1978 632477

Wade NG, Hoyt WT, Kidwell JE, et al: Efficacy of psychotherapeutic interventions to promote forgiveness: a meta-analysis. J Consult Clin Psychol 82(1):154–170, 2014 24364794

Watson D, Clark LA, Tellegen A: Development and validation of brief measures of positive and negative affect: the PANAS scales. J Pers Soc Psychol 54(6):1063–1070, 1988 3397865

Wear D, Skillicorn J: Hidden in plain sight: the formal, informal, and hidden curricula of a psychiatry clerkship. Acad Med 84(4):451–458, 2009 19318777

Winnicott DW: The theory of the parent-infant relationship. Int J Psychoanal 41:585–595, 1960 13785877

Winston A, Rosenthal RN, Pinsker H: Introduction to Supportive Psychotherapy. Washington, DC, American Psychiatric Publishing, 2004

Wood AM, Linley PA, Maltby J, et al: Using personal and psychological strengths leads to increases in well-being over time: a longitudinal study and the development of the strengths use questionnaire. Pers Individ Dif 50:15–19, 2011

Suggested Cross-References

Gratitude is discussed in Chapter 12 ("Integrating Positive Psychiatry Into Clinical Practice") and Chapter 13 ("Biology of Positive Psychiatry"). Psychotherapy is discussed in Chapter 5 ("Recovery in Mental Illnesses") and Chapter 8 ("Positive Psychotherapeutic and Behavioral Interventions"). Positive emotions are discussed in Chapter 3 ("Resilience and Posttraumatic Growth").

10

Complementary, Alternative, and Integrative Medicine Interventions

HELEN LAVRETSKY, M.D., M.S.

TAYA C. VARTERESIAN, D.O., M.S.

Western medicine tends to focus on illness and acute care rather than on prevention or wellness, which causes both patients and care providers to lose sight of their strengths and abilities. Holistic medicine and complementary, alternative, and integrative medicine (CAIM) focus on whole persons, with all their strengths and weaknesses (McBee 2008). In addition, holistic medicine tends to be preventive and wellness oriented. Health care providers will see the burgeoning number of baby boomers increasingly use Western and holistic medicine approaches for the treatment and prevention of the most common diseases of aging. CAIM therapies can be practiced mindfully to promote awareness in the practitioner and the patient. Given the widespread use of CAIM, health care providers urgently need greater awareness of and familiarity with CAIM approaches. In this chapter, we examine evidence supporting the use of CAIM approaches for enhancing resilience to prevent and treat mental disorders of aging. The major domains of CAIM therapies are defined, and relevant approaches, including biologically based therapies (omega-3 fatty acids, S-adenosyl-L-methionine (SAMe), Saint John's wort, ginkgo biloba), mind-body medicine (yoga, Tai Chi, exercise), alternative medical systems (acupuncture, Ayurveda), and other CAIM practices (religion and spirituality, expressive therapies), are discussed.

Current Utilization of CAIM

Currently, CAIM is extensively used in the United States, both to sustain well-being and to treat a wide variety of physical and mental disorders. The most recent comprehensive assessment of CAIM use in the United States, conducted as part of the 2007 National Health Interview Survey, found that roughly 40% of U.S. adults had used at least one complementary and alternative medicine (CAM) therapy within the past year (Barnes et al. 2008). The use of CAIM for treatment of mood and anxiety disorders includes acupuncture, deep breathing exercises, massage therapy, meditation, naturopathy, and yoga (Barnes et al. 2008).

An estimated 33% of adults may be using CAM therapies (Barnes et al. 2008). Principal uses of CAIM in older adults include antiaging effects for memory enhancement and alleviation of mood symptoms. With aging baby boomers expected to accelerate use of CAIM among older adults in the coming years, the importance of mental health professionals having a working knowledge of CAIM techniques intended to address late-life mood and cognitive disorders is becoming increasingly clear. The purpose of this chapter is to review the efficacy and safety of some CAIM approaches relevant to late-life mood and cognitive disorders.

Studies of CAIM Use in Late-Life Mood and Cognitive Disorders

Mood and cognitive disorders are common in older adults, with 10%–15% of patients in primary care settings having depressive symptoms and the "graying" of the population raising the number of cases of cognitive dysfunction. Alzheimer's disease (AD) is the most common cause of dementia and currently affects 5.4 million people in the United States, or roughly one in eight older adults (Alzheimer's Association 2010). By 2030, the number of people age 65 and older with AD in the United States is estimated to reach 7.7 million, which is a 50% increase (Alzheimer's Association 2010). Despite these trends, studies examining CAIM therapies for the treatment and prevention of late-life mood and cognitive disorders are limited.

A review of randomized controlled trials (RCTs) of CAIM for mood disorders in older adults found 33 trials with sufficient quality to include in the review, and a number of these studies were focused on addressing sleep and anxiety rather than mood disorders (Meeks et al. 2007). Of the 33 included trials, most had methodological limitations, and although 67% had positive outcomes, the positive studies were, on average, of lower methodological quality than the negative reports.

The National Institutes of Health funded an exhaustive review of conventional and CAM therapy approaches that was carried out by the Evidence-Based Practice Centers of the Agency for Healthcare Research and Quality; the review considered the existent clinical literature on potential risk and protective factors related to the development of AD and cognitive decline (Williams et al. 2010). The review included 25 systematic reviews and 250 primary research studies on various factors, subdivided into the following categories: nutritional factors; medical conditions and prescription and nonprescription medications; social, economic, and behavioral factors; toxic environmental factors; and genetics. Only a few factors showed a consistent association with AD or cognitive decline across multiple observational studies and the available RCTs. Factors associated with increased risk of AD and cognitive decline were diabetes, the epsilon 4 allele of the apolipoprotein E gene (*APOE4*), smoking, and depression. Factors consistently associated with a decreased risk of AD and cognitive decline were cognitive engagement and physical activity. The modification of risk for reported associations was typically small to moderate, and the currently available data were thought to be limited and generally of low strength. The overall conclusion of the review was that further research was necessary before definitive recommendations could be made regarding behavioral, lifestyle, and pharmaceutical interventions and modifications.

Nonetheless, given the current widespread use of CAIM, mental health care providers urgently need greater awareness of CAIM approaches. In this chapter, we review CAIM therapies with potential relevance for use in the treatment and prevention of late-life mood and cognitive disorders as summarized in Table 10–1.

Biologically Based Therapies and Natural Products

Omega-3 Fatty Acids

One of the most commonly used supplements is omega-3 fatty acids (Barnes et al. 2008). Sources of omega-3 fatty acids are primarily fish, but omega-3 is also present in seeds and nuts. Eicosapentaenoic acid (EPA) and docosahexaenoic acid (DHA) are two types of omega-3 requiring dietary consumption. The data support an antidepressant effect of omega-3, and deficiencies have been seen in those individuals with depression that is most likely related to membrane fluidity changes. The data supporting omega-3 supplementation in geriatric depression

Table 10–1. Integrative and holistic intervention domains and examples

Domain	Examples of interventions	Comments
Biologically based therapies	Herbal (botanical) medicines, vitamins, nonvitamin–nonmineral natural products (e.g., omega-3 fatty acids; adaptogens)	Nonvitamin–nonmineral natural products are used by 18% of U.S. adults.
Mind-body medicine	Biofeedback, meditation techniques, yoga, Tai Chi, energy therapies (e.g., light therapy, Qigong, healing touch), exercise	This domain focuses on interactions among brain, mind, body, and behavior to affect physical function and promote health.
Manipulative and body-based practices	Chiropractic spinal manipulation, massage therapies, movement therapies (e.g., pilates)	This domain focuses on structural and functional systems of the body, including bones and joints, soft tissues, and circulatory and lymphatic systems.
Alternative medical systems	Acupuncture, Ayurveda, homeopathy and naturopathy, traditional healers (e.g., American Indian healers)	This domain focuses on achieving optimal health and well-being.
Other complementary, alternative, and integrative medicine practices	Spirituality, pastoral care, expressive therapies	This domain includes approaches not formally categorized but easily accepted by individuals.

are limited but reveal positive results. One RCT of depressed older adults found omega-3 supplementation improved depression and quality of life (Rondanelli et al. 2011). The participants consisted of females living in a nursing home who had either major depressive disorder or persistent depressive disorder (dysthymia) and were not taking a standard antidepressant. The composition of omega-3 consisted of greater EPA (1.67 g) compared with DHA (0.83 g), which is consistent with what is seen in the literature for antidepressant effects. Therefore, data support the antidepressant effect of omega-3 in the geriatric population.

Supplementation with omega-3 may provide a neuroprotective role through antioxidant and anti-inflammatory effects as well as antiamyloid effects (Fotuhi et al. 2009). A review of multiple epidemiological studies shows fish consumption is related to a reduction in the risk of developing AD (Fotuhi et al. 2009). However, the data regarding omega-3 supplementation and risk reduction for dementia are mixed. A meta-analysis supports the use of omega-3 fatty acids to slow cognitive impairment in those individuals with mild cognitive impairment (MCI) but not for the treatment or prevention of dementia (Mazereeuw et al. 2012). The analysis concluded that omega-3 supplementation improved attention and processing speed in MCI (Mazereeuw et al. 2012).

However, omega-3 supplementation did not provide any improvement in older adults who were cognitively intact or who had AD. The Cochrane Database (Sydenham et al. 2012) included three RCTs that included approximately 4,000 individuals examined over a 3-year period, and researchers concluded that omega-3 supplementation does not prevent cognitively intact individuals from developing AD (Sydenham et al. 2012). Therefore, omega-3 supplementation does not appear to be effective in treating dementia or preventing its occurrence; however, it does appear to slow cognitive decline in MCI. A distinct difference exists between supplementation with omega-3 fatty acids and dietary consumption of omega-3, with dietary consumption appearing to be more effective at reducing cognitive decline in certain populations. Therefore, for the older adult wanting to prevent the development of AD, one might suggest the importance of dietary consumption of omega-3, and for the older adult with MCI, one might suggest omega-3 supplementation to improve attention and memory.

S-Adenosyl-L-Methionine

SAMe is a naturally occurring compound normally synthesized in the body formed from the amino acid L-methionine as part of a multistep metabolic pathway serving as a methyl group donor in the formation of various hormones and neurotransmitters (Mischoulon and Fava 2002). Initial oral formulations of SAMe were relatively unstable, necessitating parenteral administrations. However, the more recent development of stable oral forms of SAMe has allowed for more widespread testing and use of this compound.

SAMe is thought to play a role in depression because it is a necessary cofactor for the synthesis of serotonin, norepinephrine, and dopamine. One open trial looking exclusively at oral SAMe in a mixed age population (18–80 years old) supported its clinical benefit as an augmentation strategy in patients showing an incomplete response to conventional antidepressants (Alpert et al. 2004). Among various trials, the oral doses of SAMe ranged from 400 to 1,600 mg/day, with most trials showing benefit with dosing between 800 and 1,600 mg/day (Mischoulon and Fava 2002). Therefore, strong evidence supports the use of SAMe as an antidepressant with parenteral formulation, and support is growing for oral administration.

Saint John's Wort

Saint John's wort (*Hypericum perforatum*) is a wildflower that has been used for medicinal purposes for thousands of years. Various standardized extracts of this natural dietary supplement have been studied. The major clinical effect of Saint John's wort is that of an antidepressant.

In Europe, Saint John's wort is a commonly used antidepressant, and numerous studies have researched its use in the general adult population. Most commonly, Saint John's wort dosages range from 300 to 1,000 mg/day, with the most common dosage being 300 mg three times a day. In older adults, the available evidence base for use of Saint John's wort as an antidepressant is limited. A small RCT comparing Saint John's wort (800 mg extract LoHyp-57) and fluoxetine (20 mg) in moderately depressed older adults (60–80 years) found equivalent efficacy of these agents in reducing depression over 6 weeks (Harrer et al. 1999). Therefore, the few studies available that include older adults support the use of Saint John's wort for depression.

Ginkgo Biloba

Ginkgo biloba leaf extract is a commonly sold herbal supplement that comes from the maidenhair tree. Its effects include scavenging free radicals, lowering oxidative stress, reducing neural damage, and reducing platelet aggregation, and it has anti-inflammatory, antitumor, and antiaging activities. Its main clinical effects target cognitive disorders.

Many RCTs of ginkgo biloba in patients with various types of dementia have yielded contradictory results. A well-designed RCT called the Ginkgo Evaluation of Memory (GEM) Study evaluated, over 5 years, a large number of participants (3,072) older than 75 years with either intact cognition or MCI; the study did not show any protective effect of ginkgo biloba in preventing the development of dementia (DeKosky et al. 2008). Overall, the strongest available evidence does not support ginkgo biloba in the prevention of dementia.

Ginkgo biloba (240 mg extract EGb 761) is a multitarget compound with activity on distinct pathophysiological pathways in AD and age-related cognitive decline. Although symptomatic efficacy in dementia and MCI has been demonstrated, interpretation of data from dementia prevention trials is complicated by important methodological issues. An RCT demonstrated the efficacy of ginkgo biloba (240 mg extract EGb 761) in outpatients age 50 years or older with mild to moderate AD or vascular dementia over 24 weeks (Ihl et al. 2012). Ginkgo biloba provided a therapeutic effect on cognition, neuropsychiatric symptoms, and functional abilities. Therefore, ginkgo biloba is unlikely to prevent the development of AD but may have an impact on cognitive decline in those already afflicted with dementia. An ideal candidate to benefit from ginkgo biloba is an individual who is already experiencing dementia and would prefer an alternative approach to the pharmacological management of cognitive impairment.

Mind-Body Medicine

Mindful Physical Exercise

Mind-body medicine encompasses a number of CAIM therapies, including a group of techniques collectively known as mindful physical exercise (e.g., Qigong, yoga, and Tai Chi). Mindful physical exercise has become an increasingly employed approach for improving psychological well-being and is defined as "physical exercise executed with a profound inwardly directed contemplative focus" (La Forge 2005, p. 7). As such, mindful physical exercise contains the following key elements: 1) a noncompetitive, nonjudgmental meditative component, 2) mental focus on muscular movement and proprioceptive awareness combined with a low to moderate level of muscular activity, 3) centered breathing, 4) a focus on anatomical alignment (i.e., spine, trunk, and pelvis) and proper physical form, and 5) energy-centric awareness of individual flow of intrinsic energy, also called vital life force, qi, among others. Mindful exercise interventions have shown promise in addressing depressive symptoms in older adults. For example, a study of 82 older adult participants with depression who were randomly assigned to either 16 weeks of Qigong practice or newspaper reading groups found that Qigong participants showed significantly greater improvements in mood, self-efficacy, and personal well-being (Tsang et al. 2006).

Yoga

Widely practiced in India and beyond, yoga is an ancient multifaceted approach to health that involves multiple postures, breathing techniques, and meditation to balance the body's energy centers. Practice of yoga typically benefits from instruction by expert instructors and requires dedication to multiple weekly sessions and continual use by participants for maximal benefit. Yoga is commonly used in combination with other treatments for depression, anxiety, and stress-related disorders.

Data on the use of yoga for anxiety and depression in older adults are more limited; however, one significant study of 69 older adults in India did compare the effects of yoga with the effects of Ayurveda or a wait-list control condition on depressive symptoms (Krishnamurthy and Telles 2007). Participants in the yoga group practiced physical postures, relaxation techniques, regulated breathing, and devotional songs and attended lectures for more than 7 hours a week during the course of the 6-month trial. In particular, depressive symptoms, as measured by the short form of the Geriatric Depression Scale, decreased in the yoga group from a baseline average of 10.6 to 8.1 by 3 months and 6.7 by 6 months. Another study using the same data set looked at the practice of yoga and the effect on quality of sleep and level of depressive symptoms in the yoga group compared with the two control groups, neither of which demonstrated significant effects (Manjunath and Telles 2005). In the yoga group, the average time to fall asleep decreased by 10 minutes, and total sleep time increased by 60 minutes, which resulted in a greater feeling of being rested after 6 months.

Despite the growing body of evidence showing the effects of mindful physical exercises such as Qigong, Tai Chi, and yoga on depression, there is a dearth of studies examining mindful physical exercise and its effects on memory enhancement. An integrated approach of yoga therapy in menopausal women improved cognitive functions such as remote memory, mental balance, attention and concentration, delayed and immediate recall, verbal retention, and recognition tests (Chattha et al. 2008). In our own 8-week study comparing older caregivers of individuals with dementia who practiced 12-minute daily yogic meditation, Kirtan Kriya, with a control group who spent 12 minutes listening to instrumental music, practicing yogic meditation was associated with improved mood, mental health, cognition and brain metabolisms, telomerase levels, and gene expression (Black et al. 2013; Lavrestky 2012). In summary, both alternative and more integrative approaches combining conventional therapies with complementary use of yoga show promise for improving outcomes in geriatric depression. Response to yoga in older adults with bipolar disorder has not been examined yet, and it has not been definitively determined for older adults with cognitive disorders.

According to observations from our recent study of yogic meditation in family dementia caregivers (Lavrestky 2012), the relief from distress after 20 minutes of meditation a day can be strikingly beneficial for a person who provides around-the-clock unpaid intensive personal care to family members for many months or years. Fortunately, stress-reducing techniques can modify some of these characteristics. Many caregivers report relief in depression and insomnia and an improvement in coping ability.

Tai Chi

The practice of the Chinese marital art Tai Chi has been reported to benefit a wide variety of health conditions (Abbott and Lavretsky 2013). In a study of previously sedentary older adults, a 6-month RCT was completed to assess the impact on sleep that resulted from practicing Tai Chi three times per week compared with performing a stretching exercise (Li et al. 2004). The study found that compared with the control group, the participants in the Tai Chi group reported significantly improved sleep latency and greater total sleep duration. Although the study was not completed in a depressed population, these findings suggest a benefit of this approach for sedentary older adults struggling with sleep issues as part of their mood disturbance. In our own study comparing Tai Chi Chih (a manualized abbreviated Tai Chi) practice with health education classes in older adults with depression, the Tai Chi group demonstrated improvement in mood, cognition, physical functioning, and C-reactive protein (CRP) compared with the health education group (Lavretsky et al. 2011). Furthermore, with the appropriate accommodation for participants with physical limitations, Tai Chi can be used in a variety of settings and, for example, has been shown to improve components of physical and mental health quality of life in nursing home residents (Lee et al. 2010). Therefore, Tai Chi offers a safe and effective intervention for physical and mental well-being in older adults.

Lifestyle Interventions

Lifestyle changes can potentially improve resilience by providing better health and enhancing an individual's sense of well-being. Large-scale epidemiological studies demonstrate a strong relationship between diet and inflammation and disorders such as depression and heart disease. Diets high in refined grains, processed meat, sugar, and saturated and trans-fatty acids and low in fruits, vegetables, and whole grains promote inflammation (Kiecolt-Glaser et al. 2010). High-fat meals can increase glucose levels and triglycerides, which stimulate production of interleukin-6 and CRP (Kiecolt-Glaser et al. 2010). In contrast, higher fruit and vegetable intake is associated with lower inflammation, which may counteract proinflammatory responses to meals high in saturated fat (Kiecolt-Glaser et al. 2010). Therefore, improved nutritional intake is likely to have clinical benefit on health and well-being through anti-inflammatory pathways.

In a recent study, Payne et al. (2012) examined cross-sectional associations between clinically diagnosed depression and dietary intakes of anti-inflammatory ingredients in a cohort of older adults. Antioxidant, fruit, and vegetable intakes were assessed in 278 elderly participants (144 with depression, 134 without depression) using a Block 1998 food frequency questionnaire administered between 1999 and 2007. Vitamin C, lutein, and β-cryptoxanthin (precursor to vitamin A) intakes were significantly lower among individuals with depression than among comparison participants (P < 0.05). In addition, fruit and vegetable consumption, counted as antioxidant intake, was lower in individuals with depression. In multivariable models controlling for age, sex, education, vascular comorbidity score, body mass index, total dietary fat, and alcohol, findings showed that vitamin C, β-cryptoxanthin, fruits, and vegetables remained significant. Antioxidant, fruit, and vegetable intakes were lower in individuals with late-life depression than in comparison participants. These associations may partially explain the elevated risk of cardiovascular disease among older individuals with depression. In addition, these findings point to the importance of antioxidant food sources rather than dietary supplements. Because diet and stress both affect the immune system, the interaction of these two factors should be addressed in future studies.

Exercise

Exercise has also been shown to be important in maintaining well-being in older adults. Exercise intensity, duration, frequency, and other factors appear to play important roles in antiaging outcomes, as does the role of physical training (Salmon 2001). Human and other animal studies demonstrate that exercise targets many aspects of brain function, providing broad effects on overall brain health. The benefits of exercise have been best defined for learning and memory, protection from neurodegeneration, and alleviation of depression, particularly in elderly populations. Exercise increases synaptic plasticity by directly affecting synaptic structure and potentiating synaptic strength, as well as by strengthening the underlying systems that support plasticity, including neurogenesis, metabolism, and vascular function. Such exercise-induced structural and functional change has been documented in various brain regions but has been studied best in the hippocampus (Cotman et al. 2007).

Emerging evidence suggests that exercise has therapeutic and preventive effects on depression (Cotman et al. 2007). The prevention and treatment of depression are crucial areas to define. Depression is linked to cognitive decline and is considered to cause a worldwide health burden greater than that of ischemic heart disease, cerebrovascular disease, or tuberculosis. The therapeutic effects of exercise on depression have been most clearly established in human studies. Randomized and crossover clinical trials demonstrate the efficacy of aerobic or resistance-training exercise (2–4 months) as a treatment for depression in both young and older individuals (Blumenthal et al. 1999). The benefits are similar to those achieved with antidepressants (Blumenthal et al. 1999). Therefore, exercise appears to be a powerful intervention that has mood-enhancing effects, thereby promoting well-being and therefore resilience.

Spirituality, Meditation, and Pastoral Care

Some people prefer to seek help for mental health problems from their pastor, rabbi, or priest rather than from therapists who are not affiliated with a religious community. Counselors working within traditional faith communities are increasingly recognizing the need to incorporate psychotherapy and/or medication along with prayer and spirituality to effectively help some people with mental disorders. Both religiousness and social support have been shown to influence depression outcomes, yet some researchers have theorized that religiousness largely reflects social support. In one study, religious coping was related to social support but was independently related to depression outcomes. The authors concluded that clinicians caring for older patients with depression should consider inquiring about spirituality and religious coping as a way of improving depressive outcomes (Bosworth et al. 2003). When clinicians apply culturally sensitive assessment and interventions tailored for the individual patient, spirituality can enhance quality of life, well-being, and resilience.

Meditation is another lifestyle intervention that can affect well-being and resilience. The clinical effects of meditation influence a broad spectrum of physical and psychological symptoms and syndromes and can lead to, for example, reduced anxiety, pain, and depression; enhanced mood and self-esteem; and decreased stress. Meditation has been studied in populations with fibromyalgia, cancer, hypertension, and psoriasis. Meditation practice can positively influence the experience of chronic illness and can serve as a primary, secondary, and/or tertiary prevention strategy. Health professionals demonstrate commitment to holistic practices by asking patients about their use of meditation and can encourage this self-care activity. Simple techniques for mindfulness can be taught in clinical settings. Living mindfully with chronic illness is a fruitful area for research, and we predict that evidence will grow to support the role of consciousness in the human experience of disease. In summary, having clinicians ask about and reinforce positively held spiritual and religious beliefs appears to be an effective strategy that is complementary to routine psychotherapy and psychopharmacological management of late-life mood symptoms.

Clinical Vignette

Lena, a 65-year-old African American woman who was caring for her mother with AD and her sister with stroke-related dementia, came to participate in our meditation study. She scored 12—the moderate depression range—on the Hamilton Depression Rating Scale (HDRS). She started daily meditation and demonstrated improvement in her distress within the first 2 weeks, with an HDRS score of only 1 at the second week. Her HDRS scores fluctuated between weeks 2 and 4 and then stabilized at a low improved score at the end of the study. Lena reported an increased ability to cope and to assess her stressful situation more objectively, without the level of anger and resentment she had prior to the med-

itation experience. Lena also learned to allocate time to her own pleasurable activities and did not feel "trapped" or like a "victim of circumstances." With daily
meditation and the recognition of her own psychological needs, this stressed
caregiver increased her resilience and ability to cope with her life stressors. Also,
she felt empowered by the idea of wellness, resilience, and self-reliance. Lena's
strength was her openness and flexibility to modifying her attitudes and learning from her experiences.

Alternative Medical Systems

Acupuncture and Traditional Chinese Medicine

Acupuncture is the Chinese practice of inserting needles into the body at specific
points to manipulate the body's flow of energy to balance the endocrine system
and to regulate heart rate, body temperature, and, potentially, emotional changes.
The literature on acupuncture for depression in older adults is limited, with a pilot
study finding positive effects on measures of mood and well-being (Williams and
Graham 2006). A Chinese study of 101 adults with "post-wind stroke depression," a traditional Chinese medicine diagnosis, found that "mind-refreshing
anti-depressive" acupuncture was as effective as low-dose doxepin plus routine
acupuncture and more effective than routine acupuncture alone (Li et al. 1994).

Numerous studies have researched the use of acupuncture for depression or
stress, but only a few studies have considered the use of acupuncture for dementia. In a Chinese study, Zhou and Jin (2008) performed acupuncture on the scalp
in areas corresponding to brain regions involved in AD. Twenty-six patients with
clinically diagnosed AD underwent functional magnetic resonance imaging
while undergoing acupuncture at four acupoints. Activation occurred in both
the right main hemisphere and the left hemisphere in locations consistent with
brain regions frequently impaired in AD. These areas are closely correlated with
cognitive function (e.g., memory, reason, language, executive), providing evidence that acupuncture has a potential effect on AD. In conclusion, although
acupuncture has been used in clinics to assist people with a number of ailments,
including anxiety and depression, evidence of the efficacy of acupuncture currently remains limited, and further large, well-designed studies are needed in this
area for both mood and cognitive disorders.

Ayurveda

Ayurveda, which translates to "the science of life" and has been described as
"knowledge of how to live," is a complete natural health care system that began
in India more than 5,000 years ago and has been used within the context of mental health and aging for memory enhancement and anxiety reduction. Promoting immune system function through anti-inflammatory remedies, Ayurveda is

currently widely used in India as a system of primary health care. Because of Ayurveda's emphasis on developing an individualized regimen for patients that includes dietary, meditation, herbal, and other components, interest in using Ayurveda to treat a number of maladies, including depression, is growing worldwide. Through yoga and/or transcendental meditation techniques, Ayurveda promotes lifestyle change and education about how to release stress and tension. Furthermore, Ayurveda is geared toward treating chronic disorders associated with the aging process, and promising preliminary results related to use of Ayurveda have been found in studies of depression, anxiety, sleep disorders, hypertension, diabetes mellitus, Parkinson's disease, and AD (Sharma et al. 2007).

Other CAIM Practices: Expressive Therapies

Engagement in the creative arts holds potential as a positive coping strategy for dealing with the otherwise potentially depressive changes associated with normal aging such as retirement, lack of purpose, and social isolation (Flood and Phillips 2007). Although formal study of such activities is limited, psychological and neurobiological theories of aging support the notion that enriching and enjoyable activities have a beneficial effect on overall physical and mental health. For example, older adults enrolled in a 12-month structured chorale program reported significant improvements in overall physical health, better morale, less loneliness, and a trend toward increased overall activities (Cohen et al. 2006).

A multimodal program including components of rhythm and dance, physical and outdoor exercising, and multiple seminars on creativity, philosophy, and communication demonstrated significant effects on multiple outcome measures (Cohen et al. 2006). The 75 older adults enrolled in this 4-month program participated in multiple individual and group sessions held throughout each week of the study. Formal testing revealed that subjects reported an improved sense of purpose in life, fewer depressive symptoms, and lower levels of hypochondriasis. These gains were maintained when participants were reassessed 6 months postintervention. Thus, such interventions hold potential for older adults to experientially integrate the emotional, physical, and cognitive aspects of self that are at risk for fragmentation and decline with aging.

Summary

Late-life mood and cognitive disorders are among the most common reasons for using complementary, alternative, and integrative therapies in older adults. The amount of rigorous scientific data to support the efficacy of integrative therapies in the treatment of mood and cognitive disorders is still extremely limited in younger adults and is often essentially nonexistent in older adults.

There is a need for further research involving larger, well-designed RCTs to determine the efficacy of CAIM therapies in the treatment of mood and cognitive disorders during late life. The ultimate goal is development of effective, well-tolerated, and safe treatment approaches to prevent these serious and disabling conditions and to enhance resilience to stress, well-being, and positive aging.

Clinical Key Points

- Complementary, alternative, and integrative medicine is a holistic and integrative approach to wellness and balance of mind, body, and spirit and includes multifaceted interventions such as mind-body medicine and the use of natural products and supplements.

- Lifestyle factors such as diet, exercise, and spirituality can enhance resilience and positive aging by creating physical and mental well-being.

- Careful evaluation and judicious use of supplements and herbs can promote wellness while minimizing side effects.

- The impact of mindful physical exercise goes beyond physical improvements to include psychosocial benefits as well.

References

Abbott R, Lavretsky H: Tai Chi and Qigong for the treatment and prevention of mental disorders. Psychiatr Clin North Am 36(1):109–119, 2013 23538081

Alpert JE, Papakostas G, Mischoulon D, et al: S-adenosyl-L-methionine (SAMe) as an adjunct for resistant major depressive disorder: an open trial following partial or nonresponse to selective serotonin reuptake inhibitors or venlafaxine. J Clin Psychopharmacol 24(6):661–664, 2004 15538131

Alzheimer's Association: 2010 Alzheimer's disease facts and figures. Alzheimers Dement 6(2):158–194, 2010 20298981

Barnes PM, Bloom B, Nahin RL: Complementary and alternative medicine use among adults and children: United States, 2007. Natl Health Stat Rep 12(12):1–23, 2008 19361005

Black DS, Cole SW, Irwin MR, et al: Yogic meditation reverses NF-κB and IRF-related transcriptome dynamics in leukocytes of family dementia caregivers in a randomized controlled trial. Psychoneuroendocrinology 38(3):348–355, 2013 22795617

Blumenthal JA, Babyak MA, Moore KA, et al: Effects of exercise training on older patients with major depression. Arch Intern Med 159(19):2349–2356, 1999 10547175

Bosworth HB, Park KS, McQuoid DR, et al: The impact of religious practice and religious coping on geriatric depression. Int J Geriatr Psychiatry 18(10):905–914, 2003 14533123

Chattha R, Nagarathna R, Padmalatha V, et al: Effect of yoga on cognitive functions in climacteric syndrome: a randomised control study. BJOG 115(8):991–1000, 2008 18503578

Cohen GD, Perlstein S, Chapline J, et al: The impact of professionally conducted cultural programs on the physical health, mental health, and social functioning of older adults. Gerontologist 46(6):726–734, 2006 17169928

Cotman CW, Berchtold NC, Christie LA: Exercise builds brain health: key roles of growth factor cascades and inflammation. Trends Neurosci 30(9):464–472, 2007 17765329

DeKosky ST, Williamson JD, Fitzpatrick AL, et al; Ginkgo Evaluation of Memory (GEM) Study Investigators: Ginkgo biloba for prevention of dementia: a randomized controlled trial. JAMA 300(19):2253–2262, 2008 19017911

Flood M, Phillips KD: Creativity in older adults: a plethora of possibilities. Issues Ment Health Nurs 28(4):389–411, 2007 17454290

Fotuhi M, Mohassel P, Yaffe K: Fish consumption, long-chain omega-3 fatty acids and risk of cognitive decline or Alzheimer disease: a complex association. Nat Clin Pract Neurol 5(3):140–152, 2009 19262590

Harrer G, Schmidt U, Kuhn U, et al: Comparison of equivalence between the St. John's wort extract LoHyp-57 and fluoxetine. Arzneimittelforschung 49(4):289–296, 1999 10337446

Ihl R, Tribanek M, Bachinskaya N; GOTADAY Study Group: Efficacy and tolerability of a once daily formulation of Ginkgo biloba extract EGb 761* in Alzheimer's disease and vascular dementia: results from a randomised controlled trial. Pharmacopsychiatry 45(2):41–46, 2012 22086747

Kiecolt-Glaser JK, Christian L, Preston H, et al: Stress, inflammation, and yoga practice. Psychosom Med 72(2):113–121, 2010 20064902

Krishnamurthy MN, Telles S: Assessing depression following two ancient Indian interventions: effects of yoga and ayurveda on older adults in a residential home. J Gerontol Nurs 33(2):17–23, 2007 17310659

La Forge L: Aligning mind and body: exploring the disciplines of mindful exercise. ACSM's Health and Fitness Journal 9:7–14, 2005

Lavretsky H: Resilience, stress, and late life mood disorders. Annu Rev Gerontol Geriatr 32:49–72, 2012

Lavretsky H, Alstein LL, Olmstead RE, et al: Complementary use of tai chi chih augments escitalopram treatment of geriatric depression: a randomized controlled trial. Am J Geriatr Psychiatry 19(10):839–850, 2011 21358389

Lee LY, Lee DT, Woo J: The psychosocial effect of Tai Chi on nursing home residents. J Clin Nurs 19(7–8):927–938, 2010 20492037

Li C, Huang Y, Li Y, et al: Treating post-stroke depression with "mind-refreshing antidepressive" acupuncture therapy: a clinical study of 21 cases. International Journal of Clinical Acupuncture 5:389–393, 1994

Li F, Fisher KJ, Harmer P, et al: Tai chi and self-rated quality of sleep and daytime sleepiness in older adults: a randomized controlled trial. J Am Geriatr Soc 52(6):892–900, 2004 15161452

Manjunath NK, Telles S: Influence of yoga and Ayurveda on self-rated sleep in a geriatric population. Indian J Med Res 121(5):683–690, 2005 15937373

Mazereeuw G, Lanctôt KL, Chau SA, et al: Effects of ω-3 fatty acids on cognitive performance: a meta-analysis. Neurobiol Aging 33(7):e17–e29, 2012 22305186

McBee L: Mindfulness-Based Elder Care. New York, Springer, 2008

Meeks TW, Wetherell JL, Irwin MR, et al: Complementary and alternative treatments for late-life depression, anxiety, and sleep disturbance: a review of randomized controlled trials. J Clin Psychiatry 68(10):1461–1471, 2007 17960959

Mischoulon D, Fava M: Role of S-adenosyl-L-methionine in the treatment of depression: a review of the evidence. Am J Clin Nutr 76(5):1158S–1161S, 2002 12420702

Payne ME, Steck SE, George RR, et al: Fruit, vegetable, and antioxidant intakes are lower in older adults with depression. J Acad Nutr Diet 112(12):2022–2027, 2012 23174689

Rondanelli M, Giacosa A, Opizzi A, et al: Long chain omega 3 polyunsaturated fatty acids supplementation in the treatment of elderly depression: effects on depressive symptoms, on phospholipids fatty acids profile and on health-related quality of life. J Nutr Health Aging 15(1):37–44, 2011 21267525

Salmon P: Effects of physical exercise on anxiety, depression, and sensitivity to stress: a unifying theory. Clin Psychol Rev 21(1):33–61, 2001 11148895

Sharma H, Chandola HM, Singh G, et al: Utilization of Ayurveda in health care: an approach for prevention, health promotion, and treatment of disease. Part 1—Ayurveda, the science of life. J Altern Complement Med 13(9):1011–1019, 2007 18047449

Sydenham E, Dangour AD, Lim WS: Omega 3 fatty acid for the prevention of cognitive decline and dementia. Cochrane Database Syst Rev 6:CD005379, 2012 22696350

Tsang HW, Fung KM, Chan AS, et al: Effect of a qigong exercise programme on elderly with depression. Int J Geriatr Psychiatry 21(9):890–897, 2006 16955451

Williams J, Graham C: Acupuncture for older adults with depression-a pilot study to assess acceptability and feasibility. Int J Geriatr Psychiatry 21(6):599–600, 2006 16783799

Williams JW, Plassman BL, Burke J, et al: Preventing Alzheimer's Disease and Cognitive Decline. Evidence Report/Technology Assessment No 193 (Prepared by the Duke Evidence-Based Practice Center under Contract No. HHSA 290-2007-10066-I; AHRQ Publ No 10-E005). Rockville, MD, Agency for Healthcare Research and Quality, 2010

Zhou Y, Jin J: Effect of acupuncture given at the HT 7, ST 36, ST 40 and KI 3 acupoints on various parts of the brains of Alzheimer' s disease patients. Acupunct Electrother Res 33(1–2):9–17, 2008 18672741

Suggested Cross-References

Meditation and yoga are discussed in Chapter 12 ("Integrating Positive Psychiatry Into Clinical Practice"). Spirituality is discussed in Chapter 2 ("Positive Psychological Traits") and Chapter 13 ("Biology of Positive Psychiatry").

Suggested Readings

Abbott R, Lavretsky H: Tai Chi and Qigong for the treatment and prevention of mental disorders. Psychiatr Clin North Am 36(1):109–119, 2013 23538081

Barnes PM, Bloom B, Nahin RL: Complementary and alternative medicine use among adults and children: United States, 2007. Natl Health Stat Rep 12(12):1–23, 2008 19361005

Blumenthal JA, Babyak MA, Moore KA, et al: Effects of exercise training on older patients with major depression. Arch Intern Med 159(19):2349–2356, 1999 10547175

Williams JW, Plassman BL, Burke J, et al: Preventing Alzheimer's Disease and Cognitive Decline. Evidence Report/Technology Assessment No 193 (Prepared by the Duke Evidence-based Practice Center under Contract No. HHSA 290-2007-10066-I; AHRQ Publ No 10-E005). Rockville, MD, Agency for Healthcare Research and Quality, 2010

11

Preventive Interventions

CARL C. BELL, M.D., DLFAPA, FACPSYCH

It is easier to build strong children than to repair broken men.

Frederick Douglass

In traditional medicine, if a patient goes to a physician for treatment of a rat bite, the physician cleans the bite, dresses it, gives antibiotics, and administers a tetanus shot. The physician who is also practicing public health would give our imaginary patient the same treatment but would go a step further; he or she would arrange for someone to go into the patient's community and set rattraps. Accordingly, in this chapter, I discuss principally psychiatric prevention interventions and psychiatric public health for individuals and populations.

In this chapter, I focus primarily on universal preventive interventions that are targeted to the public or a whole population group that has not been identified because of individual risk (O'Connell et al. 2009); this strategy is also known as *primary prevention*, that is, the efforts in public health to prevent the disease before symptom onset. I cover some general strategies for prevention and then look at some specific prevention interventions for children and adults. Indicated preventive interventions that have a huge potential impact on public health and health disparities are also covered. These interventions are those directed at high-risk individuals who are identified as having minimal but detectable signs or symptoms that foreshadow mental, emotional, or behavioral disorders and preventive interventions that focus on biological markers that indicate a person has a predisposition for such a disorder but does not meet diagnostic criteria at the time of the intervention (O'Connell et al. 2009). This level of prevention is very similar to the older secondary prevention referring to the reduction or cessation of symptom progression once symptoms have appeared. The emphasis on early prevention is not meant to belittle *selective prevention,* that is, preventive interventions that are targeted to individuals or a subgroup of the population whose risk of developing mental, emotional, or behavioral disorders is significantly higher than average (O'Connell et al. 2009); selective prevention is similar to *tertiary prevention,* which refers to a treatment designed to halt the progression of the disease once it has been established. In this chapter, I underscore preventive strategies for mental, emotional, and behavioral disorders because, unfortunately, some people do not know prevention is possible in psychiatry.

Strategies for Preventive Interventions

In public health, two types of interventions prevent illnesses—biotechnical and psychosocial—and of the two, the biotechnical interventions are the easiest to implement. For example, in the United States, a condition called *cretinism,* which is caused by a lack of iodine in the diet, resulted in brain damage from hypothyroidism. (Iodine is a trace element necessary for the production of thyroid hormones.) The biotechnical intervention of putting iodine in common table salt has solved this physical and mental health problem in the United States. Psychosocial interventions are more difficult to implement because such interventions involve a change in people's behavior, and changing behavior is not an easy task. Behavior is complex and multidetermined, and in their efforts to prevent behaviors that result in physical, mental, and spiritual illness, mental health professionals must understand the causes of such behaviors. However, because the causes of behavior can be intuitive and counterintuitive, mental health professionals need science to ferret out the multiple, true causes of behavior.

Conceptual Framework for Behavioral Prevention: Theory of Triadic Influence

One scientific strategy that is feasible for preventing behaviors generating physical, mental, and spiritual illness and maintaining well-being is the theory of triadic influence (TTI) (Flay et al. 2009). TTI takes into account cultural and environmental, social and familial, and personality and biological causes of behavior and provides a scientific framework to experiment and learn efficacious and effective methods of health behavior change (Bell et al. 2002). Typically, complex behavior change theories are difficult to implement and apply in the public domain, making both individual- and population-based behavior changes difficult (O'Connell et al. 2009). Accordingly, it became necessary to translate TTI into a form that would be readily acceptable and easy to use by the public; thus, seven universal community field principles were developed from the TTI (Bell et al. 2002).

Seven Community Field Principles for Cultivating Resiliency and Health Behavior Change

Rebuilding the Village/Constructing Social Fabric

Human beings are social animals, and from conception to death, humans need other people to do well in their lives, that is, to "live long and prosper"; people need what the ancients called *village* and what modern scientists call *social fabric* or *collective efficacy* (Sampson et al. 1997). If this necessity of life is missing or has become frayed, humans would do well to construct or rebuild it. A hundred years ago when Chicago experienced a rash of juvenile delinquency in recently immigrated southern and eastern Europeans, Nobel Prize–winning social worker Jane Addams spearheaded community-organizing efforts (rebuilding the village). She was also instrumental in establishing the first juvenile court, an example of older psychosocial technology, which was designed to be a family-strengthening institution to decrease delinquency (Beuttler and Bell 2010). Efforts that are more recent involve establishing block clubs that encourage neighbors to get to know one another and their families to provide a sense of village that encourages all of the adults on the block to assist one another in monitoring everyone in the community (adults and youths) to be supportive of healthy development. For example, the formation of youth sports activities (e.g., American Youth Soccer Organization soccer activities; www.ayso.org/) allows parents and youths to come together in a healthy environment to support learning social and emotional skills, building self-esteem, and providing an adult protective shield nurturing and strengthening youths. In another example, Chicago Public Schools (CPS) supported religious school–community partnership networks in each of the CPS regions, and these collaborations provided tutoring, family-strengthening services, and social services. By collaborating with the religious community, CPS increased attendance, improved school environments, provided positive role models, and created prosocial activities for youths. Through these partnerships, CPS helped coordinate antiviolence marches with religious communities throughout the city. In addition, the network of secular and nonsecular organizations provided assistance in mentoring programs, off-site detention and community service programs, after-school homework centers, school-community activities, and youth outreach workers, and it developed a "walking school bus" (i.e., recruiting adults to walk children to and from school) and held antiviolence workshops. Thus, CPS was able to increase village in Chicago neighborhoods, which reduced violence (Bell et al. 2001).

Social support can be real or virtual. Internet-based social group support offers the prospect of enhancing curricular-based interventions through one of several mechanisms: 1) increasing use of the curricular-based prevention, 2) providing opportunities to discuss contents and increase sociocultural relevance, and 3) directing increasing social support (Jeste and Bell 2011). For example, ReachOut in Australia has demonstrated considerable appeal to the public, showing that online groups can sustain individual membership for as long as a year (Jeste and Bell 2011).

Providing Access to Ancient and Modern Medical Technology (Biotechnical and Psychosocial)

An excellent example of an ancient and recently rediscovered "modern" biotechnical prevention intervention is the omega-3 polyunsaturated fatty acids. Consider the ancient aphorism that "fish is brain food" and the modern evidence that omega-3 fatty acids may be protective of brain competency (Jeste and Bell 2011). Modern science has also documented another ancient practice, three-ball cascade juggling, which increases neuroconnectivity in the brain (Boyke et al. 2008). Of course, we are all wondering where our new virtual village—the Internet—is going to lead, because it is a way for people to be monitored and connected.

Improving Bonding, Attachment, and Connectedness Dynamics

Being social animals, humans need to be connected to others, and this connectedness is protective during all phases of life. Likewise, as with other human needs, connectedness can be nurtured. Unfortunately, humans have progressed so much that they need social service programs to do what people used to do naturally when there were more intact villages; fortunately, informal home visitation and social clubs also continue to support families and their children.

Improving Self-Esteem

Bean (1992) spelled out the various characteristics of *self-esteem* as 1) a sense of power (also known as self-efficacy or having confidence in your ability for mastery), 2) a sense of models (e.g., understanding how things work makes people feel good and builds self-esteem because it provides the ah-ha feeling that everyone likes), 3) a sense of uniqueness (e.g., ethnic, racial, or cultural identity), and 4) a sense of connectedness. There are multiple and varying ways to support the development of self-esteem.

Increasing Social and Emotional Skills

Having social skills allows one to be welcomed into social groups, and having the emotional skill of affect regulation helps prevent one's default of getting upset when things go bad, which ultimately makes the situation worse (Bell and McBride 2010). The absent emotional skill of self-control is the most obvious characteristic of teenagers and delinquents. The problems of poor frustration tolerance, temper outbursts, self-destructive behavior, and poor relationships with others are diagnosed with many different psychiatric labels. Youths, by definition, are still immature, and this immaturity has its origins in the path brain development takes toward maturity. Although extraordinarily complex, two important brain systems exist: the survival (flight, fight, or freeze) and the thinking (judgment, wisdom, and discernment) systems of the brain, which are generally located in the limbic system and the frontal lobes, respectively. The way that nature works is that the limbic system, or survival parts of the brain, fully develops first, and then the frontal lobes, or thinking part of the brain, fully develop last. Rather than get technical about how the brain works, a simple analogy is to think of youths as cars with mainly gasoline, no brakes or steering wheels (Bell and McBride 2010). Accordingly, adults and the community have the responsibility to help youths develop brakes and a steering wheel, that is, affect regulation.

Reestablishing the Adult Protective Shield and Monitoring

Knowing that someone is shielding you and monitoring your behavior is a very protective mechanism because it ensures that you will have support to keep yourself out of harm's way. People who hold each other accountable for certain standards of behavior always do better in life. Adults can teach youths self-control. Adults need to provide youths with brakes and a steering wheel to keep them safe and headed in the right direction until they "mature," which is the field principle of adult protective shield, which needs a village. The brain usually matures around age 26 when the frontal lobes fully come online and youths develop some affect regulation, or self-control, that puts them in a better position to think before they act because they have the capacity to consider the consequences of their behavior (National Academy of Sciences 2013).

Youths involved with juvenile justice are prone to have more problems with self-control. Such youths may often come from environments where brakes and steering wheels, that is, responsible adults and communities, are not predominant in their lives or where life is so hard it damages rather than nurtures youths. Until youths develop some self-control, it is imperative that society protect itself and protect the youths from themselves and various out-of-control, risky, youthful behaviors. However, the need to protect society coupled with research revealing brain and child development calls for a different approach to juvenile delinquency, and the response to delinquency becomes more complex than simply taking a punitive, after-the-crime approach. The heavy focus on protecting society with the absence of recognition of child development is preventing the shift from a punitive to a child welfare juvenile justice system, reflective of how the system first began 100 years ago (Beuttler and Bell 2010). Juvenile justice has erred in focusing too much on retribution and punishment in its approach to youths, and this approach is counterproductive, but the rationale and call for reform in juvenile justice are growing (National Academy of Sciences 2013).

Minimizing the Residual Effects of Trauma and Creating a Sense of Mastery or Self-Efficacy

Stress, distress, and traumatic stress are unavoidable in life; however, these occurrences in and of themselves are usually not harmful; what is problematic is the helplessness an individual feels when confronted with them, especially in the case of traumatic stress (Bell 2001). Experiences of traumatic stress are common findings in juvenile justice and foster care. Abram et al. (2004) assert that exposure to trauma is a fact of life for delinquent youths because more than 56.8% of their sample were exposed to trauma six or more times. Thus, institutions that have youths in confinement must be aware of how to take a *trauma-informed* approach to such youths. Additionally, because, by definition, youths in child protective services and foster care experience trauma in the form of abandonment, neglect, and abuse, the National Child Traumatic Stress Network (2014) has advocated *psychological first aid* as a basic skill needed in juvenile detention centers and foster care. The core features of psychological first aid are easily adapted (Table 11–1) and implemented in large organizations that care for traumatized youths (Jeste and Bell 2011). Helping youths in foster care to overcome early abuse and neglect is an admirable goal, and helping them to build coping skills to confront future adverse experiences is fruitful. Although some youths naturally have more protective factors, abused and neglected youths can be assisted in becoming more resilient by infusing protective factors into their lives (Jeste and Bell 2011). Thus, risk factors do not become predictive factors if youths develop and have protective factors. The prevention of trauma in youths in foster care is akin to prevention of trauma in youths in various disasters. Thus, from a public health perspective, it is important to help people cultivate resiliency when they find themselves in difficult situations such as foster care, juvenile justice, and disasters (Hobfoll et al. 2007; Jeste and Bell 2011; National Academy of Sciences 2013).

Applying the Seven Community Field Principles

Examples of specific activities to actualize each of the seven community field principles are provided in Table 11–2. Youths and adults who are involved with one risky behavior are likely to be involved in more than one perilous behavior.

Table 11–1. Core features of psychological first aid for children: challenge and first aid application in three grade categories

Preschool		Grades 3–5		Grade 6 and higher (adolescents)	
Challenge	Application	Challenge	Application	Challenge	Application
Helplessness and passivity	Provide support, rest, comfort, food, and an opportunity to play	Preoccupation with their actions during the event	Help them express secret imaginations about the event	Detachment, shame, and guilt	Encourage discussion of the event and realistic expectations of what could have been done
Generalized fear	Reestablish adult protective shield	Specific fears from traumatic reminders	Help them identify and articulate traumatic reminders and encourage them not to generalize	Self-consciousness about fear, sense of vulnerability	Help them understand the adult nature of these feelings and encourage peer understanding and support
Cognitive confusion	Give repeated concrete clarifications	Traumatic play	Give permission to talk or act it out, address distortions, and acknowledge normality of feelings and reactions	Posttraumatic acting up: drug use, delinquency, sexual behavior	Help them understand the acting up as an effort to numb their responses or to voice their anger about the event
Lack of verbalization	Help them verbalize general feelings and complaints	Fear of being overwhelmed	Encourage the expression of their feelings in a supportive environment	Self-destructive or accident-prone behavior	Address the impulse toward reckless behavior and link it to the challenge for impulse control associated with violence

Table 11–1. Core features of psychological first aid for children: challenge and first aid application in three grade categories *(continued)*

	Preschool		Grades 3–5		Grade 6 and higher (adolescents)	
Challenge	Challenge	Application	Challenge	Application	Challenge	Application
Sleep disturbances	Sleep disturbances	Encourage them to let their parents and teachers know	Impaired concentration and learning	Encourage them to let their parents and teachers know when intrusions interfere with learning	Abrupt shifts in relationships	Discuss the expectable strain on relationships with family and peers
Anxious attachment		Provide consistent caregiving	Sleep disturbances	Encourage them in reporting their dreams and explain why people have bad dreams	Desires and plans for revenge	Elicit actual plans of revenge, address realistic consequences of these actions, and encourage constructive alternatives that lessen the sense of traumatic helplessness
Regressive symptoms		Tolerate regressive symptoms in a time-limited manner	Concerns about safety of self and others	Help them share worries and reassure them with realistic information	Change in life attitudes	Link attitude changes to the event's impact

Table 11–1. Core features of psychological first aid for children: challenge and first aid application in three grade categories *(continued)*

Preschool		Grades 3–5		Grade 6 and higher (adolescents)	
Challenge	Application	Challenge	Application	Challenge	Application
Anxiety about death	Give explanations about the physical reality of death	Aggression and recklessness	Help them cope with the challenge of their own impulse control	Premature entry into adulthood	Encourage postponing radical decisions in order to process the response to the event and grief
		Somatic complaints	Help them identify the physical sensations they felt during the event		
		Concerns about parents	Help them tell their parents how they are feeling		
		Concern for victims	Encourage constructive activities on behalf of the injured or deceased		
		Grief	Help them retain positive memories as they work through the more intrusive, traumatic memories		

Source. Adapted from Pynoos and Nader 1988.

As several preventive population-based interventions have shown (Bell and Mc-Bride 2011; Bell et al. 2001, 2008; Redd et al. 2005), prevention interventions add protective factors to youths' lives, insulating them from multiple risk factors that have the potential to negatively affect well-being. In parallel but separate research, Jeste and Bell (2011) showed that the three characteristics of resilient children of depressed parents are the capacity to be deeply engaged in relationships (connectedness), the ability to accomplish age-appropriate developmental tasks (creating self-esteem), and the capacity for self-reflection and self-understanding (social and emotional skills). Youths who engage in risky sexual behaviors are also likely to engage in risky behaviors involving substances, violence, suicide, truancy, and dropping out of school (Flay et al. 2009). It is important to understand that like the various systems of the human body (e.g., respiratory, circulatory, digestive, and nervous systems), which all must work together for optimal functioning, the seven universal community field principles all work together in an interdependent manner to prevent physical, mental, and spiritual illness and promote well-being. These principles are valuable for strengthening multiple large-scale preventive interventions (Bell and McBride 2011). These seven universal community field principles of behavior change have been found to be effective in guiding other prevention research and in promoting resiliency and behavior change in youths and adults (Breland-Noble et al. 2006; Kaslow et al. 2010; Redd et al. 2005). The principles are deemed universal because they can be used in various contexts, and despite being somewhat generic, they are directionally correct. At the same time, they offer flexibility, allowing them to be shaped to a specific cultural context.

Finally, the TTI model and field principles can be successfully applied to all age groups, young and old alike (Flay et al. 2009). Specific prevention interventions are designed for children and adults at the individual and group levels, and a careful examination of the core principles driving these efforts will reveal that they easily fit into the schemata of the seven universal community field principles of health behavior change. The following two sections will cover specific preventive interventions for youths and adults at the individual and group levels. The reader may notice specific preventive interventions may emphasize one field principle more heavily than the others; the reality is that unless all the principles are actively used, the likelihood of success will be diminished. Another important reality is that regardless of the purpose—universal, selected, or indicated prevention—people do better if they have village, access to technology, connectedness, social and emotional skills, self-esteem, safety, and hope in their lives. As David Satcher, the sixteenth surgeon general of the United States, once noted, if the vaccine for HIV were developed (a biotechnical intervention), without a village to inform its members of the advance and get them the vaccine, at best, the community members would get the vaccine late and, at worst, they would not get it at all.

Table 11–2. Seven field principles derived from the theory of triadic influence

Field principle	Activities to actualize principles
Rebuilding the village/constructing social fabric	Bring stakeholders together to agree on a shared vision of developing social capital (social networks, relations, trust, and power as a function of either the individual or a geographical entity, e.g., a city neighborhood) to create an interdependent network of people, functions, and services designed to create connectedness among stakeholders, safety, security, and synergy.
Providing access to modern and ancient technology (biotechnical and psychosocial)	Transport evidence-based technology to care for individuals, families, and groups (e.g., multiple-family groups, psychological first aid, frameworks for empowerment evaluation and related enabling activities, stages and tasks of coalition development technologies).
Improving bonding, attachment, and connectedness dynamics	Facilitate attachment of youths to caregivers, caregivers to youths, youths to schools, caregivers to schools, and caregivers to their neighbors and their communities; attach stakeholders to positive, proactive community and organizational systems to improve self-esteem.
Improving self-esteem	Foster improvement in an individual's sense of power (self-efficacy), uniqueness, models, and connectedness.
Increasing social and emotional skills (e.g., affect regulation)	Teach and encourage communication skills (e.g., "I messages"), parenting skills, refusal skills, negotiation skills, leadership and management skills, etc.
Reestablishing the adult protective shield and monitoring, creating safety	Develop caregiver monitoring systems for youths and develop community systems that protect youths.
Minimizing the residual effects of trauma and creating a sense of mastery or self-efficacy, creating hope	Develop an individual's sense of self-efficacy; create a sense of safety, social networks, and social fabric; turn "learned helplessness" into "learned helpfulness."

Population-Based Clinical Vignette: Using the Seven Field Principles to Create Common Ground and Shared Vision to Facilitate Change

In 2000, it was learned that in McLean and Peoria counties in Illinois, the removal of African American children from their homes was 23/1,000 and 24/1,000, respectively, and the Illinois statewide average was 4.3/1,000 (Redd et al. 2005). A project to decrease the rate of removal began with an assessment of the service environment and contextual factors in the target community. Using the seven field principles as a conceptual guide, project staff developed a business plan to improve the quality of existing service systems and to introduce new services. Two years after the intervention began, the number of African American children removed from their homes decreased by more than half (11.1/1,000).

Specific Prevention Interventions in Children at the Individual and Group Levels

Several preventive interventions have been shown to be effective in preventing school failure, antisocial behavior and juvenile delinquency, depression in adolescents, risky sexual behaviors, and trauma- and stressor-related disorders (O'Connell et al. 2009). They all, officially or unofficially, involve one or more aspects of the seven universal community field principles designed to promote health behavior change and increase resiliency by cultivating protective factors for children at the individual and group levels. Thus, they prevent risk factors from becoming predictive of bad outcomes.

Fetal Alcohol Spectrum Disorders

School failure is a major concern of parents. One of the largest preventable public issues responsible for school failure is the exposure of children to alcohol while they are in their mother's womb. The leading known preventable cause of speech and language disorders, specific learning disorders, attention-deficit/hyperactivity disorder, and intellectual disability is *fetal alcohol spectrum disorders* (FASD) (Stratton et al. 1996). The prevalence of this preventable public mental health problem is 100/1,000 (May and Gossage 2001). Recently, the problem of FASD— or, as it is called in DSM-5, *neurobehavioral disorder associated with prenatal alcohol exposure* (NDA-PAE)—has been designated as a "condition for further study" (American Psychiatric Association 2013). This designation is important because as Bell (2014) observed, more than one-third of the African American psychiatric patients seen in a poor African American community in Chicago's South Side had symptoms that fit the criteria for NDA-PAE. NDA-PAE is most likely the largest preventable public health problem in poor African American and American Indian communities. Although some women do not understand or care about the dangers of drinking while pregnant, most women do not know they are pregnant and drink until they learn they are pregnant, at which point they stop, but the damage has been done.

Ancient models of psychosocial efforts to prevent women from drinking while pregnant are as old as the story of Samson's mother in the Old Testament of the Bible (Judges 13:3–5), and multiple psychosocial prevention interventions to change pregnant women's drinking behavior exist. A "modern" biotechnical prevention intervention is the use of vitamins to prevent brain damage from alcohol use. Modern neuroscience research is accumulating evidence that the biotechnical preventive intervention of giving pregnant women high doses of choline (reclassified as a B vitamin), folate, and vitamin A may prevent their children from developing NDA-PAE (Bell 2014). Furthermore, research is ongoing about how postnatal choline for children with NDA-PAE may ameliorate the condition (Bell 2014).

Clinical Vignette: Over-the-Counter Nutrients and Reduction in Affect Dysregulation

An 18-year-old man, Ron, was brought to a family medicine clinic by his grandmother, who reported that she had guardianship of her grandson; because of her daughter's problem drinking, child protective services found her daughter to be an "unfit" parent. A psychiatric evaluation revealed that Ron had problems with impulse control; frustration tolerance; affect regulation; hyperactive behavior; reading, math, and comprehension skills; judgment; social perception; and memory. In addition, Ron had vestiges of skin folds at the inner corner of his eyes, small eye openings, a flat midface, an indistinct philthrum, a thin upper lip, and strabismus. The grandmother also reported that Ron was born prematurely and with a heart murmur. He was diagnosed with bipolar disorder in his early teens and was treated with various mood stabilizers without much success. He is currently taking mood stabilizer medication (valproic acid) but is still having temper outbursts several times a week. Ron and his grandmother were told that given his history, he most likely had a NDA-PAE. On the basis of clinical experience, the clinician suggested that Ron purchase over-the-counter vitamins and nutrients and take choline 500 mg twice a day, folate 400 µg twice a day, vitamin A 7,000 units daily, and omega-3 500 mg twice a day. After 6 months on the suggested nutrient supplement regime and while still taking valproic acid, he seemed calmer (i.e., less hyperactive) and was reported to be less impulsive, in better control of his affect, and less prone to frustration. His grandmother reported the difference was like "night and day." Of course, a vignette of one patient does not qualify as science, but solid clinical observations often precede good scientific clinical research.

Psychosocial Prevention of School Failure

The Good Behavior Game (GBG) is a well-researched universal prevention program provided to young children to help them practice social and emotional skills
in elementary school (Jeste and Bell 2011). Because the game encourages development of these skills early in life, children learn to curb aggressive behavior
that will cause them problems in life. In the game, if classroom teams are able
complete team assignments by working together in a cooperative group manner
and fulfilling known teacher expectations, they win token rewards for good behavior (Jeste and Bell 2011). This strategy has significantly reduced disruptive
behavior, leaving more time for academic learning. Multiple large-scale, long-
term research studies in U.S. schools (in Baltimore) revealed GBG reduced aggressive and disruptive behavior during first grade, and for boys who were constantly aggressive, GBG reduced the likelihood that they would receive a
diagnosis of conduct disorder in adolescence or antisocial personality disorder
in later life (O'Connell et al. 2009). The GBG has reduced suicidal behavior and
the risk of alcohol or illegal drug use and has also reduced the use of mental health
and drug treatment services. The benefits of the GBG exceed its costs (O'Connell
et al. 2009), and schools in Manitoba, Canada, are implementing the GBG in all
of their first-grade classrooms (Manitoba 2011).

Prevention of Antisocial Behavior and Delinquency

Home Visitation
One antisocial and delinquency prevention strategy, home visitation, is an intensive intervention that seeks to encourage successful pregnancy and infant
development. Because of the problems with fidelity in implementation, home
visiting programs can be done in a variety of ways, but the main tactic is for a
nurse or paraprofessional to visit women during or after their pregnancies (or
both); these visits may continue until after the child is a toddler. Parenting, child
development, social support, good parent-child relationships, case management, and human services access are the major foci of home visitation programs
(O'Connell et al. 2009). The evaluation of home visitation programs shows that
families and children receiving these programs do better with social and emotional functioning than those who do not and that the programs are cost-effective
(Bell and McBride 2010).

The most researched home visitation program is the Nurse-Family Partnership (NFP). NFP is an effective intervention that targets several causes of delinquency (e.g., mother-infant bond, parental smoking), which directly influences
later affect regulation of the offspring. The NFP has been shown to improve pregnancy outcomes, maternal caregiving, and maternal life course and prevented
antisocial behavior in offspring (O'Connell et al. 2009). A randomized controlled

study called the Healthy Families New York program suggested that the use of paraprofessionals to do home visiting can achieve prevention benefits similar to those of NFP when targeting women during their first pregnancy (O'Connell et al. 2009). Similar to NFP, Healthy Families New York had a greater impact on mothers who were psychologically vulnerable.

Parenting Programs

Adolescents who perceive their parents do not care about them, have difficulty talking to parents about problems, and make critical decisions on the basis of peers' advice compromise their behavioral and emotional health (Bell and Mc-Bride 2011); these difficulties result in a lack of connectedness, social and emotional skills, and adult protective shield, respectively. Accordingly, social and emotional skills training that improves connectedness in families in the form of parenting programs has demonstrated long-term outcomes with decreased aggressive and antisocial behaviors.

Prevention of Adolescent Depression

Clinical depression is a serious, disabling psychiatric mood disorder that is persistent for at least 2 solid weeks. People commonly misreport unhappiness as depression. Clinical depression is rare in children. It increases when youths reach adolescence; in any given year, about 5% of adolescents may experience a clinical depression, and about 20% have an episode of clinical depression during their adolescent phase of life—about the same rate as adults (O'Connell et al. 2009). Interventions to prevent clinical depression in young people have focused on three main risk factors: depressed parents (adolescents with depressed parents are three to four times more likely to become depressed); a negative, ruminating, pessimistic, powerless, depressed way of thinking; and elevated levels of depressive symptoms or a history of depression (Beardslee et al. 2011). The most common methods of preventing depression are teaching social and emotional skills (i.e., cognitive-behavioral strategies) and giving at-risk people models in family-based approaches (e.g., a sense of models to understand and avoid helplessness in the face of a problem). For adolescents of depressed parents, educational approaches about depression involving both parents and adolescents have prevented these at-risk youths from developing depressive symptoms.

Beardslee et al. (2011) pointed out that social and emotional skills training aimed at helping adolescents with depressed parents understand that their parents had an illness for which the adolescents were not responsible, thus freeing the adolescents to go on with their own lives, is helpful. Beardslee et al. found that parenting programs reduce depressive symptoms among youths and reduce the incidence of depressive disorders. Because of the popularity of the Internet, interest in using the Internet to prevent adolescent depression is growing. There are six Internet-based studies with an effect size (a statistical measure of the strength of a variable being studied) of small to medium impact for preventing depression. For example, Project CATCH-IT (Competent Adulthood Transition with Cognitive-Behavioral, Humanistic Interpersonal Training) is a primary care–based Web site that focuses on the prevention of depression in adolescents through the integration of cognitive-behavioral therapy, interpersonal psychotherapy, and behavioral activation (all social and emotional skills) and interacts with its users through homework assignments and short narratives (Jeste and Bell 2011). Another study, the Penn Resiliency Program (Gillham and Reivich 2014), which was delivered in schools, produced a good level of success by using methods to challenge negative depressed ways of thinking in diverse groups of adolescents (O'Connell et al. 2009).

Prevention of Risky Sexual Behaviors

Teenage pregnancies have been decreasing for the last 30 years (Kost and Henshaw 2008); however, the research on prevention of teenage pregnancy is poorly studied (O'Connell et al. 2009). Researchers rarely study success. Risky sexual behaviors result in teenage pregnancy and sexually transmitted diseases. Bell and McBride (2011) reviewed research showing parental monitoring and an authoritative parenting style, that is, an adult protective shield, are associated with adolescents who engage in less risky sexual behavior and have fewer sexual partners and pregnancies and increased condom use. These family-based prevention interventions focus on 1) improving supportive parental and community behaviors, 2) improving parent-child communication (e.g., teaching how to use "I messages," which is a model for how to communicate hard-to-talk-about topics), and 3) increasing parental monitoring and limit setting by using principles of rebuilding village, connectedness, a sense of models, and adult protective shield, respectively (Bell et al. 2008). In addition, sophisticated analysis of multiple different family-based interventions to increase maternal sensitivity and infant attachment (connectedness) have been shown to be effective in contributing to social and emotional learning and resilience and reducing the risk for psychopathology (Bell and McBride 2011).

Another strategy using the universal community field principle of increasing bonding, attachment, and connectedness dynamics to decrease risky sexual behavior is the Cradle to Classroom program in CPS (Bell et al. 2001). This long-range prevention strategy teaches teenage mothers the parenting skills needed to bond with and parent their babies and how to access community resources. Assuming a practical and resource-oriented philosophy, Cradle to Classroom provides counseling about domestic violence and access to prenatal, nutritional, medical, social, and child care services. In CPS in 2002, of 495 seniors with babies, 100% graduated, 78% enrolled in a 2- or 4-year college, and only 5 seniors had a repeat pregnancy (Bell and McBride 2011). Similarly, the

Seattle Social Development Project delivered an intervention that simultaneously involved parents, teachers, and schoolchildren during the grammar school years. This intervention has shown long-term positive effects on mental health more than a decade later (O'Connell et al. 2009).

Prevention of Trauma- and Stressor-Related Disorders in Youths

From Freud's observations to earlier community-based studies on children exposed to violence and to more recent large-scale studies on adverse childhood experiences (Centers for Disease Control and Prevention 2010), psychiatric observations have consistently shown that traumatic stress and distress drive a multitude of risky behaviors. Clearly, universal/primary prevention of trauma- and stressor-related disorders in youths is paramount, but it is a relatively new area of scientific investigation. The universal concept cultivating resilience in youths as a prevention strategy has significant merit (Bell 2001). Although it is difficult to do randomized controlled trials in this area, an expert consensus panel looked at five essential elements (developed from the seven universal field principles) of immediate and middle-term trauma intervention (Hobfoll et al. 2007): 1) a sense of safety, 2) calming, 3) a sense of self- and community efficacy, 4) connectedness, and 5) hope. The literature on resilience is very diverse because many different disciplines (e.g., psychiatric, psychological, sociological, biochemical, cultural, spiritual) have explored this protective factor in life. Reviewing these perspectives on resilience, Bell (2011) suggested that factors involved in resilience include 1) biological factors (intellectual and physical ability, toughness), 2) psychological factors (adaptive mechanisms such as ego resilience, emotional attributes such as emotional well-being, and cognitive attributes such as cognitive styles), 3) spiritual attributes, 4) attributes of posttraumatic growth, 5) social attributes (interpersonal skills, interpersonal relationships, connectedness, and social support), and 6) environmental factors (positive life events and socioeconomic status). Some studies show that optimism can buffer the effects of life stress and enable some individuals to mobilize protective factors such as adaptive coping skills, increased self-efficacy, ways of reinterpreting adverse experiences in a positive manner, and strategies for seeking social support. Thus, formal research to improve psychosocial functioning and resilience is being conducted, which will help the various disciplines find some common ground on the issue of resilience; in the interim, mental health professionals and parents can look to ancient technology to strengthen youths, for example, training "heart" in sports (Bell 2011).

Special Education, Juvenile Justice, and Child Protective Services

David Satcher, when he was the 16th U.S. surgeon general, suggested that if the United States wanted to have an impact on prevention for children, the nation needed to address the needs of children in special education, juvenile justice, and child protective services (U.S. Public Health Service 2000). Because the issues of prevention of school failure (i.e., the children who would be in special education) and child protective services were addressed earlier in this chapter (e.g., see subsections "Fetal Alcohol Spectrum Disorders, "Psychosocial Prevention of School Failure" and "Minimizing the Residual Effects of Trauma and Creating a Sense of Mastery or Self-Efficacy"), in this section, I look at the issue of preventive interventions for children in juvenile justice because children are often traumatized by involvement with this system.

The recent report by the National Academy of Sciences (2013) underscores the need to hold youths accountable for wrongdoing, prevent further offending, and treat youths fairly. On the basis of the science in this report, the manner of juvenile justice reform being advocated is to shift from a punitive model that condemns, controls, and confines for lengthy periods to a model that encourages restorative justice, social and emotional skills building (such as evidence-based "affective regulation" practices), prosocial behavior (providing self-esteem), and immersion in environments that support youth development. Research highlights that adolescents are less likely to get on or stay on a delinquent path if they have a parent or parent figure to whom they are strongly connected and who supports their successful development, are involved with peer groups that actualize prosocial behavior and academic success, and are involved with activities that strengthen autonomous decision making and critical thinking (National Academy of Sciences 2013).

Specific Prevention Interventions in Adults at the Individual and Group Levels

By observing mental, emotional, and behavioral disorders, psychiatrists understand that some disorders characteristically occur during childhood development (e.g., autism spectrum disorders, which are classified as neurodevelopmental disorders in DSM-5) and others begin in adulthood or elderhood (e.g., Alzheimer's disease). It should be noted that sometimes adult psychiatrists with an adult patient who has a neurodevelopmental disorder (that began in childhood) do not realize the patient's illness began in childhood and misclassify it as one of the psychiatric disorders of adulthood. Until psychiatrists get a better understanding of the mechanisms that cause these disorders, they must work with what little they know now and do their best to prevent illness and treat people.

True adult mental, emotional, and behavioral disorders may start in adolescence or later but may not become clinically significant (i.e., interfere with a person's ability to function in social, occupational, or other important activities) until adulthood or elderhood. This reality makes prevention tricky because it is difficult to connect the early beginning of an illness with a very distant presentation.

Prevention of Trauma- and Stressor-Related Disorders in Adults

Culture, Insight, and Mindfulness

Considering that stress, distress, and, at the far end of the spectrum, traumatic stress are extraordinarily common in life (Jeste and Bell 2011), the prevention of trauma- and stressor-related disorders is an important area of exploration. Clearly, a universal prevention strategy would be to prevent exposure to traumatic events; for example, reducing fatal or devastating automobile accidents using the biotechnical strategy of seat belts and air bags would accomplish part of this goal. Bell (2011) emphasized the protective aspects of culture and briefly reviewed the protective factors found in various cultures; thus, coherent cultural practices may be an ancient technology universally preventing trauma- and stressor-related disorders. Another common aspect of life that makes prevention more feasible for adults is the knowledge of self that psychiatrists know as a social and emotional skill called *insight*. Simply put, the more a person knows about himself or herself, the easier it is for that person to use his or her will to adapt and control his or her behavior. Currently, Western cultures are using modern science to confirm the universal ancient wisdom of knowing oneself or developing insight (in Eastern cultures, this social and emotional skill is *mindfulness*). Researchers are beginning to understand these skills are overarching methods of cultivating resiliency and protecting against trauma and stressor-related disorders (Bell 2001). Davidson and McEwen (2012) outlined the neuropsychiatric changes that meditation and mindfulness cultivate. The current research into mindfulness is another example of modern neuroscience validating ancient technology and wisdom.

Posttraumatic Stress Disorder

Selective/secondary prevention efforts have been suggested for people who are at great risk for developing a well-known trauma-related disorder: posttraumatic stress disorder (PTSD). The diagnosis of acute stress disorder (ASD) was developed in the hopes that such a diagnosis would facilitate ways to prevent PTSD. However, after exploring the relationship between ASD and PTSD, researchers found that people with ASD did not automatically progress to developing PTSD; in fact, developing PTSD from ASD was the exception, not the rule. It turns out that major predictors of who will develop PTSD are making catastrophic interpretations of events and having a sense of low self-efficacy (Bell 2011; Jeste and Bell 2011). These characteristics can be altered with the awareness of negative emotional and mental habits. By using will, one can change these negative expectations into more positive, protective expectations.

Although psychosocial methods have been shown to be successful once PTSD is present, psychosocial interventions to prevent PTSD have shown mixed research results (Jeste and Bell 2011). The immediate, single-session approach (i.e., psychological debriefing) that has been tested the most is *critical incident stress debriefing* (CISD). In CISD, a mental health professional typically spends 3–4 hours with victims of a traumatic event to seek to normalize stress responses, provide education, teach coping skills, and help victims ventilate about their experience. However, research shows that CISD is, at best, ineffective and, at worst, harmful (Jeste and Bell 2011). However, variations of trauma-focused, cognitive-behavioral therapy (essentially, the development of social and emotional skills) and prolonged exposure therapy in individuals with ASD demonstrate effectiveness. Matching the patient's intensity of treatment to his or her level of anxiety is another approach that may help prevent PTSD. What is clear is that the least effective approaches involve interventions that occur within a few days after the event, whereas the more effective approaches are those implemented after a brief delay (several weeks or months after the event) and in multiple sessions (Jeste and Bell 2011). Biotechnical, pharmacological approaches to preventing PTSD have been suggested (e.g., propranolol, clonidine, or guanfacine to block adrenergic receptors in the brain; opioids; cortisol; or selective serotonin reuptake inhibitors); however, recruiting and retaining subjects exposed to trauma for a randomized controlled trial is difficult.

Prevention of First-Episode Psychosis

Although the evidence is not complete, research provides some evidence that psychosis can be prevented. An Institute of Medicine report (O'Connell et al. 2009) observes that about half of patients with psychoses experience their first psychotic symptoms in their early teen years but are not diagnosed and treated until years later. The time between the onset of psychotic symptoms and the start of treatment may be 1–2 years, and the duration of untreated psychosis has a negative impact on the prognosis of psychotic illness (Jeste and Bell 2011). Here again our European and Australian psychiatric colleagues are way ahead of the U.S. curve. One screening instrument, the Bonn Scale for the Assessment of Basic Symptoms, can accurately detect early signs of psychosis (Jeste and Bell 2011). Research on adolescents and young adults with early signs of psychosis and who are at ultrahigh risk for developing a psychotic disorder suggests the biotechnical intervention of giving them omega-3 fatty acids reduced the development of psychosis (Jeste and Bell 2011).

Studies show that medication and/or psychosocial treatment can prevent conversion from preclinical signs and symptoms of psychosis to actual psychosis by half the expected rate (Jeste and Bell 2011). The difficulty with this approach is that patients with psychoses tend to lack insight into the nature of their difficulties and usually maintain that nothing is wrong with them; in fact, many clinicians suggest that patients' lack of insight into the nature of their illness is a cardinal feature of schizophrenia. For example, Yale's Prevention through Risk Identification, Management, and Education (PRIME) preventive intervention uses medication to prevent conversion to psychosis; despite participants showing a 50% decrease in the conversion to psychosis, the program has had a difficult time recruiting and retaining patients for the study (Jeste and Bell 2011). Hopefully, a definitive, objective laboratory test will be discovered, and the public will become less skittish about preventive intervention for these devastating illnesses.

Prevention of Postpartum Depression

Screening and Risk Factors

Postpartum depression generally occurs in the postpartum period, which usually lasts up to 6 weeks after a mother gives birth, and is relatively easy to screen for using the Edinburgh Postnatal Depression Scale (Gibson et al. 2009), a 10-item patient self-report scale with excellent validity for this period. This scale is readily available on the Internet, takes 1–5 minutes to complete, and is easy to score; as a result, it is used in many obstetrical units in hospitals to identify potential postpartum depression. Prospective studies reveal that anxiety and mood symptoms during pregnancy increase the risk for postpartum depression (American Psychiatric Association 2013, p. 187). Thus, many women who develop postpartum depression actually develop symptoms in the last month of pregnancy during the peripartum period (i.e., occurring during the last month of gestation or the first few months after delivery) (American Psychiatric Association 2013, p. 186). However, although this scale is a valuable public health intervention, it does not constitute strict prevention (i.e., universal/primary prevention) because this intervention is selective/secondary prevention or indicated/tertiary prevention. Using the modern technology of the Internet, universal postpartum depression prevention interventions have recently been explored. One example of such an intervention is the Mothers and Babies Internet Project (University of California San Francisco 2014). Such investigations have the advantage of being able to obtain a large number of participants for this area of inquiry, and they are easy to implement.

Regarding universal prevention of postpartum depression, in the absence of a widely validated screening tool, clinical assessment is the best strategy for early identification of women at risk for developing postpartum depression (Jeste and Bell 2011). Such a clinical assessment obtains a history of any depressive episodes, premenstrual dysphoric symptoms, current and past stressors, and a history of any family depression. In addition, very importantly, the assessment obtains an inventory of social supports, that is, people who are in a position to offer practical assistance with the care of the baby, which is essentially assessing the village available to the new mother (Jeste and Bell 2011).

Social Support and Postpartum Depression

With the exception of using public health nurses or midwives, it is not clear whether formal social support systems are effective for preventing postpartum depression. Most studies of informal or natural social support systems (i.e., the protective support systems that are inherent in family, community, and culture) indicate that such systems reduce the risk of developing postpartum depression, and in many coherent cultures, postpartum depression is unknown (Jeste and Bell 2011). Thus, helping women rebuild their villages during pregnancy may be a more fruitful prevention approach.

Nutrients, Exercise, and Sleep

The standing hypothesis is that the dramatic postpartum shift in the body's chemistry is a risk factor for postpartum depression. Accordingly, having a healthy brain and body is essential to optimum resilience, and nutrients that support brain functioning (omega-3 fatty acids, choline, folate, vitamin B_{12}, iron, and vitamin D) may be protective; the research is clear that deficiencies in these nutrients are associated with more depression. It is also clear that maternal physiology is designed to shunt these nutrients into the fetus and breast milk to support the baby's development, potentially draining the mother of these necessities. Diets high in seafood that is rich in omega-3 fatty acids lead to lower rates of postpartum depression (Jeste and Bell 2011). Furthermore, exercise and sleep are certainly old standbys in the area of resiliency.

Prevention of Depression in Later Life

Depression in later life is a major public health problem because of high prevalence rates; the association with excess mortality after cerebrovascular accident, myocardial infarction, and cancer; the risk for suicide; and its recalcitrant nature. Older adults (age 65 and older) face the challenge of having integrity or despair, and the resolution, or virtue, to be obtained in this stage of life is wisdom. Wisdom allows for the establishment of an existential identity, or a sense of integrity that helps an individual weather the physical deterioration of old age. Clearly, although promising prevention interventions that address the issue of depression in the elderly are being developed (Jeste and Bell 2011), the universal/

primary preventive intervention for depression in later life is limited because it would have to be started earlier in life, and mental health professionals have just begun to explore these issues. However, interventions promoting self-efficacy and resilience appear to be promising prevention strategies for depression. Moreover, using innovative, modern approaches (i.e., biotechnical technological strategies available from the Internet) may be fruitful (Jeste and Bell 2011). Accordingly, these explorations also fit quite well within the context of the seven universal field principles. Most depression prevention strategies have been modeled after depression treatments, and they are indicated/secondary or selected/tertiary interventions. Again, the emphasis on universal/primary prevention is not to disparage the other forms of prevention. Depression in the elderly is a serious problem because it is associated with higher death rates from heart failure, myocardial infarction, bypass surgery, cerebrovascular accident (depression occurs in at least a third of stroke patients), and cancer; ergo, effective screening for depression and effective treatment of depression would have a huge impact on public health (Jeste and Bell 2011).

Despite the rarity of such prevention interventions, some solid leads are being explored for the development of preventive interventions for depression in the elderly. The issues of poor sleep, loneliness, and poor health in the elderly are prime areas of investigation. Similarly, mild cognitive impairment, bereavement, increased or decreased body mass index, poor ambulation, chronic pain, and lack of exercise are all thought to be risk factors related to depression.

Research investigating problem-solving therapy is currently under way (Jeste and Bell 2011). In addition, there is research under way that shows the effectiveness of stepped-care prevention implemented by mental health nurses; stepped-care prevention consists of watchful waiting, bibliotherapy, and problem-solving therapy and, if these steps fail, referral to a primary care physician for treatment if the symptoms of depression persist. Finally, the Prevention of Suicide in Primary Care Elderly: Collaborative Trial (PROSPECT) study illustrates how treatment by primary care physicians decreases suicidal ideation in the elderly by twofold (Jeste and Bell 2011).

Prevention of Dementia

Alzheimer's Disease

The most common form of dementia, a degenerative neuropsychiatric condition characterized by cognitive decline (most notably, memory loss) in earlier states and physical impairment in later states, is Alzheimer's disease, which can be definitively diagnosed only during autopsy. Because the world's population is aging and it is predicted that Alzheimer's disease will dramatically increase in prevalence, a serious race is taking place to find biomarkers to identify the disorder earlier than autopsy and to prevent the illness from devastating the elderly.

Unfortunately, in 2010, the National Institutes of Health issued a state-of-the-science conference statement (Daviglus et al. 2010) that opined the research on prevention of Alzheimer's disease was of low quality. The gold standard of randomized control trials may not be the best approach to learn the causes of chronic multifactorial diseases, which may be better studied using population-based follow-up studies. The authors and critics of the report both agreed that interventions for preventing Alzheimer's disease that target multiple adjustable risk factors would be more fruitful and that the current preventive interventions were likely started too late in the course of the illness to have much impact. They also agreed on using population-based follow-up studies to try to get a fix on how to prevent this devastating illness that could ravage the United States if health care professionals do not get a handle on it (Jeste and Bell 2011).

Biological Approaches to Dementia Prevention

Intervening in the biological risk factors associated with dementia (e.g., diabetes mellitus, current smoking, depression, the apolipoprotein E gene, vascular cognitive impairment from multi-infarct dementia, hypertension, other less common neurological dementias, and the recently recognized, by the public, dementia from head injury) is very appealing to physicians who are devotees of biotechnical preventive interventions, that is, medications. Unfortunately, the National Institutes of Health review found no substantiation of the value of dietary or herbal supplements, diet, physical activity, or drugs (prescription or over-the-counter) for the prevention of Alzheimer's disease or cognitive decline. Research on physical activity and a diet that is low in saturated fat and high in vegetables showed some weak evidence for being protective against Alzheimer's disease and cognitive decline (Daviglus et al. 2010; Jeste and Bell 2011).

Psychosocial Approaches to Dementia Prevention

Being reclusive and not participating in social activities and maintaining social connections (i.e., actively living in the village) has been studied as a risk factor for the development of cognitive decline and Alzheimer's disease. However, the evidence for these relationships and the evidence for living alone or living with a partner in relation to the risk for developing cognitive decline or Alzheimer's disease are mixed (Jeste and Bell 2011). Part of the difficulty is determining which came first, the cognitive decline or the social isolation. Similarly, evidence suggesting that increased involvement in intellectual activities and cognitive training in later life are associated with less cognitive decline, resulting in less risk of mild cognitive impairment, is limited; unfortunately, this evidence is also contradictory. Similar to the evidence for biological approaches, the evidence for psychosocial approaches for the prevention of Alzheimer's disease is considered to be of low quality (Daviglus et al. 2010; Jeste and Bell 2011).

Summary

Fortunately, multiple evidence-based preventive interventions can be adapted to various age ranges, cultures, and contexts. Unfortunately, limited space prohibits listing all of the available programs. If a preventive intervention has elements of the seven universal community field principles and if the intervention is supported by ancient knowledge, personal experience, and modern science, then the chances are good that it is an efficacious and efficient intervention that can be implemented. It is not that mental health professionals lack scientific evidence that preventive interventions work; it is the dearth of individual and political will that keeps them from implementing what they know works.

The other major issue that is important to keep in mind is that "public health is like plowing water" (C. Lopez, Chairperson, Chicago Board of Health, personal communication, May 2013). Accordingly, once a problem is fixed and a public health preventive intervention is in place, it is important to ensure that the intervention is institutionalized. When the various human cultures were more intact and cohesive, families were more protected by ancient practices developed over the centuries to support human development; however, at the same time, there were mental, emotional, and behavioral disorders that were not understood and were left untreated. As always, humans struggle with balancing the old and the new—the challenge is not to throw the baby out with the bath water but to use science and natural protective resources to improve the human condition.

The United States has difficulty implementing biotechnical or psychosocial evidence-based interventions. Institutionalizing preventive interventions requires a strong evidence base; a vehicle to adapt, disseminate, and implement the intervention; and the political will to do it. Health care professionals have the evidence, and the Affordable Care Act is providing them with the mechanism, but the political will to implement what health care professionals already know is lacking (Bell and McBride 2010).

Clinical Key Points

- What mental health professionals have learned is frequently what they already know but do not practice.

- Maintaining good sleep hygiene, getting regular exercise for both the body and the mind, developing discipline and will, seeking wisdom, cultivating good relationships, being safe, and living in intact villages are all protective.

- The difficulty in changing behavior is implementation of efficacious psychosocial interventions.

- Biotechnical interventions are easier than psychosocial interventions, but both are important.

- By using the seven universal community field principles, health care professionals are able to give people an easy to understand model that is based on sound scientific evidence to help enlist their will to change their health behaviors.

- Prevention is possible in psychiatry.

References

Abram KM, Teplin LA, Charles DR, et al: Posttraumatic stress disorder and trauma in youth in juvenile detention. Arch Gen Psychiatry 61(4):403–410, 2004 15066899
American Psychiatric Association: Diagnostic and Statistical Manual of Mental Disorders, 5th Edition. Arlington, VA, American Psychiatric Association, 2013
Bean R: The Four Conditions of Self-Esteem: A New Approach for Elementary and Middle Schools, 2nd Edition. Santa Cruz, CA, ETR Associates, 1992
Beardslee WR, Chien PL, Bell CC: Prevention of mental disorders, substance abuse, and problem behaviors: a developmental perspective. Psychiatr Serv 62(3):247–254, 2011 21363895
Bell CC: Cultivating resiliency in youth. J Adolesc Health 29(5):375–381, 2001 11691598
Bell CC: Trauma, culture, and resiliency, in Resiliency in Psychiatric Clinical Practice. Edited by Southwick S, Charney D, Litz B, Friedman M. Cambridge, UK, Cambridge University Press, 2011, pp 176–188
Bell CC: Fetal alcohol exposure among African Americans. Psychiatr Serv 65(5):569, 2014 24788732
Bell CC, McBride DF: Affect regulation and prevention of risky behaviors. JAMA 304(5):565–566, 2010 20682937
Bell CC, McBride DF: Family as the model for prevention of mental and physical health problems, in Family and HIV/AIDS: Cultural and Contextual Issues in Prevention and Treatment. Edited by Prequegnat W, Bell CC. New York, Springer, 2011, pp 47–68
Bell CC, Gamm S, Vallas P, et al: Strategies for the prevention of youth violence in Chicago public schools, in School Violence: Contributing Factors, Management, and Prevention. Edited by Shafii M, Shafii S. Washington, DC, American Psychiatric Press, 2001, pp 251–272
Bell CC, Faly B, Paikoff R: Strategies for health behavioral change, in The Health Behavioral Change Imperatives: Theory, Education, and Practice in Diverse Populations. Edited by Chunn J. New York, Kluwer Academic/Plenum Publishers, 2002, pp 17–40
Bell CC, Bhana A, Petersen I, et al: Building protective factors to offset sexually risky behaviors among black youths: a randomized control trial. J Natl Med Assoc 100(8):936–944, 2008 18717144
Beuttler FW, Bell CC: For the Welfare of Every Child—A Brief History of the Institute for Juvenile Research, 1909–2010. Chicago, University of Illinois, 2010
Boyke J, Driemeyer J, Gaser C, et al: Training-induced brain structure changes in the elderly. J Neurosci 28(28):7031–7035, 2008 18614670

Breland-Noble AM, Bell CC, Nicholas G: Family First: The development of an evidence based family intervention for increasing participation in psychiatric clinical care and research in depressed African American adolescents. Family Process 45(2):153–169, 2006

Centers for Disease Control and Prevention (CDC): Adverse childhood experiences reported by adults—five states, 2009. MMWR Morb Mortal Wkly Rep 59(49):1609–1613, 2010 21160456

Davidson RJ, McEwen BS: Social influences on neuroplasticity: stress and interventions to promote well-being. Nat Neurosci 15(5):689–695, 2012 22534579

Daviglus ML, Bell CC, Berrettini W, et al: National Institutes of Health State-of-the-Science Conference statement: preventing alzheimer disease and cognitive decline. Ann Intern Med 153(3):176–181, 2010 20547888

Flay BR, Snyder F, Petraitis J: The theory of triadic influence, in Emerging Theories in Health Promotion Practice and Research, 2nd Edition. Edited by DiGlemente RJ, Kegler MC, Crosby RA. New York, Jossey-Bass, 2009, pp 451–510

Gibson J, McKenzie-McHarg K, Shakespeare J, et al: A systematic review of studies validating the Edinburg Postnatal Depression Scale in antepartum and postpartum women. Acta Psychiatr Scand 119(5):350–364, 2009 19298573

Gillham J, Reivich K: Building resilience in children: The Penn Resiliency Project. 2014. Available at: http://www.ppc.sas.upenn.edu/gillhampowerpoint.pdf. Accessed August 26, 2014.

Hobfoll SE, Watson P, Bell CC, et al: Five essential elements of immediate and mid-term mass trauma intervention: empirical evidence. Psychiatry 70(4):283–315, discussion 316–369, 2007 18181708

Jeste DV, Bell CC: Preface prevention in mental health: lifespan perspective. Psychiatr Clin North Am 34(1):xiii–xvi, 2011 21333835

Kaslow NJ, Leiner AS, Reviere S, et al: Suicidal, abused African American women's response to a culturally informed intervention. J Consult Clin Psychol 78(4):449–458, 2010 20658802

Kost K, Henshaw S: U.S. teenage pregnancies, births, and abortions, 2008: national trends by age, race, and ethnicity. 2008. Available at: http://www.guttmacher.org/pubs/USTPtrends08.pdf. Accessed August 26, 2014.

Manitoba: Rising to the challenge: a strategic plan for the mental health and well-being of Manitobans. Summary report of achievements: year one. 2011. Available at: http://www.gov.mb.ca/healthyliving/mh/docs/challenge_report_of_achievements.pdf. Accessed August 26, 2014.

May PA, Gossage JP: Estimating the prevalence of fetal alcohol syndrome: a summary. Alcohol Res Health 25(3):159–167, 2001 11810953

National Academy of Sciences: Reforming Juvenile Justice: A Developmental Approach. Washington, DC, National Academy of Sciences Press, 2013

National Child Traumatic Stress Network: Psychological first aid. 2014. Available at: http://www.nctsn.org/content/psychological-first-aid. Accessed August 26, 2014.

O'Connell ME, Boat T, Warner KE: Preventing Mental, Emotional, and Behavioral Disorders Among Young People: Progress and Possibilities. Washington, DC, National Academies Press, 2009

Pynoos R, Nader K: Psychological first aid for children who witness community violence. J Trauma Stress 1:445–473, 1988

Redd J, Suggs H, Gibbons R, et al: A plan to strengthen systems and reduce the number of African-American children in child welfare. Illinois Child Welfare 2:34–46, 2005

Sampson RJ, Raudenbush SW, Earls F: Neighborhoods and violent crime: a multilevel study of collective efficacy. Science 277(5328):918–924, 1997 9252316

Stratton K, Howe C, Battaglia F: Fetal Alcohol Syndrome: Diagnosis, Epidemiology, Prevention, and Treatment. Washington, DC, National Academies Press, 1996

University of California San Francisco: The Mothers and Babies Internet Project. 2014. Available at: https://ihrc.ucsf.edu/interventionConsole/Default.aspx?ConsoleName= MothersAndBabiesandLanguage=es. Accessed August 26, 2014.

U.S. Public Health Service: Report of The Surgeon General's Conference on Children's Mental Health: A National Action Agenda. Washington, DC, U.S. Department of Health and Human Services, 2000

Suggested Cross-References

Social factors are discussed in Chapter 3 ("Resilience and Posttraumatic Growth"), Chapter 4 ("Positive Social Psychiatry"), Chapter 5 ("Recovery in Mental Illnesses"), Chapter 12 ("Integrating Positive Psychiatry Into Clinical Practice"), and Chapter 16 ("Bioethics of Positive Psychiatry"). Sleep is discussed in Chapter 12 and Chapter 14 ("Positive Child Psychiatry"). Self-efficacy is discussed in Chapter 2 ("Positive Psychological Traits").

Suggested Readings

Bell CC, McBride DF: Family as the model for prevention of mental and physical health problems, in Family and HIV/AIDS: Cultural and Contextual Issues in Prevention and Treatment. Edited by Pequegnat W, Bell CC. New York, Springer, 2011, pp 47–68

Hobfoll SE, Watson P, Bell CC, et al: Five essential elements of immediate and mid-term trauma intervention: empirical evidence. Focus 7:221–242, 2009

Jeste DV, Bell CC: Preface prevention in mental health: lifespan perspective. Psychiatr Clin North Am 34(1):xiii–xvi, 2011 21333835

National Academy of Sciences: Reforming Juvenile Justice: A Developmental Approach. Edited by Bonnie RJ, Chemers BM, Schuck J. Washington, DC, National Academy of Sciences Press, 2013

O'Connell ME, Boat T, Warner KE (eds): Preventing Mental, Emotional, and Behavioral Disorders Among Young People: Progress and Possibilities. Washington, DC, National Academies Press, 2009

Integrating Positive Psychiatry Into Clinical Practice

SAMANTHA BOARDMAN, M.D.

P. MURALI DORAISWAMY, M.D.

In his 2012 American Psychiatric Association presidential address, Dilip Jeste, M.D., called for a new era of "positive psychiatry" that focuses on mental wellness:

> We should not be satisfied merely with treating patients with mental illness but with improving their overall well-being. There are many studies that have shown that positive traits like optimism and social engagement are associated with significant decreases in mortality, and I think as psychiatrists, we are in a good position to incorporate these into psychotherapy and psychosocial interventions. (qtd. in Cassels 2012)

The goal of this chapter is to provide a pragmatic summary of the relevant literature and practical tools and tips for integrating positive psychiatry into everyday practice.

Background

The fields of sociology, psychology, and psychiatry have been formally studying positive traits and interventions for decades, but *positive psychology* as an umbrella term describing the theories and scientific research about what makes life worth living rose to prominence in the late 1990s (Seligman and Csikszentmihalyi 2000). In comparison with traditional psychiatry and psychology, which focuses mainly on mental illness and pathology, positive psychology focuses on human strengths and wellness. As Seligman argues, "mental health is so much more than the mere absence of mental illness" (see Fowler et al. 1999). Instead of focusing exclusively on what's wrong, positive psychology asks an equally important but often overlooked question: What's right?

Over the past decade, research has shown the efficacy of positive psychology interventions such as counting one's blessings (Seligman et al. 2005), practicing kindness, setting personal goals expressing gratitude (Sheldon and Lyubomirsky 2006), and using character strengths can enhance well-being and in some cases relieve depressive symptoms. Positive psychiatry, which incorporates positive psychology's insights, thus expands psychiatrists' perspective and broadens the way they think about mental health and treatment options. A more balanced understanding of the range of human experience that better integrates existing knowledge about mental illness with knowledge about positive mental health benefits therapists and their patients alike.

Balanced Approach

If therapists' exclusive aim is to reduce depression, anxiety, and anger, they miss out on the opportunity to explore their patients' strengths and potential (Duckworth et al. 2005). Moreover, even if treatment is successful and they are able to relieve their patients' negative symptoms, this success does not automatically translate into well-being and happiness. Building positive resources such as positive emotions, character strengths, and social connections and helping clients find meaningful work has benefits, including counteracting negative symptoms and buffering them against future reoccurrence (Kobau et al. 2011).

Certainly, those with mental illness could benefit from a model of mental health that explores and develops a patient's optimal functioning in addition to providing symptom relief. Getting the fullest picture of who a patient is not only at his or her worst but also at his or her best is critical. By deepening their understanding of their patient's emotional scaffolding, therapists are better positioned to treat patients in a meaningful and impactful way. Indeed, the job of the therapist of the future may not simply be to provide symptom relief but may also be to help clients recognize, build, and bolster their strengths and then use these strengths to navigate around their weaknesses (Duckworth et al. 2005).

Positive Psychiatry Tools: Fix What's Wrong and Build What's Strong

Abraham Maslow (1966/2002) famously said, "I suppose it is tempting, if the only tool you have is a hammer, to treat everything as if it were a nail." Perhaps not every problem needs a hammer, nor is every problem a nail. In addition to medication and traditional therapy (e.g., cognitive-behavioral therapy, interpersonal psychotherapy, supportive therapy), clinicians can add a number of well-documented positive psychiatry tools to their toolbox.

Resilience

One of these tools is resilience. Reivich and Shatte's (2002) research in this area illustrated how important resilience is for well-being and, moreover, that it can be taught. They defined *resilience* as the capacity to respond to adversity in healthy and productive ways. However, it is important to keep in mind that there is more to resilience than recovering from serious setbacks. The skills of resilience are as important to broadening and enriching one's everyday life as they are to dealing with major disappointments. It is a mind-set that enables one to think accurately, flexibly, and thoroughly.

Mental illness and resilience have a bidirectional relationship. Mental flexibility and optimism are essential components of resilience, and resilience in turn lowers risk for major depression, suicidality, posttraumatic stress disorder, and substance use in adults exposed to traumatic experiences. The 10-item Connor-Davidson Resilience Scale (CD-RISC; Connor and Davidson 2003) is one example of a tool that clinicians can use in their practice both at intake and posttreatment; scores for the U.S. population overall and scores for psychiatric samples are available. The two-item CD-RISC 2 is an even shorter version to measure a person's "bounce back" (Vaishnavi et al. 2007).

Currently, as part of a $145 million initiative to enhance the psychological fitness of soldiers, resilience skills are being taught in the U.S. Army as part of the Comprehensive Soldier Fitness program. The Master Resilience Training (MRT) Course is the foundation of this endeavor (Reivich et al. 2011). During a 10-day MRT course, sergeants are trained to use resilience skills on the basis of a curriculum developed by the University of Pennsylvania, the Penn Resilience Program, and other empirically validated work in the field of positive psychology. It is a "train the trainer model": sergeants trained in MRT teach the skills they have learned to their soldiers.

The overarching aim of such programs is to improve social and emotional fitness and flexible thinking (Table 12–1). These skills have broader applications and can be taught in schools, on sports fields, in business settings, and in therapists' offices.

Table 12–1.   Six core competencies of resilience

Self-awareness	Identifying one's thoughts, emotions, and behaviors and patterns in each that are counterproductive
Self-regulation	The ability to regulate impulses, thinking, emotions, and behaviors to achieve goals, as well as the willingness and ability to express emotions
Optimism	Noticing the goodness in self and others, identifying what is controllable, remaining wedded to reality, and challenging counterproductive beliefs
Mental agility	Thinking flexibility and accurately, perspective taking, and willingness to try new strategies
Character strengths	Identifying the top strengths in oneself and others, relying on one's strengths to overcome challenges and meet goals, and cultivating a strength approach in one's unit
Connection	Building strong relationships through positive and effective communication, empathy, willingness to ask for help, and willingness to offer help

Source.   Adapted from Reivich et al. 2011.

An optimistic thinking style is a key feature of resilience (Reivich and Shatte 2002). Research shows optimistic people are happier, healthier, and more productive; have better relationships; succeed more; are better problem solvers; and are less likely to become depressed than pessimistic people. By integrating concepts such as resilience and optimism into clinical work, therapists might gain a more complete understanding of the human experience—both positive and negative experiences (Kobau et al. 2011).

Positive Activity Interventions

Layous and Lyubomirsky (2012) showed that volitional activities, known as *positive activity interventions,* can make a difference in terms of an individual's well-being, even in individuals with a mental illness. In the scientific literature, positive interventions are formally defined as "treatment methods or intentional activities that aim to cultivate positive feelings, behaviors, or cognitions" (Sin and Lyubomirsky 2009). They are evidence-based intentional exercises that are designed to increase well-being and enhance flourishing. Although positive interventions were originally studied as activities for nonclinical populations and for helping healthy people thrive, they are increasingly being valued for their therapeutic role in treating psychopathology (Seligman et al. 2006).

One study showed that people can alleviate depressive symptoms and increase well-being by practicing certain intentional activities (Layous and Lyubomirsky

2012). Positive exercises such as using one's signature strengths, counting one's blessings, and writing letters of gratitude have been tested in randomized controlled trials. Sin and Lyubomirsky (2009) conducted a meta-analysis examining 51 positive interventions. Results indicated that these positive interventions significantly improved well-being (effect size of 0.29) and decreased depressive symptoms (a moderate effect size of 0.31), which is an impressive finding considering that many of these interventions were brief and self-administered. To put this finding into perspective, the effect size of antidepressants for mild to moderate depression is thought to be around 0.31 or *lower.*

Additional interventions, such as performing acts of kindness, meditating on positive feelings, and practicing optimism, also might be useful in the clinical setting. Rather than aiming solely to decrease depressed symptoms, these interventions aim to cultivate positive thoughts, feelings, and experiences.

The positive activities discussed below promote positive feelings, thoughts, and behaviors, and therapists may want to consider "prescribing" the right ones for the right patients.

Gratitude

Writing down three good things that happened and why these things are good has been shown to be an effective tool in promoting well-being and reducing depressive symptoms (Seligman et al. 2005). A conscious focus on blessings has been shown to enhance personal and interpersonal benefits (Emmons and Mc-Cullough 2003).

Prosocial Activities

Kindness and everyday happiness are closely associated, and therapists may want to encourage patients to explicitly engage prosocial activities. As studies show, performing and recording acts of kindness promote happiness. Volunteering, for example, is one of the most important prosocial activities and is linked with life satisfaction. People who donate their time feel more socially connected and live longer (Jenkinson et al. 2013). High-quality relationships matter in everyday life and during periods of stress. Supportive others can, in fact, alter the perception of everyday events so that they are not perceived as threats or stressors. For example, one study showed that observers perceived a hill they would have to climb to be less steep if they were with a friend rather than alone (Schnall et al. 2008). Research on the biological underpinnings of close relationships further illustrates the benefits of close social ties. In a study of pain perception, the presence of a loved one reduced the perception of physical pain in response to a painful stimulus (Coan et al. 2006). Another study showed similar reduction and pain attenuation at the neural level in those holding the hands of loved ones (Gable and Gosnell 2011). Helping patients cultivate social support, enhance interpersonal relations, and foster community ties is important for their psychological well-being.

Clinical Vignette

Lawrence is a 72-year-old retired librarian in good physical health who lost his wife to cancer 10 years ago. His children and grandchildren live across the country. He has a history of depression and mild anxiety. He presented to a psychiatrist 6 months ago in the midst of a depressive episode; symptoms included poor sleep, reduced appetite, low energy, lack of interest in life, passive suicidal ideation, low mood, and difficulty concentrating. He was prescribed a selective serotonin reuptake inhibitor. He noticed a remarkable improvement overall but still does not feel like "himself." Lawrence's therapist recommended the following positive interventions: 1) taking a half-hour walk every morning to pick up the newspaper rather than driving, 2) joining a book club at the local senior center, and 3) volunteering to work with high school juniors and seniors on their college essays.

Lawrence felt better while taking the medication, but he continued to experience residual symptoms. By engaging in these positive interventions, he began to feel more connected to his community, and he made new friends and renewed old friendships. He found working with the high school students to be particularly meaningful and invigorating.

Writing as a Tool

Visualizing and writing about one's best possible self at a time in the future leads to increases in optimism, hope, and well-being. Therapist-supervised or -recommended writing exercises may be an effective tool to help patients focus on positive emotions and experiences.

Signature Strengths

"So, tell me what's bothering you…" is a common icebreaker at the beginning of a therapy session. This model of treatment largely overlooks the psychological strengths and positive aspects of behavior that might be useful in therapy. Although therapy is an opportunity for clients to discuss their problems and distress, it can also be a time for them to identify their strengths and learn how to use them. The VIA (Values in Action) survey (University of Pennsylvania 2014) measures and classifies 24 character strengths (Peterson and Seligman 2004), including emotional intelligence, kindness, leadership, and perseverance. The questionnaire determines an individual's top five strengths. In one study (Seligman et al. 2005), participants who were asked to use their strengths in novel and creative ways showed increases in happiness and decreases in depression scores.

Lifestyle Tools

Physical Activity

Exercise has an immediate and positive effect on mood. Even a single "dose" of exercise—30 minutes of walking on a treadmill—has been shown to lift the mood of a patient with major depressive disorder. Moreover, exercise has been shown to be as effective as medication for patients with mild major depressive disorder and to potentially have lasting results (Blumenthal et al. 2007). Moderate exercise may also prevent depression (see Mammen and Faulkner 2013). Exercise has also been shown to enhance executive cognitive abilities in older adults and to provide benefits for patients with anxiety (see Pontifex et al. 2013). Moreover, physical activity has been shown to optimize learning by improving impulse control, attention, and arousal and reducing learned helplessness. In addition to reducing symptom severity, research shows that physical activity enhances well-being and improves quality of life.

Clinical Vignette

John is a 56-year-old businessman with no past psychiatric history. He underwent knee surgery 4 weeks before presenting to a therapist's office. He complains of difficulty concentrating, irritability, restlessness, difficulty initiating and completing tasks at work, and difficulty sleeping. He denies being in any pain and denies taking any pain medication. John's symptoms are consistent with adult attention-deficit/hyperactivity disorder (ADHD) except that he does not have a history of ADHD.

On further evaluation, John reveals that up until his knee surgery, he had run 5 miles each day since high school. He describes how running helped clear his head and keep him focused. Evidence shows that physical activity provides benefits to patients with ADHD (Pontifex et al. 2013), and it is possible that unbeknownst to John, he had been "self-medicating" with exercise all his life. Since his surgery, he had not engaged in any physical activity. His therapist recommends that he swim laps several days a week. The swimming is helpful for the physical recovery of his knee, and he begins feeling better almost immediately.

Meditation and Yoga

Mindfulness meditation enhances positive affect and decreases anxiety and negative affect (see Keng et al. 2011). Even those new to meditation can experience the benefits of mindfulness meditation in as short as 5 days (Tang et al. 2009). Likewise, yoga, Tai Chi, and other forms of meditative practices are equally helpful, and a systematic review of studies researching yoga found potential benefits across a range of psychiatric conditions (Balasubramaniam et al. 2013).

Prioritizing Sleep

Sleep is vital for clearance of neurotoxins via the glymphatic system and for cognitive consolidation. Therapists tend to think of sleep problems as symptoms, but sleep problems also contribute to mental health issues (Krystal 2006). Lifestyle and behavioral interventions can make a difference in quality of sleep and quality of life. For example, decreasing alcohol, nicotine, and caffeine intake; increasing physical activity; and keeping the bedroom dark and free of distractions such as a cell phone are strategies to improve sleep.

Technology

Advances in technology offer many possible mental health–enhancing tools, including Web-based interventions, apps, and games. Discussion groups are a particularly helpful tool because they enhance social connection. Online sites such as PatientsLikeMe.com offer patients tools to track mental health–related symptoms and enhance peer learning and social support.

Healthy Habits

Another strategy therapists may want to encourage in patients is the creation of good habits. This strategy is much easier with a *build what's strong* approach than with a *fix what's wrong* approach (Duckworth et al. 2005). Most people assume that emotion and mood lead to certain behaviors, but the opposite is true too. William James (1897) always stressed the importance of actions and their influence on emotion, and studies bear out this idea. For example, faking a smile has been shown to boost a person's mood and relieve stress (Kraft and Pressman 2012), and good posture has been shown to increase feelings of power (Carney et al. 2010). In other words, employing a "fake it till you make it" strategy may be useful for certain patients in the right context. These strategies empower patients to become better problem solvers on their own. When a patient is able to discipline himself or herself with regard to mastering one healthy habit (e.g., not drinking more than two glasses of alcohol in 1 day), that discipline then leads to a positive cascade of disciplinary improvements in many other routine habits (e.g., waking up early to exercise), the so-called keystone habit effect.

Clinical Vignette

Andrea is a married 38-year-old woman, former lawyer, and mother of three children younger than 12. Her internist referred her for treatment because she was complaining of stress, low energy, and feeling overwhelmed. She is not sleeping well or eating well; she reports eating "too much garbage" and never losing the baby weight from her pregnancies. She describes herself as irritable and short-tempered with her kids and husband and expresses concern that she is not a good mother or wife. She denies any suicidal ideation. She denies any substance abuse. She has never sought treatment before or been diagnosed with a mental illness. Her chief complaint is "I'm permanently in a bad mood."

Andrea's presentation meets the diagnostic criteria for a major depressive episode. She does not want to take medication. The therapist prescribes the following positive interventions to provide another approach: gratitude, signature strengths, physical activity, meditation, and prosocial activities. First, the therapist suggests that Andrea write down three things that went well and why at the end of each day (Emmons and McCullough 2003; Seligman et al. 2005; Sheldon and Lyubomirsky 2006) and consider using this exercise to play a game at night with her husband and kids. Second, Andrea is asked to take the Signature Strengths Questionnaire and use her strengths in new ways. Third, Andrea was on the track team in college and likes the idea of joining a running group to incorporate exercise. Tracking her moods before and after workouts helps her maintain motivation. Fourth, the therapist advises Andrea that meditating for just 5 minutes a day can make a difference. Fifth, Andrea has not worked since the birth of her second child and decides to do some pro bono legal work for 3 hours a week. Rather than focusing exclusively on what is going wrong in Andrea's life, these interventions enable the therapist to build on her strengths and potential. Moreover, the interventions engage Andrea in the treatment process.

As a result, Andrea reports that her mood has improved significantly and that she feels calmer and less irritable. Subsequently, she feels her relationship with her children and husband has improved and reports finding more meaning and purpose in her life. She also remarks she is proud of herself for helping find her way out of "the hole" she had fallen into. Andrea considers the skills she has learned from positive intervention to be lifelong skills that she will continue to use even when treatment ends.

Nutrition and Diet

Although therapists are trained to ask about daily intake in the context of eating disorders and about appetite in the context of depression, what patients actually eat is not a major focus of treatment. According to preliminary research, a healthy diet may reduce the risk of severe depression, and junk food, sugar, and processed meats may increase depressive symptoms. The Mediterranean diet, which emphasizes consumption of plant-based foods, limits red meat, and replaces butter with olive oil, is associated with decreased risk of late-life depression and cognitive dysfunction (Sánchez-Villegas et al. 2009). Evidence shows that a diet high in saturated fat may contribute to ADHD and impair brain function in the U.S. context (although it must also be stressed that a child's brain needs all types of fats to develop normally). Likewise, because many psychotropics are associated with weight gain, counseling patients on healthy dietary habits is now an essential part of positive psychiatry.

Nature

The positive benefits of a natural environment include increased self-confidence, improved self-esteem, and improved quality of social relationships. Nature provides a restorative environment and can be therapeutic (see Bratman et al. 2012). Walking through a forest has been shown to activate the cortex, lower blood cortisol and blood pressure levels, strengthen immunity, and promote muscle relaxation (Park et al. 2007).

Additional Tools

Mindfulness-Based Cognitive Therapy

Mindfulness-based cognitive therapy (MBCT) is based on mindfulness-based stress reduction. Randomized clinical trials show that MBCT reduces rates of relapse by 50% among patients who have recurrent depression and that it is also effective for the treatment of generalized anxiety disorder (see Evans et al. 2008). MBCT combines cognitive therapy–based exercises with information and mindfulness and focuses on how thinking affects emotions, enabling patients to recognize negative thought patterns and let them go. The goal is to help patients gain more effective skills to manage stress as well as a greater capacity for relaxation.

Development of a Comprehensive Positive Psychiatry Treatment Plan

Positive psychotherapy is a term that has been used to define a comprehensive treatment plan for patients that is based on positive psychology approaches (Figure 12–1). It has been studied primarily for effectiveness in patients with depression (Seligman et al. 2006). Positive psychotherapy is predicated on identifying a patient's strengths and applying them (Table 12–2). The goal is to increase positive emotions, engagement, and meaning in life, rather than directly targeting depressive symptoms.

Tailoring of Positive Psychiatry for Specific Disorders

Broadly beneficial interventions such as resilience building, social support, exercise, diet, yoga, meditation, sleep, and stress reduction have been reported to benefit a broad range of psychiatric disorders; hence, their application is not necessarily disorder specific. Most effectiveness studies of positive psychology and positive psychotherapy have been in patients with depressive or anxiety disorders, but emerging evidence shows the value of positive psychology and positive psychotherapy even in conditions such as schizophrenia. For example, a pilot study found that group-based positive psychotherapy may improve psychological well-being, hope, savoring, psychological recovery, self-esteem, and psychiatric symptoms in patients with schizophrenia (Meyer et al. 2012). Positive psychiatry therapies may also hold promise for the ability of patients with schizophrenia to manage negative symptoms that are often refractory to conventional medications. Likewise, positive psychology administered via computer games can be useful to treat youths with psychiatric or conduct disorders (Ahmed and Boisvert 2006). Clearly, a person's personality may influence the application of positive psychiatry approaches because personality traits are known predictors of happiness. Thus, traits such as neuroticism (a strong negative predictor of happiness) may signal to clinicians a need for positive psychology interventions more so than a trait such as extraversion.

Engagement

Instead of viewing patients as passive recipients of an intervention strategy that is predetermined by their doctor, engaging patients as "active seekers of health" (Keyes and Lopez 2002, p. 49) will likely lead to better outcomes. Encouraging

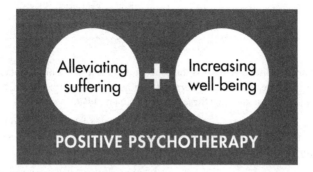

FIGURE 12–1. Positive psychotherapy

patients to take an active role in their treatment enables them to become better problem solvers and to take responsibility for their health. Taking medication and showing up for appointments is not enough. A belief you can accomplish what you set your mind to is a key determinant of behavior, perseverance, and effort. Opportunities to gain a greater sense of self-efficacy abound in positive psychology interventions. As Aristotle reportedly said, "Happiness is not something that happens to you." Encouraging patients to be more proactive in their care is especially beneficial in the mental health setting.

By adding positive interventions to their toolbox, psychiatrists can expand their range of treatment options and, more importantly, better engage patients in the treatment process. By definition, these interventions are not for patients or for therapists who are interested in a "quick fix." The interventions are for patients who want to engage and participate in and shape their experience. As William James (1892) said, it is up to us to "make our nervous system our ally instead of our enemy" (p. 133). Therapists can help patients do just that.

A Strategic Approach: Psychological Mechanisms Underlying Interventions

What makes positive interventions effective? Exploring the psychological factors underlying these interventions is worthwhile. Positive interventions are thought to decrease depressive symptoms, increase well-being, and foster positive outcomes in relationships, work, and health (Layous et al. 2011). The critical mediating variables are increases in positive emotions, behaviors, and thoughts. Positive emotions then trigger upward spirals toward greater flourishing, resilience, and well-being.

A belief in one's capabilities to produce desired effects through one's own actions (Maddux and Galinsky 2009) is at the core of self-efficacy theory and is a key element of positive interventions. The three sentences "I think I can. I think I can. I think I can." from the beloved children's book *The Little Engine That Could* (Piper 1930, p. 3) capture the essence of self-efficacy theory. It is predicated on the notion that individuals are active participants rather than passive reactors in

Table 12–2.   An overview of the 14 sessions of positive
                   psychotherapy

Session 1:

The client and the therapist discuss the concept that the absence or lack of positive resources (positive emotions, character strengths, and meaning) can cause and maintain depression and how these can create an empty life.

Homework: The client writes a one-page (roughly 300 words) positive introduction, in which he or she tells a concrete story showing him or her at his or her best and illustrating how he or she used his or her highest character strengths.

Session 2:

The client identifies his or her character strengths from the positive introduction and discusses situations in which these character strengths have helped him or her previously.

Homework: The client completes the VIA questionnaire online to identify his or her character strengths.

Session 3:

The client and therapist focus on specific situations in which character strengths may facilitate cultivation of pleasure, engagement, and meaning.

Homework: The client starts a blessings journal, in which he or she writes, every night, three good things (big or small) that happened that day. (This homework continues through the entire course of therapy.)

Session 4:

The client and therapist discuss the roles of good and bad memories in maintaining depression. Holding onto anger and bitterness maintains depression and undermines well-being.

Homework: The client writes about feelings of anger and bitterness and how they feed his or her depression.

Session 5:

The therapist introduces forgiveness as a powerful tool that can transform feelings of anger and bitterness into neutrality or even, for some, into positive emotions.

Homework: The client writes a forgiveness letter describing a transgression and related emotions and pledges to forgive the transgressor (if appropriate) but does not deliver the letter.

Session 6:

The client and therapist discuss gratitude as enduring thankfulness.

Homework: The client writes a gratitude letter to someone he or she never properly thanked and is urged to deliver it in person.

Session 7:

The client and therapist review the importance of cultivating positive emotions through writing in the blessings journal and the use of character strengths.

Table 12–2. An overview of the 14 sessions of positive psychotherapy *(continued)*

Session 8:

The client and therapist discuss the fact that *satisficers* ("this is good enough") have better well-being than *maximizers* ("I must find the perfect wife, dishwasher, or vacation spot"). Satisficing is encouraged over maximizing.

Homework: The client reviews ways to increase satisficing and devises a personal satisficing plan.

Session 9:

The client and therapist discuss optimism and hope, using explanatory style: the optimistic style is to see bad events as temporary, changeable, and local.

Homework: The client thinks of three doors that closed on him or her and considers what doors have opened.

Session 10:

The client is invited to recognize character strengths of a significant other(s).

Homework: The therapist coaches the client to respond actively and constructively to positive events reported by others, and the client arranges a date that celebrates his or her character strengths and those of his or her significant other.

Session 11:

The client and therapist discuss how to recognize the character strengths of family members and where the client's own character strengths originated.

Homework: The client asks family members to take the VIA questionnaire online and then draws a tree that includes the character strengths of all members of the family

Session 12:

The therapist introduces savoring as a technique to increase the intensity and duration of positive emotion.

Homework: The client plans pleasurable activities and carries them out as planned. The client is provided with a list of specific savoring techniques.

Session 13:

The client and therapist discuss the idea that the client has the power to give one of the greatest gifts of all—the gift of time.

Homework: The client is to give the gift of time by doing something that requires a fair amount of time and calls on his or her character strengths.

Session 14:

The client and therapist discuss that a full life integrates pleasure, engagement, and meaning.

Source. Adapted from Seligman et al. 2006.

their experience and that they have a role in shaping their environment. This is a key concept for patients.

Motivation and Fit

Another important factor for therapists to consider is motivation. Intrinsic motivation is important for positive interventions to work and complements a patient's sense of self-efficacy. Behavior that is self-generated, volitional, and motivated from within is considered to be self-determined and autonomous (Brown and Ryan 2004). It is differentiated from behavior that is motivated by external controls or pressure. For example, if a patient is told by a therapist to write a gratitude letter but has no intrinsic motivation or lacks a sense of competence, the intervention is unlikely to be as successful as it would be for a motivated and self-determined individual. The key is choosing the right intervention for the right patient.

Goal setting is an excellent strategy for motivating patients. Goal-setting theory (Locke 1996) focuses on harnessing beliefs that translate thoughts into action. Locke defines *goals* as "the object or aim of an action" (Locke 1996, p. 118) with internal and external components—the internal aspect is the idea or feeling underlying the goal, and the external aspect is the actual condition or object sought. Goals that are both specific and difficult lead to the highest performance. For example, vague advice such as "do your best" is less effective than "try to get more than 80% correct." A belief in one's ability to succeed is critical in goal-setting theory; it matters for level of goals chosen, for sustaining commitment to goals, and for response to feedback. It helps to clearly define what to focus on and how to use attention bandwidth most effectively. When considering treatment options, therapists may want to keep goal setting in mind. It is important for patients to have specific treatment-related goals. Therapists can help patients articulate their goals explicitly.

Therapists also play a key role in helping patients find an appropriate intervention. Motivation is a critical factor because levels of effort to practice an intervention and continued practice result in greater improvement of depressive symptoms. A therapist's clinical judgment certainly matters for these decisions. For example, prescribing the three blessings exercise to a suicidal patient in the midst of a major depressive episode would be inappropriate and unsuitable. As the patient gets better, depending on his or her individual strengths, interests, and context, the three blessings exercise might be a good fit.

As the literature suggests, choosing the right intervention is an important consideration for clinical practice. However, although what an individual patient wants and prefers matters, what an individual needs may be the most important consideration of all (Layous and Lyubomirsky 2012). Therapists are uniquely positioned to weigh in on these decisions.

Special Cases

Positive interventions may be especially useful for patients who are potential candidates for medication but who are reluctant or ambivalent about taking it. There are a number of limitations associated with taking medications, including stigma, lack of efficacy, financial burden, patient noncompliance, and undesirable side effects. Because positive interventions teach patients ways to increase positive emotions, behaviors, and cognitions without professional help, they may limit the need and cost of ongoing treatment, may serve as tools to prevent relapse in the face of triggers such as stress, and may lead a greater sense of self-efficacy. Significantly, patients practicing positive interventions may attribute improvement in their mood and symptoms to their own doing rather than an external agent such as medication or a therapist and thereby improve their sense of autonomy. Furthermore, positive interventions can complement medication or therapy when a patient has only a partial response to those treatments.

Positive Psychiatry Versus Pharmacotherapy

Although, to date, no multicenter studies compare positive psychiatry and pharmacotherapy approaches directly or study their effects in combination, we envision these approaches as complementary. In theory, positive psychology could target many areas not well addressed by available psychotropics, such as negative symptoms, cognition, functioning, and relapse prevention. Ultimately, the combination of medication and positive psychology may lead to greater recovery rates, higher societal functioning, and better quality of life.

Interpretative Caveats and Potential Risks of Positive Psychology

Clinicians should bear in mind many caveats in this field. The vast majority of studies of positive psychology have been in either healthy individuals or subjects with mild depression or anxiety. We are not aware of any multicenter randomized controlled trials testing the efficacy or safety of positive psychology for any major psychiatric disorder. Indeed, the U.S. military's adoption of positive psychology has been criticized by some as not being fully evidence based. Thus, it is not our intent to recommend positive psychology as a substitute for psychiatric evaluation or traditional treatment methods but, rather, for it to be viewed as an emerging adjunctive approach. Of note, positive psychology exercises may be harmful for some patients (Sergeant and Mongrain 2011). In an Internet study of 772 volunteers, participants who were described as needy experienced *reductions* in self-esteem following gratitude and exercises that involved listening to uplifting music. Therefore, it is important to choose interventions with care and with individual patients in mind. Scheduling follow-up visits with these patients would be important to monitor compliance, to reassess whether the correct intervention was chosen for the individual patient, and to decide whether ongoing treatment is necessary.

Summary

Positive psychiatry envisions a mental health model that thinks more broadly about the range and richness of human experience and about the context, rather than just focusing on illness symptoms or neurobiology. It is not our intent that psychotropics or existing psychotherapies be replaced by positive psychology, but rather that these be viewed as complementary therapies. Although much of the research done to date in positive psychology has been with healthy populations, increasing evidence suggests these approaches can help people with a range of mental illnesses. Clearly, the evidence base should be increased through additional randomized trials examining the efficacy of positive psychology interventions both as monotherapy for preventing illness and in combination with existing therapies to reduce recidivism.

A biological, genetic, and neural model of psychiatry may be promising for the future, but we await major insights and breakthroughs. In the meantime, therapists should focus on what they know and what is best for their patients. A therapeutic approach that focuses on strength and resilience as much as it does on symptoms may be just what the doctor ordered.

Clinical Key Points

- Expand treatment options and consider interventions beyond traditional therapy and medication.

- Build what is strong. Teach patients how to live with their mental illness while optimizing their well-being by emphasizing strengths and focusing on what is possible.

- Engage patients in the therapeutic process. Showing up is not enough; patients need to play an active role in treatment.

- Emphasize connection to others and community.

- Create upward spirals: Positive activities build positive emotions, thoughts, and behaviors. They are thought to decrease depressive symptoms, increase well-being, and foster positive outcomes in relationships, work, and health.

References

Ahmed M, Boisvert CM: Using positive psychology with special mental health populations. Am Psychol 61(4):333–335, 2006 16719682

Balasubramaniam M, Telles S, Doraiswamy PM: Yoga on our minds: a systematic review of yoga for neuropsychiatric disorders. Front Psychiatry Jan 25 3:117, 2013 23355825

Blumenthal JA, Babyak MA, Doraiswamy PM, et al: Exercise and pharmacotherapy in the treatment of major depressive disorder. Psychosom Med 69(7):587–596, 2007 17846259

Bratman GN, Hamilton JP, Daily GC: The impacts of nature experience on human cognitive function and mental health. Ann N Y Acad Sci 1249:118–136, 2012 22320203

Brown KW, Ryan RM: Fostering healthy self-regulation from within and without: a self-determination theory perspective, in Positive Psychology in Practice. Edited by Linley PA, Joseph S. Hoboken, NJ, Wiley, 2004, pp 105–124

Carney DR, Cuddy AJ, Yap AJ: Power posing: brief nonverbal displays affect neuroendocrine levels and risk tolerance. Psychol Sci 21(10):1363–1368, 2010 20855902

Cassels C: "Positive psychiatry" focus of new APA president's term. MedScape Medical News, May 2012

Coan JA, Schaefer HS, Davidson RJ: Lending a hand: social regulation of the neural response to threat. Psychol Sci 17(12):1032–1039, 2006 17201784

Connor KM, Davidson JR: Development of a new resilience scale: the Connor-Davidson Resilience Scale (CD-RISC). Depress Anxiety 18(2):76–82, 2003 12964174

Duckworth AL, Steen TA, Seligman MEP: Positive psychology in clinical practice. Annu Rev Clin Psychol 1:629–651, 2005 17716102

Emmons RA, McCullough ME: Counting blessings versus burdens: an experimental investigation of gratitude and subjective well-being in daily life. J Pers Soc Psychol 84(2):377–389, 2003 12585811

Evans S, Ferrando S, Findler M, et al: Mindfulness-based cognitive therapy for generalized anxiety disorder. J Anxiety Disord 22(4):716–721, 2008 17765453

Fowler RD, Seligman MEP, Koocher GP: The APA 1998 Annual Report. Am Psychologist 54(8):537–568, 1999

Gable SL, Gosnell CL: The positive side of close relationships, in Designing Positive Psychology: Taking Stock and Moving Forward. Edited by Sheldon KM, Kashdan TB, Steger MF. New York, Oxford University Press, 2011, pp 265–279

James W: The stream of consciousness, in Psychology (Chapter XI), 1892, pp 125–138

James W: The Will to Believe and Other Essays. London, Longmans, Green, & Co, 1897

Jenkinson CE, Dickens AP, Jones K, et al: Is volunteering a public health intervention? A systematic review and meta-analysis of the health and survival of volunteers. BMC Public Health 13:773, 2013 23968220

Jeste DV: A fulfilling year of APA presidency: from DSM-5 to positive psychiatry. Am J Psychiatry 170(10):1102–1105, 2013 24084815

Keng SL, Smoski MJ, Robins CJ: Effects of mindfulness on psychological health: a review of empirical studies. Clin Psychol Rev 31(6):1041–1056, 2011 21802619

Keyes CLM, Lopez SJ: Toward a science of mental health: positive directions in diagnosis and interventions, in Handbook of Positive Psychology. Edited by Snyder CR, Lopez SJ. New York, Oxford University Press, 2002, pp 45–59

Kobau R, Seligman ME, Peterson C, et al: Mental health promotion in public health: perspectives and strategies from positive psychology. Am J Public Health 101(8):e1–e9, 2011 21680918

Kraft TL, Pressman SD: Grin and bear it: the influence of manipulated facial expression on the stress response. Psychol Sci 23(11):1372–1378, 2012 23012270

Krystal AD: Sleep and psychiatric disorders: future directions. Psychiatr Clin North Am 29(4):1115–1130, abstract xi, 2006 17118285

Layous K, Lyubomirsky S: The how, who, what, when, and why of happiness: mechanisms underlying the success of positive interventions, in Light and Dark Side of Positive Emotion. Edited by Gruber J, Moskowitz J. Oxford, UK, Oxford University Press, 2012, pp 474–495

Layous K, Chancellor J, Lyubomirsky S, et al: Delivering happiness: translating positive psychology intervention research for treating major and minor depressive disorders. J Altern Complement Med 17(8):675–683, 2011 21721928

Locke EA: Motivation through conscious goal-setting. Appl Prev Psychol 5:124, 1996

Maddux WW, Galinsky AD: Cultural borders and mental barriers: the relationship between living abroad and creativity. J Pers Soc Psychol 96(5):1047–1061, 2009 19379035

Mammen G, Faulkner G: Physical activity and the prevention of depression: a systematic review of prospective studies. Am J Prev Med 45(5):649–657, 2013 24139780

Maslow AH: The Psychology of Science: A Reconnaissance (1966). Chapel Hill, NC, Maurice Bassett Publishing, 2002

Meyer PS, Johnson DP, Parks A, et al: Positive Living: a pilot study of group positive psychotherapy for people with schizophrenia. J Posit Psychol 7:239–248, 2012

Park BJ, Tsunetsugu Y, Kasetani T, et al: Physiological effects of Shinrin-yoku (taking in the atmosphere of the forest)—using salivary cortisol and cerebral activity as indicators. J Physiol Anthropol 26(2):123–128, 2007 17435354

Peterson C, Seligman MEP: Character Strengths and Virtues: A Handbook and Classification. New York, Oxford University Press, 2004

Piper W: The Little Engine That Could. New York, The Platt & Munk Co, 1930

Pontifex MB, Saliba BJ, Raine LB, et al: Exercise improves behavioral, neurocognitive, and scholastic performance in children with attention-deficit/hyperactivity disorder. J Pediatr 162(3):543–551, 2013 23084704

Reivich K, Shatte A: The Resilience Factor: 7 Essential Skills for Overcoming Life's Inevitable Obstacles. New York, Broadway Books, 2002

Reivich KJ, Seligman ME, McBride S: Master resilience training in the U.S. Army. Am Psychol 66(1):25–34, 2011 21219045

Sánchez-Villegas A, Delgado-Rodríguez M, Alonso A, et al: Association of the Mediterranean dietary pattern with the incidence of depression: the Seguimiento Universidad de Navarra/University of Navarra follow-up (SUN) cohort. Arch Gen Psychiatry 66(10):1090–1098, 2009 19805699

Schnall S, Harber KD, Stefanucci JK, et al: Social support and the perception of geographical slant. J Exp Soc Psychol 44(5):1246–1255, 2008 22389520

Seligman MEP: Authentic Happiness: Using the New Positive Psychology to Realize Your Potential for Lasting Fulfillment. New York, Free Press, 2002

Seligman ME, Csikszentmihalyi M: Positive psychology: an introduction. Am Psychol 55(1):5–14, 2000 11392865

Seligman ME, Steen TA, Park N, et al: Positive psychology progress: empirical validation of interventions. Am Psychol 60(5):410–421, 2005 16045394

Seligman ME, Rashid T, Parks AC: Positive psychotherapy. Am Psychol 61(8):774–788, 2006 17115810

Sergeant S, Mongrain M: Are positive psychology exercises helpful for people with depressive personality styles? J Posit Psychol 6:260–272, 2011

Sheldon KM, Lyubomirsky S: How to increase and sustain positive emotion: the effects of expressing gratitude and visualizing best possible selves. J Posit Psychol 1:73–82, 2006

Sin NL, Lyubomirsky S: Enhancing well-being and alleviating depressive symptoms with positive psychology interventions: a practice-friendly meta-analysis. J Clin Psychol 65(5):467–487, 2009 19301241

Tang YY, Ma Y, Fan Y, et al: Central and autonomic nervous system interaction is altered by short-term meditation. Proc Natl Acad Sci USA 106(22):8865–8870, 2009 19451642

University of Pennsylvania: Authentic Happiness Questionnaire. 2014. Available at: http://www.authentichappiness.sas.upenn.edu/questionnaires.aspx. Accessed August 26, 2014.

Vaishnavi S, Connor K, Davidson JRT: An abbreviated version of the Connor-Davidson Resilience Scale (CD-RISC), the CD-RISC2: psychometric properties and applications in psychopharmacological trials. Psychiatry Res 152(2–3):293–297, 2007 17459488

Suggested Cross-References

Social factors are discussed in Chapter 3 ("Resilience and Posttraumatic Growth"), Chapter 4 ("Positive Social Psychiatry"), Chapter 5 ("Recovery in Mental Illnesses"), Chapter 11 ("Preventive Interventions"), and Chapter 16 ("Bioethics of Positive Psychiatry"). Sleep is discussed in chapters 11 and 14 ("Positive Child Psychiatry"). Meditation and yoga are discussed in Chapter 10 ("Complementary, Alternative, and Integrative Medicine Interventions"). Gratitude is discussed in Chapter 9 ("Positivity in Supportive and Psychodynamic Therapy") and Chapter 13 ("Biology of Positive Psychiatry"). Resilience is discussed in chapters 3 and 13. Nutrition is discussed in Chapter 14.

PART IV

SPECIAL TOPICS IN
POSITIVE PSYCHIATRY

13

Biology of Positive Psychiatry

RAEANNE C. MOORE, PH.D.

LISA T. EYLER, PH.D.

PAUL J. MILLS, PH.D.

RUTH M. O'HARA, PH.D.

KATHERINE WACHMANN, PH.D.

HELEN LAVRETSKY, M.D., M.S.

Although the field of neuroscience has historically focused on disease, impairment, disability, and the harmful effects of stress and trauma, the growing field of positive neuroscience focuses on studying what the brain does well. Positive neuroscience is a blend of positive psychology and neuroscience, and positive neuroscientists are interested in the neural mechanisms that serve to enrich a person's life and potentially provide a buffering effect against negative

We thank Monte Buchsbaum, M.D., Marc Norman, M.D., and David Salmon, M.D., for providing the clinical vignettes used in this chapter. This work was supported, in part, by National Institutes of Health grant T32 MH019934 and by the University of California, San Diego Center for Healthy Aging and Sam and Rose Stein Institute for Research on Aging.

psychological functioning (i.e., depression, anxiety, and other mental health disorders). In this chapter, we focus on the neurobiology, as well as other biological mechanisms, that underpins several positive psychological traits. The commonalities among the brain regions involved in the various psychological traits are striking; for example, the anterior cingulate cortex is implicated in empathy, resilience, optimism, creativity, spirituality, wisdom, and social decision making. Similar commonalities are found among the genetic markers and among the blood and saliva markers involved in the various positive traits. To emphasize these commonalities, we have chosen to organize this chapter by biological mechanisms instead of by positive psychological traits. Specifically, we discuss the following three biological mechanisms: 1) the neurocircuitry of the positive psychological traits with the most empirical support, including empathy and compassion, resilience, optimism, and creativity; 2) the genetic bases of positive psychological traits; and 3) blood and saliva biomarkers associated with positive psychological traits.

Neurocircuitry of Positive Psychological Traits

Measurement of Brain Function

Many studies on positive neuroscience use advanced neuroimaging tools, such as functional magnetic resonance imaging (fMRI). fMRI can be used to measure brain activity during tasks thought to directly measure a particular psychological trait (e.g., measuring empathy by showing the participant a video of someone suffering) or to monitor brain activity during emotional or cognitive tests (such as a facial affect matching task) known to activate the brain regions of interest, which can then be examined for correlations with positive psychological traits outside of the scanner. Furthermore, a more traditional neuropsychological approach has also been used to understand the neurological impairments and/or changes in positive traits after neuronal injury.

Another approach examines the potential therapeutic effects of brain stimulation on improving positive psychological traits. Transcranial direct current stimulation uses static direct electrical currents to stimulate the brain. It is safe, painless, noninvasive, and inexpensive. Novel work by Professor Snyder and colleagues at the Centre for the Mind in Sydney, Australia, has demonstrated that by using transcranial direct current stimulation to "turn off" certain parts of the brain, other skills such as problem solving, insight, and creativity can be enhanced (Chi and Snyder 2012). These various techniques for measuring the neural mechanisms of positive psychological traits have helped scientists discover brain regions implicated in several positive psychological traits, as described in the subsection "Empathy and Compassion" (and shown in Figure 13–1 later in this section).

Empathy and Compassion

Empathy

A general consensus in the literature on the neurocircuitry of empathy is that of *shared networks* or *shared representations*. This theory posits that sharing the emotions of others activates neural structures similar to those activated by experiencing the same emotions firsthand. Empathic responding appears to be context specific and dependent on information available in the environment. The anterior insula and medial and anterior cingulate cortex have frequently been implicated as being consistently activated in empathy. At least two forms of empathy have been identified: affective-perceptual (feeling with) and cognitive-evaluative (perspective taking) components, with these dimensions thought to have overlapping but nonidentical neural bases. In a meta-analysis of the relevant fMRI literature, Fan et al. (2011) found that the left anterior midcingulate cortex was activated more frequently when a person was engaging in the cognitive-evaluative form of empathy, whereas greater activation in the right interior insula was found when a person was engaging in affective-perceptual empathy. The left anterior insula was active in both forms of empathy, and the researchers concluded that the bilateral insula, dorsal anterior cingulate cortex, anterior midcingulate cortex, and supplementary motor area form a core neural network of empathy. This core neural network was observed when research participants were empathizing with a variety of different emotions, including pain, fear, disgust, anxiety, and happiness, implying that this neural network is relevant to empathy in general and is not emotion specific. Other brain regions that have been implicated in the empathy network include the anterior temporal cortex, sensorimotor cortex, the inferior frontal gyrus (IFG), the prefrontal cortex (PFC, including medial orbitofrontal PFC, dorsomedial PFC, and dorsolateral PFC), the superior temporal sulcus and gyrus, and temporal-parietal cortex areas.

Brain activity during emotion processing appears to change with age, with older adults demonstrating less neural activity with negative stimuli, a positivity bias for remembering positive information better than negative information, and an ability to ignore irrelevant negative stimuli. Researchers call this the "emotion paradox in the aging brain" and interpret the age-related brain changes to emotional responding as improved emotional control and regulation in late life (for a comprehensive review, see Mather 2012). Our group examined the neural correlates of emotional and cognitive empathy in healthy older adults (mean age=79) and found more deactivation in the bilateral amygdala and right insula during a working memory task among older adults with higher levels of affective-perceptual empathy (Moore et al., in press). We also found greater bilateral insula and right frontal activation during a response inhibition task and greater midline precuneus activation during an affective facial matching task in older adults with higher cognitive empathy. Our preliminary findings speak to the possibility of differential relationships for the different forms of empathy in old age and provide support for the emotion paradox theory.

Compassion

The neural circuitry of compassion is less well understood. Compassion can be defined as an outward behavioral response of empathy, with the intention of reducing another's perceived suffering. Given that having an empathic response is a precursor to compassionate behavior, it is probable that empathy-related neural processes are activated during personal experiences of compassion. In one of the few fMRI studies specifically examining neural activation during the experience of compassion, Simon-Thomas and colleagues (2012) found that when they induced compassion in their undergraduate research participants during scanning, the midbrain periaqueductal gray was activated. They also found that self-reports of compassion were related to activation in a region near the periaqueductal gray and in the right IFG.

Central Function of Brain Regions Involved in Empathy and Compassion

The anterior insula and anterior and midcingulate cortex have consistently been shown to be involved in experiences of direct pain. The same regions are activated when one takes the perspective of another person and feels someone else's pain, which lends support to the shared-network perspective on empathy. Empathy-related insular and cingulate activity may represent a link between interoceptive (data from within the body, such as blood oxygen levels, muscle tension, and blood pressure) and exteroceptive (data from the outside world) stimuli, but this proposed linkage is speculative at this time.

Resilience

The study of the neurocircuitry of resilience has received considerable attention in the scientific literature. Scientists have attempted to elucidate both the psychological and the neurobiological underpinnings of resilience, which has been difficult given the complex nature of this construct. To date, neuroimaging studies of resilience have focused on brain regions involved in emotion and stress regulation circuitry. Other regions believed to be critical to resilience include pathways involved in attention, learning and memory, speed of recovery from stress, positive versus negative outlook, response to fear, and adaptive social behaviors. Across review papers, the PFC has consistently been implicated as a critical brain region for resilience. The PFC is involved in intentional emotion regulation, which can help with the self-regulation of stress. Inhibition of subcortical regions by the PFC is heightened among depressed individuals, which can result in a reduced capacity to regulate stress-related emotions.

Evidence also shows a role for the insular cortex in resilience. At the OptiBrain Center at the University of California, San Diego, cognitive neuroscientists have conducted multiple studies examining the neural pathways believed to be critical to resilience in elite athletes (e.g., Olympic athletes, marines, adventure racers). Elite athletes are thought to have ultraresilient brains and therefore have been able to provide researchers with insight into optimal resilience performance. Paulus and colleagues' work at the OptiBrain Center used fMRI methods to probe interoceptive distress (e.g., the sensation of increased difficulty breathing in air) in elite athletes and "normal" participants and found group differences in resilience in the insular cortex, with the elite athletes having an attenuated insular cortex activation during an aversive experience (Paulus et al. 2012). Similar insular patterns were found by this research group in elite military personnel, providing evidence for the role of the insular cortex in handling stress, or, said another way, having resilience under extreme environmental conditions. The literature has mixed evidence for the role of the hippocampus, amygdala, anterior cingulate cortex, hypothalamic-pituitary-adrenal (HPA) axis reward circuitry, and somatic nervous system in resilience.

Overall, the literature points to a relationship between resilience and core emotion-processing regions (i.e., amygdala, insula) in younger adults. In an unpublished study examining the association between resilience and emotion processing among older adults, we did not find any relationship between resilience and amygdala or insular cortex response. However, dorsolateral PFC response was greater in high-resilience older adults, indicating that older adults who are more resilient may have more dorsolateral PFC responses during an affective task, whereas their younger counterparts may have more amygdala and insular responses. Whether these differences are reflective of cognitive coping strategies, changes in emotion regulation, other processing differences, or are simply due to sampling differences is currently unknown.

Optimism

The majority of studies examining the neurocircuitry of optimism have been done exploring the *optimism bias*. The optimism bias is defined as the tendency for people to overestimate the likelihood of experiencing good events in their life and to underestimate the likelihood of experiencing bad events. In the Affective Brain Lab at the University College London, Sharot and colleagues found that trait optimism was related to enhanced activation in the rostral anterior cingulate cortex (rACC) and that the optimism bias was also related to enhanced activation in the rACC as well as the amygdala (Sharot et al. 2007). They also found a strong correspondence between brain responses in the rACC and amygdala when people were imagining future positive events and less correspondence of brain activation between these two structures when people were imagining future negative events. In another study, Sharot et al. (2011) found activation of the left IFG among optimists and pessimists alike when responding to positive information. However, when responding to negative information, the right IFG of more optimistic people was less likely to respond than the right IFG of less optimistic and pessimistic people. The researchers interpreted these findings as the brains of the optimistic people failing to integrate undesirable information about the future, which is related to increased happiness and well-being. In other words, the brains of optimistic people appear to be wearing "rose-tinted glasses."

Given what researchers know about the emotion paradox of the aging brain, older adults would be expected to demonstrate a greater positivity bias in their brains compared with younger adults. Chowdhury et al. (2013) examined age-related neural differences in response to biases about future negative events (termed an "update bias"). Compared with the younger adults, the older adults exhibited a greater update bias, and this update bias was related to activation of the dorsal anterior cingulate cortex in the older group but not the younger group. In a study examining individual differences in optimism among older adults, we found that older adults who had greater optimism showed reduced activation in their fusiform and frontal regions when viewing fearful faces (Bangen et al. 2014). These results may reflect a decreased salience of negative stimuli and/or better emotion regulation in optimistic older adults.

Creativity

Because of the complexity (and perhaps vagueness) of the construct and measurement difficulties in laboratory environments, the neural underpinnings of creativity are largely unknown. In a review of 72 experiments, Dietrich and Kanso (2010) found creative cognition to be broadly divided into three categories: divergent thinking, artistic creativity, and insight. Inconsistent findings were found for divergent thinking and artistic creativity, but for both creative constructs it is evident that no single brain region is sufficient. In terms of *divergent thinking*, defined as coming up with multiple solutions to a problem, the only consistency among neuroimaging studies was a finding of diffuse prefrontal activation. Studies examining artistic creativity have generally found activation in the motor and temporoparietal regions. Imaging studies examining the neural mechanisms of insight (also known as having an "aha" moment) have been more reliable. The researchers did not find support for right brain dominance despite a popular belief that "right brain thinking" underlies insight. There is convergent evidence for the involvement of the superior temporal gyrus and the anterior cingulate cortex in insight. The superior temporal gyrus appears to help with successful solutions of problems by making remote verbal associations, whereas the anterior cingulate cortex appears to help with cognitive flexibility. The role of prefrontal regions in moments of insight is unknown.

Much of what is known about creativity in the brain comes from lesion studies. The most compelling studies have come from patients with localized lesions to their left language areas, including the left IFG, left temporoparietal region, and left inferior parietal lobe. These regions are largely responsible for logical thinking, verbal communication, and comprehension, and theory posits that these regions may be inhibiting the formation of creative thought. By inactivating these regions and their potential inhibitory links to other parts of the frontal cortex, some think that the right PFC has an enhanced ability to generate novel creative thoughts and solutions. Examples of acquired savant syndrome in patients with lesions to these regions date back to the 1970s, with patients developing extraordinary artistic, mathematical, and memory skills. It is interesting to consider that "exceptional abilities" may lie in all of us but are being inhibited by the logical and verbal centers in our brains. However, we must also consider what costs might come from disabling these abilities in the hopes of unlocking hidden creativity.

Other Positive Traits

The neurocircuitry of other positive traits, including spirituality, humor, wisdom, and social decision making, has been studied in enough depth for at least one review paper to have been written on each trait. A summary of the brain regions that have been implicated in each of these traits is provided in Table 13–1. We chose to report findings from what we deemed the most comprehensive review paper for a particular trait. Empathy, resilience, optimism, and creativity are also included in the table for comparison purposes. Additionally, the numbering system that is used in Figure 13–1 is cross-referenced in Table 13–1 to highlight the overlap between traits in the regions noted in the figure. Interestingly, as Table 13–1 shows, considerable overlap occurs among the regions thought to be involved in these various traits. Please note, however, that support is mixed for these traits, and the brain regions presented have not been consistently found across studies.

Summary of Brain Regions Involved in Neurocircuitry of Positive Psychological Traits

Although the neurocircuitry of the various positive psychological traits we have described varies depending on the specific trait, the population, and the methods used to measure them, considerable overlap in the brain regions involved exists. Figure 13–1 depicts a broad neural model of positive psychological traits.

Table 13–1. Summary of brain regions with general support for positive psychological traits

	Frontal and prefrontal cortex	Temporal lobe	Limbic system	Parietal lobe	Other
Empathy	Dorsolateral PFC [4]; dorsomedial PFC [1]; supplementary motor area[a]; inferior frontal gyrus; medial orbitofrontal PFC	Insula[a] [5]; anterior temporal cortex; superior temporal sulcus and gyrus	Anterior cingulate cortex[a] [1]; anterior midcingulate cortex[a]	Temporoparietal junction [6]; sensorimotor cortex	—
Resilience	PFC[b] [4]	Insula[b] [5]	Anterior cingulate cortex [1]; amygdala [3]; hippocampus; hypothalamic–pituitary–adrenal axis reward circuitry	—	—
Optimism	Inferior frontal gyrus	Fusiform gyrus	Anterior cingulate cortex [1]; amygdala [3]	—	—
Creativity	Diffuse prefrontal regions [4]	Superior temporal gyrus	Anterior cingulate cortex [1]	Temporoparietal junction [6]; motor cortex	—
Spirituality[c]	Dorsolateral PFC [4]; ventrolateral PFC [4]; ventromedial PFC [2]; medial orbitofrontal cortex	Insula [5]; ventromedial temporal lobe; middle temporal cortex	Anterior cingulate cortex [1]; posterior cingulate cortex; amygdala; nucleus accumbens and striatum	Temporoparietal junction [6]; posterior superior parietal lobule; medial parietal cortex; inferior parietal lobule; angular gyrus	Brain stem

Table 13–1. Summary of brain regions with general support for positive psychological traits *(continued)*

	Frontal and prefrontal cortex	Temporal lobe	Limbic system	Parietal lobe	Other
Humor[d]	Inferior frontal cortex	Insula [5]; posterior temporal cortex	Amygdala [3]; hippocampus; parahippocampal cortex; nucleus accumbens and striatum	—	Midbrain
Wisdom[e]	Dorsomedial PFC [1]; ventromedial PFC [2]; medial PFC; inferior frontal gyrus; medial orbitofrontal cortex	Superior temporal gyrus	Anterior cingulate cortex [1]; posterior cingulate cortex; amygdala; nucleus accumbens and striatum	Parietal association cortex	—
Social decision making[f]	Dorsolateral PFC [4]; ventrolateral PFC [4]; dorsomedial PFC [1]; ventromedial PFC [2]; frontal pole, inferior frontal cortex, medial orbitofrontal cortex	Insula [5]; superior temporal gyrus	Anterior cingulate cortex [1]; amygdala [3]; posterior cingulate cortex; nucleus accumbens and striatum; caudate nucleus	Temporoparietal junction [6]; inferior parietal cortex	—

Note. Numbers in brackets correspond to brain regions denoted in Figure 13–1. Dashes indicate a particular region is not involved in the neurocircuitry of a particular trait. PFC = prefrontal cortex.

[a]Components of the core neural network of empathy (Fan et al. 2011). [b]Most support in the resilience literature. [c]Spirituality data from review by Fingelkurts and Fingelkurts (2009). [d]Humor data from review by Taber et al. (2007). [e]Wisdom data from review by Meeks and Jeste (2009). [f]Social decision-making data from review by Rilling and Sanfey (2011).

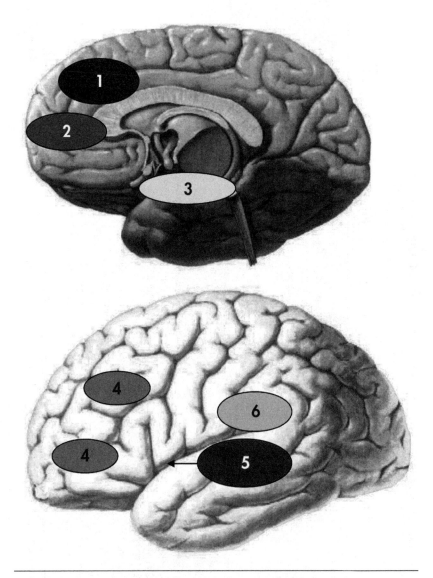

FIGURE 13–1. Broad neural model of positive psychological traits.

Medial (*upper*) and lateral (*lower*) surfaces of the cerebral cortex are depicted. Brain regions are numbered on the basis of function and are cross-referenced accordingly in Table 13–1.

1) Dorsomedial prefrontal cortex (PFC) and the dorsal anterior cingulate cortex (intentional and automatic emotion regulation and self/other pain avoidance motivation). 2) Ventromedial PFC (automatic emotion regulation). 3) Amygdala (emotion identification). 4) Dorsolateral PFC and ventrolateral PFC (intentional emotion regulation and cognitive reappraisal). 5) Anterior insula (self/other awareness of subjective state). 6) Temporoparietal junction (self/other distinction processes and theory of mind).

Source. Adapted from Meeks and Jeste 2009.

Figure 13–1 shows six brain functions seen across the various traits: 1) dorsal medial PFC and the dorsal anterior cingulate cortex (intentional and automatic emotion regulation and self/other pain avoidance motivation), 2) ventromedial PFC (automatic emotion regulation), 3) amygdala (emotion identification), 4) dorsolateral PFC and ventrolateral PFC (intentional emotion regulation and cognitive reappraisals), 5) anterior insula (self/other awareness of subjective state), and 6) temporoparietal junction (self/other distinction processes and theory of mind). As can be seen, the majority of the neural circuits for positive psychological traits lie in the PFC and the interplay between the PFC and structures of the limbic system. The PFC, particularly the ventrolateral PFC, is what scientists believe makes humans different from their closest nonhuman (i.e., primate) relatives. As the following clinical vignettes demonstrate, damage to the PFC can cause significant personality and behavioral changes. However, it is highly likely that it is not just the PFC that makes human brains unique but, rather, the communication between the PFC and other brain regions. The brain networks that we have described in relation to the various positive psychological traits include integration of neural activity of higher-order cortical brain regions with lower-level sensory and motor regions, which can result in advanced emotional functioning, adaptive responses to stress, and novel and complex goal-directed problem solving. There is clearly much researchers still do not know about the brain systems involved in positive psychological traits. However, science is continuing to make considerable advances in understanding the neural circuitry of the brain (see the Human Connectome Project's Web site, www.humanconnectomeproject.org), which will hopefully continue to lead to novel targets for enhancing quality of life.

Illustrative Vignettes

Positive psychological characteristics are typically considered to be traitlike in nature and rather stable over time. They do not generally fluctuate on the basis of mood, stress levels, or changes to one's external environment. However, these characteristics may change in people with long-lasting health problems or acute infection (such as a state of delirium) and in people with brain lesions. The involvement of particular brain regions in these acute changes is additional evidence for the centrality of some regions to the expression of these positive traits.

Clinical Vignette 1

At age 48, Martin, a married and formerly successful, responsible architect, was let go from his job for progressive troublesome behavioral changes, namely, obsessively shutting off the lights in the offices of his coworkers. His new obsession with conserving energy was pervasive, and he also went around his home turning off all the lights and made his wife stop the car ignition at stop signs and stop lights. Martin also became obsessed with license plates, trash on the side of the road, and consuming excessive amounts of candy, and at age 49, Martin was diagnosed with psychosis. He continued to develop additional obsessions and rituals, including fixations on killing ants, his own hygiene (including shaving and showering five times per day despite wearing the same clothing every day), and food, to the extent that he was consuming so much food and soda his wife was forced to put a lock on the refrigerator. Martin also developed personality changes. He became disinhibited, impulsive, and mildly apathetic and had inappropriate manners. He began calling people names and developed a serious dislike for people who were overweight and for people with tattoos. According to his wife, Martin had a loss of empathy and was unable to connect with other people's emotions as he was previously able to do. For example, she stated that when she would cry, he would not show any emotional response but would tell her in a neutral voice not to cry and to be happy. He also reportedly failed to show an emotional response when his 1-year-old baby fell.

Neuropsychological testing, conducted when Martin was 50, revealed significant impairment in the frontal executive domains, yet his memory and visuospatial function were relatively spared. Functional brain imaging showed hypometabolism in the frontal lobes. At that time, Martin was accurately diagnosed with behavioral-variant frontotemporal dementia, and his bizarre behaviors, neuropsychological functioning, and personality changes progressively worsened over time.

Clinical Vignette 2

Julia, a 48-year-old woman with brain cancer, underwent two right frontal craniotomies with tumor resections over the course of 8 years. The tumor recurrence after the first surgery was more invasive than the original tumor and had infiltrated the patient's bilateral frontal lobes and anterior temporal lobes (right more than left), as well as the right frontal horn of her right lateral ventricle. Following the second surgery, Julia denied any changes to her cognitive functioning (except diminished concentration, which she attributed to poor sleep), personality, or everyday functional behaviors. She also denied any past or present depression or anxiety. However, according to Julia's daughter, her mother had changes in cognition, personality, and behaviors after the second surgery. Julia's daughter stated that her mother had been experiencing confusion, language problems (repetitive speech), and memory problems, such as forgetfulness and getting lost in familiar places. Additionally, her daughter reported significant personality changes and stated that her mother became more dramatic and prone to yelling and verbal altercations when she became frustrated and that she was "short-tempered" and "sometimes mean." Collateral information was obtained from a close friend of Julia's, who stated that the patient's personality changes began 1 year before the first tumor was diagnosed. According to the friend, Julia's personality changes progressed over the years and had worsened since the second surgery. Primary changes included verbal and physical aggressive behaviors and frequent threats to harm others. The friend described an incident in which Julia, unprovoked, became enraged with her hair stylist while getting her hair done and stabbed the stylist in the leg with a pencil. Another time, the police had to be called to resolve a dispute between Julia and her roommate. Julia's friend also reported changes in short-term memory and executive functions (i.e., decreased multitasking, poor planning, and reduced judgment).

Neuropsychological testing revealed relatively intact executive functions and some impairment in learning and memory. Clearly, however, the personality and social changes caused by the tumor were leading to the greatest impairments in everyday functioning in this patient.

Genetic Bases of Positive Traits

Another approach to understanding the biology of positive traits is through examination of their genetic associations. Genetic markers can both identify individuals who are more likely to display a specific psychological trait and point to the potential etiological pathway that may lead to the development of the trait. Cumulatively, the range of genetic studies examining positive traits suggests that these traits likely have a moderate to strong genetic basis. The consideration of the genetic underpinnings of positive psychological traits is a new area of research, and only a few studies conducted to date have addressed these issues. Furthermore, positive traits are typically considered in the context of examining a specific psychiatric disorder or a specific genetic marker, rather than the trait itself being the focus of the investigation. Even if genetic markers are identified, it is not yet clear that such markers are both sensitive to and specific for positive psychological traits. Definitions of positive traits themselves vary, and thus, the phenotype under investigation can vary across studies of the same positive trait. More broad-based, non-hypothesis-driven, agnostic genome-wide association studies (GWASs) targeted to understanding the genetic basis of positive traits are rare.

Heritability of Genetic Traits: Twin Studies

Twin studies are one way to understand the extent to which a trait is heritable by comparing the trait in monozygotic (MZ) versus dizygotic (DZ) twins. Approximately 50% of the genome is shared in DZ twins, whereas the genome is shared entirely in MZ twins. Factors that are more concordant in MZ twins than in DZ twins may have a stronger genetic basis, whereas factors associated with similar rates of concordance in MZ and DZ twin pairs suggest that there are both genetic and environmental factors at play. Estimates of the genetic heritability of positive traits using twin studies have suggested 31%–36% heritability for resilience to stressful life events (Amstadter et al. 2014) and for optimism (Mosing et al. 2009); the heritability of empathy may be as high as 46% in some age groups (Knafo et al. 2008), and heritability may be 30%–40% for subjective well-being. Overall, these studies suggest that there is a considerable genetic contribution to a range of positive traits.

Candidate Genetic Markers and Positive Traits

Inferences about the genetic basis of positive traits often come from studies of candidate genetic markers. One genetic risk factor associated with the development of psychopathological response to stress is the serotonin transporter promoter polymorphism (5HTTLPR). Therefore, several investigators have considered it to be an ideal target for studying the genetic basis of several positive traits, particularly resilience. The short or deletion form (the S allele) is associated with reduced transcription and reuptake efficiency within the serotonergic system, whereas the long form (the L allele) is considered to confer increased resilience and thus is protective against negative outcomes such as depression and anxiety in the presence of stress. In a sample of 423 undergraduates, Stein et al. (2009) found S allele carriers had reduced resilience to stress, whereas carriers of the L allele had higher levels of resilience, suggesting that a more efficient serotoninergic system may confer increased resiliency to stress. This genetic marker was not found to be associated with resilience in an older adult sample, suggesting the association of 5HTTLPR with resilience attenuates with age (O'Hara et al. 2012). Additional candidate genes found to be associated with different aspects of resiliency include the monoamine oxidase A (*MAOA*), neuropeptide Y (*NPY*), brain-derived neurotrophic factor (*BDNF*), corticotropin-releasing hormone receptor 1 (*CRHR1*), FK506-binding protein 5 (*FKBP5*), 5HTTLPR, catechol O-methyltransferase (*COMT*), and nerve growth factor inducible (*NGFI-A*) genes.

Although the physiological basis of positive traits can be indicated by their genetic basis, their biological basis can sometimes be the starting point for understanding their genetic underpinnings. Oxytocin is one hormone documented to be involved in positive traits such as good social communication skills and has been associated with increased levels of trust and generosity. Many investigators have suggested that genetic variation in the oxytocin receptor gene (*OXTR*) may have a role in empathy modulation. Located on 3p25, *OXTR* spans 17 kb, contains four exons and three introns, and has many polymorphic sites. Several studies have identified various single nucleotide polymorphisms (SNPs) or haplotypes (combinations of polymorphisms) associated with different types of empathy (e.g., Wu et al. 2012). Because *OXTR* has also been associated with levels of optimism, this gene may play a key role in the regulation of many positive traits.

Another candidate marker for positive traits is calcium channel, voltage-dependent, L type, alpha 1C subunit (*CACNA1C*), with Strohmaier et al. (2013) finding that genetic variation in *CACNA1C* was related to lower levels of optimism as well as resilience. *CACNA1C* is a member of a family of genes implicated in calcium channels and is considered to be key for normal function of both heart and brain cells. However, although findings are mixed, many investigations have found *CACNA1C* to be associated with a range of psychiatric disorders, including schizophrenia, depressive disorders, and bipolar disorders. This finding raises a critical issue pertinent to understanding the genetic basis of positive traits. It may be that any genotype associated with a negative outcome, such as a specific psychiatric disorder, will likely have a genotype that is also associated with positive traits that characterize the absence of the disorder. As such, these genetic markers may be nonspecific for positive traits per se but are associated with a range of positive traits by virtue of not being associated with the negative traits integral to mental health disorders. For example, in our own investigation (O'Hara et al. 2012), the 5HTTLPR L allele was not associated with resilience but was instead associated with better cognitive performance and self-rated successful aging. Thus, resilience may actually be a proxy variable for cognitive function, with which the 5HTTLPR L allele is well documented to be associated. In another investigation, our group found decreased neuroconnectivity among 5HTTLPR S allele carriers (Waring et al. 2013), suggesting a neurobiological basis for increased resilience. Indeed, it is interesting to note that other candidate genes found to be associated with resiliency, including *BDNF* and *COMT*, have been implicated in brain neurocircuitry that is thought to subserve emotional regulation and other potential aspects of positive psychological traits. Because candidate genetic marker studies of positive traits are often conducted only in the context of psychiatric disorders, the interpretation that researchers can make with respect to their true association with positive traits is limited. Non-hypothesis-testing, agnostic, data-driven GWAS investigations of positive traits are required to more fully understand if there are specific markers that have high penetrance for specific positive traits, but to date, such investigations are few in number.

Multigene Association Studies

McGrath et al. (2013) performed a GWAS of the mental and physical components of health-related quality of life across diagnosis (1.6 million SNPs), adjusting for psychiatric symptom severity. After controlling for diagnostic category and symptom severity, they found that the strongest evidence of genetic association was between variants in ADAM metallopeptidase with thrombospondin type 1 motif, 16 (*ADAMTS16*) and physical functioning, but no other positive markers were identified. In one of the few other investigations to explore a range of genetic markers associated with positive traits, Rana et al. (2014) examined 426 women from the Women's Health Initiative study. On the basis of a literature review, they examined 65 candidate gene SNPs judged to be related to predisposition to resilience and optimism. Following correction for type I errors, they found no significant associations of resilience and optimism with any of the specific gene SNPs in single-locus analyses. The authors concluded that positive psychological traits are likely to be genetically complex, such that many loci, rather than one specific gene or SNP, have small effects that contribute to the phenotypic variation.

Blood- and Saliva-Based Biomarkers Associated With Positive Psychological Traits

When one scans the literature on the topic of blood- and saliva-based biomarkers of positive psychological traits, one finds that the domains of resilience, optimism, and well-being have been the most heavily researched. The next most frequently researched topics are compassion and mindfulness, happiness, spirituality, and gratitude. Biomarkers examined in the context of these traits have focused on telomere protection of the chromosomes; autonomic measures, including catecholamines and cortisol; and commonly measured biomarkers of inflammation such as interleukin-6 (IL-6) and C-reactive protein (CRP).

Resilience

In terms of resilience, telomere length, considered a proxy for cellular aging, and telomerase, the enzyme that regulates telomere length, have received the most empirical attention. Resilience is associated with less HPA axis activation to stress. In turn, greater stress (in terms of both early life stress and the chronicity of stress) is associated with shorter telomere length. Epel et al. (2006) describe resilience as a composite of multiple factors such as psychological stress resilience, healthy lifestyle factors, and social connections and show that higher resilience is associated with longer telomere length and that each aspect of resilience acts as a protective factor from stress-induced telomere shortening. One of the routes through which stressors affect telomere length and telomerase activity is through autonomic activation as seen via elevated catecholamine and cortisol levels.

Optimism and Well-Being

Like individuals with high resilience, individuals with more optimism show less HPA activation in response to stressors (e.g., Lai et al. 2005). Similar findings have been reported for inflammatory biomarkers. Brydon et al. (2009), for example, examined linkages between dispositional optimism and the immune system in healthy young men and found that optimism was inversely related to IL-6 levels, such that men with higher optimism showed reduced IL-6 responses to acute stress independent of resting IL-6 levels, BMI, age, or depression. Similar findings with IL-6, as well as links between optimism and general immune responsiveness and antioxidant levels, have been reported in the literature.

A unique study on this topic of biomarkers and well-being also examined if ill-being showed biomarkers distinct from those of well-being. Among the measured biomarkers were endocrine (i.e., cortisol, epinephrine, norepinephrine, dihydroepiandrosterone sulfate (DHEA-S) and cardiovascular (i.e., high-density lipoprotein [HDL] cholesterol, total/HDL cholesterol, systolic blood pressure, waist-hip ratio, glycosylated hemoglobin) markers. Well-being was found to be significantly associated with lower cortisol, epinephrine, and norepinephrine levels. Further analysis revealed that higher personal growth and purpose influenced daily slopes of salivary cortisol (Ryff et al. 2006).

The relationship between optimism and well-being is not always straightforward, however. It has been described as a complex relationship that is dependent on the duration and type of stressor involved and is potentially influenced by gender, such that not all studies report a protective effect of optimism on stress-induced immune changes. Studies on healthy elderly men and postmenopausal women, for example, have not found any significant associations between telomere length and optimism or have found that the effects are restricted to women (O'Donovan et al. 2009).

Compassion and Mindfulness

Studies on the domains of compassion and mindfulness examine not only existing trait levels but also levels influenced by the practice of different forms of meditation. A meditation practice that fosters compassion, for example, has been shown to influence stress-induced IL-6 levels, with the effects being dependent on the degree of engagement with the practice. In these studies, individuals who regularly practice compassion meditation and/or participate in compassion training have lower IL-6 responses to stress (e.g., Pace et al. 2009). Similarly, individuals who have high trait self-compassion have lower resting CRP levels.

Mindfulness has received increasing attention over the past decade because of the increase in research on mindfulness meditation techniques. Some research suggests that mindfulness influences the endocrine response to stress such that individuals with higher mindfulness show lower cortisol levels in acute stress conditions (Brown et al. 2012). We conducted an exploratory study in healthy individuals to examine different components of mindfulness in relationship to inflammation and found that the mindfulness components of observing and nonreactivity were associated with lower IL-6 levels.

Happiness

In heart failure, a condition with marked severe and chronic inflammation, patients with more positive affect show lower levels of tumor necrosis factor–α, soluble tumor necrosis factor receptor 2, and IL-6 (Brouwers et al. 2013). Such effects of happiness on inflammatory profile have also been reported in healthy individuals, with those having more happiness showing lower levels of interferon-γ. In addition, several studies have examined the HPA axis in the context of happiness. In the large Whitehall II study of nearly 3,000 individuals, for example, more positive affect was associated with lower cortisol levels (Steptoe et al. 2008).

Spirituality and Gratitude

The potential effects of spirituality and religiousness on health and mortality have been actively researched for decades. Only a small subset of those studies, however, has examined potential biomarkers associated with such effects. Similar to individuals in studies on resilience and happiness, individuals who report greater spiritual wellness have lower levels of CRP (Holt-Lunstad et al. 2011). This effect might be mediated by lower stress and HPA activation because several studies showed that higher self-reported spirituality or well-being is associated with lower cortisol levels. These findings have been reported in various other populations, including healthy individuals, people living with HIV, and military veterans with posttraumatic stress disorder. Some of the authors of this chapter have been studying inflammatory profiles in different stages of heart failure development. We have found that in patients with New York Heart Association stages II and III heart failure, those with high trait spirituality and high trait gratitude have lower levels of the cardiac biomarker soluble ST2, which is a member of the IL-1 receptor family and is secreted by cardiac muscle cells under mechanical stress. Thus, heart failure patients with more trait spirituality as well as more trait gratitude show a more favorable profile of an important prognostic biomarker of heart failure.

Interventions to Improve Positive Psychological Traits: A Biological Perspective

The clinical implications for understanding the neurocircuitry, biomarkers, and genetics of positive psychiatry are vast. A better understanding of the biological mechanisms underlying positive psychological traits can lead to the development of novel interventions to alter and/or increase these traits. For example, methodologies to target specific neural circuits, including fMRI neurofeedback, mindfulness meditation, mental training exercises, and cognitive reappraisal training are promising noninvasive techniques that can possibly stimulate and strengthen emotion regulation. In particular, mindfulness meditation and cognitive reappraisals may be two methods that can be used to enhance resilience through the mechanism of enhancing PFC regulation of limbic and brain-stem systems. Interfering with certain brain circuits using magnetic stimulation might also be a way of influencing behaviors, such as the optimism bias. Novel pharmaceuticals or natural compounds may also be able to regulate executive and limbic function and may lead to increases in positive psychological traits. For instance, medications that improve regulation of the HPA axis and the sympathetic nervous system in response to stress may be able to improve function in the PFC and regulate limbic reactivity to stress, which could potentially lead to improvements in resilience. As another example, giving oxytocin to people while they are engaged in compassion training versus completing compassion training alone may serve to bolster the results of compassion training. To our knowledge, these therapeutic treatment targets have yet to be empirically tested, and they provide interesting avenues for future research.

Summary

In this chapter, we pull together the growing evidence for the biological basis of positive psychological traits. To date, the majority of clinical research has focused on identifying the neurobiology of these traits, but ongoing research on the genetic markers and blood and saliva markers involved in these traits is under way. There are exciting treatment opportunities to enhance positive psychological traits through our existing knowledge of the neurocircuitry, biomarkers, and genetics of positive psychiatry. However, a caveat is that current scientific assessment methods are limited to assessing these mechanisms from a single biological perspective (neurocircuitry, genetic, or blood and saliva markers), and integrated research is needed to develop novel interventions aimed at concurrently strengthening the neural networks and other biological mechanisms associated with positive psychological traits. An emerging trend in academic research has been to bridge the knowledge gap and share research across multiple disciplines, and multidisciplinary research teams of engineers, software architects, experimental psychologists, neurologists, physicians, and others are working together to design and implement novel approaches to capturing, storing, and analyzing data on biological mechanisms. These collaborative efforts will greatly enhance the ability to measure, and eventually improve, the biology of positive psychological traits.

Clinical Key Points

- Positive psychological traits are a function of various neural networks throughout the brain; these traits are not localized to discrete brain structures, lobes, or hemispheres.

- Research has shown that strengthening the neural connections between certain brain structures can improve certain traits (e.g., empathy, resilience), whereas suppressing the neural connections between structures may improve other traits (e.g., creativity).

- Data suggest that positive psychological traits likely have a moderate to strong genetic basis; however, literature is limited regarding specific genetic markers subserving these traits.

- Research has also demonstrated relationships between positive psychological traits and saliva- and blood-based biomarkers; particularly notable are reduced hypothalamic-pituitary-adrenal axis activation and reduced inflammatory biomarker responses to stress in individuals with greater positive psychological traits.

- Treatments aimed at strengthening these neural networks and other biological mechanisms, through either pharmacological or nonpharmacological means or a combination of both, have the potential to improve positive psychological traits.

References

Amstadter AB, Myers JM, Kendler KS: Psychiatric resilience: longitudinal twin study. Br J Psychiatry 205(4):275–280, 2014 24723629

Bangen KJ, Bergheim M, Kaup AR, et al: Brains of optimistic older adults respond less to fearful faces. J Neuropsychiatry Clin Neurosci 26(2):155–163, 2014 24275797

Brouwers C, Mommersteeg PM, Nyklíček I, et al: Positive affect dimensions and their association with inflammatory biomarkers in patients with chronic heart failure. Biol Psychol 92(2):220–226, 2013 23085133

Brown KW, Weinstein N, Creswell JD: Trait mindfulness modulates neuroendocrine and affective responses to social evaluative threat. Psychoneuroendocrinology 37(12):2037–2041, 2012 22626868

Brydon L, Walker C, Wawrzyniak AJ, et al: Dispositional optimism and stress-induced changes in immunity and negative mood. Brain Behav Immun 23(6):810–816, 2009 19272441

Chi RP, Snyder AW: Brain stimulation enables the solution of an inherently difficult problem. Neurosci Lett 515(2):121–124, 2012 22440856

Chowdhury R, Sharot T, Wolfe T, et al: Optimistic update bias increases in older age. Psychol Med 4:1–10, 2013 24180676

Dietrich A, Kanso R: A review of EEG, ERP, and neuroimaging studies of creativity and insight. Psychol Bull 136(5):822–848, 2010 20804237

Epel ES, Lin J, Wilhelm FH, et al: Cell aging in relation to stress arousal and cardiovascular disease risk factors. Psychoneuroendocrinology 31(3):277–287, 2006 16298085

Fan Y, Duncan NW, de Greck M, et al: Is there a core neural network in empathy? An fMRI based quantitative meta-analysis. Neurosci Biobehav Rev 35(3):903–911, 2011 20974173

Fingelkurts AA, Fingelkurts AA: Is our brain hardwired to produce God, or is our brain hardwired to perceive God? A systematic review on the role of the brain in mediating religious experience. Cogn Process 10(4):293–326, 2009 19471985

Holt-Lunstad J, Steffen PR, Sandberg J, Jensen B: Understanding the connection between spiritual well-being and physical health: an examination of ambulatory blood pressure, inflammation, blood lipids and fasting glucose. J Behav Med 34(6):477–488, 2011 21487720

Knafo A, Zahn-Waxler C, Van Hulle C, et al: The developmental origins of a disposition toward empathy: genetic and environmental contributions. Emotion 8(6):737–752, 2008 19102585

Lai JC, Evans PD, Ng SH, et al: Optimism, positive affectivity, and salivary cortisol. Br J Health Psychol 10(Pt 4):467–484, 2005 16238860

Mather M: The emotion paradox in the aging brain. Ann N Y Acad Sci 1251:33–49, 2012 22409159

McGrath LM, Cornelis MC, Lee PH, et al: Genetic predictors of risk and resilience in psychiatric disorders: a cross-disorder genome-wide association study of functional impairment in major depressive disorder, bipolar disorder, and schizophrenia. Am J Med Genet B Neuropsychiatr Genet 162B(8):779–788, 2013 24039173

Meeks TW, Jeste DV: Neurobiology of wisdom: a literature overview. Arch Gen Psychiatry 66(4):355–365, 2009 19349305

Moore RC, Dev SI, Jeste DV, et al: Distinct neural correlates of emotional and cognitive empathy in older adults. Psychiatry Research: Neuroimaging (in press)

Mosing MA, Zietsch BP, Shekar SN, et al: Genetic and environmental influences on optimism and its relationship to mental and self-rated health: a study of aging twins. Behav Genet 39(6):597–604, 2009 19618259

O'Donovan A, Lin J, Tillie J, et al: Pessimism correlates with leukocyte telomere shortness and elevated interleukin-6 in post-menopausal women. Brain Behav Immun 23(4):446–449, 2009 19111922

O'Hara R, Marcus P, Thompson WK, et al: 5-HTTLPR short allele, resilience, and successful aging in older adults. Am J Geriatr Psychiatry 20:452–456, 2012 22233775

Pace TW, Negi LT, Adame DD, et al: Effect of compassion meditation on neuroendocrine, innate immune and behavioral responses to psychosocial stress. Psychoneuroendocrinology 34(1):87–98, 2009 18835662

Paulus MP, Flagan T, Simmons AN, et al: Subjecting elite athletes to inspiratory breathing load reveals behavioral and neural signatures of optimal performers in extreme environments. PLoS ONE 7(1):e29394, 2012 22276111

Rana BK, Darst BF, Bloss C, et al: Candidate SNP associations of optimism and resilience in older adults: exploratory study of 935 community-dwelling adults. March 26, 2014. Available at: http://www.sciencedirect.com/science/article/pii/S1064748114001092. Accessed August 27, 2014.

Rilling JK, Sanfey AG: The neuroscience of social decision-making. Annu Rev Psychol 62:23–48, 2011 20822437

Ryff CD, Dienberg Love G, Urry HL, et al: Psychological well-being and ill-being: do they have distinct or mirrored biological correlates? Psychother Psychosom 75(2):85–95, 2006 16508343

Sharot T, Riccardi AM, Raio CM, et al: Neural mechanisms mediating optimism bias. Nature 450(7166):102–105, 2007 17960136

Sharot T, Korn CW, Dolan RJ: How unrealistic optimism is maintained in the face of reality. Nat Neurosci 14(11):1475–1479, 2011 21983684

Simon-Thomas ER, Godzik J, Castle E, et al: An fMRI study of caring vs self-focus during induced compassion and pride. Soc Cogn Affect Neurosci 7(6):635–648, 2012 21896494

Stein MB, Campbell-Sills L, Gelernter J: Genetic variation in 5HTTLPR is associated with emotional resilience. Am J Med Genet B Neuropsychiatr Genet 150B(7):900–906, 2009 19152387

Steptoe A, O'Donnell K, Badrick E, et al: Neuroendocrine and inflammatory factors associated with positive affect in healthy men and women: the Whitehall II study. Am J Epidemiol 167(1):96–102, 2008 17916595

Strohmaier J, Amelang M, Hothorn LA, et al: The psychiatric vulnerability gene CACNA1C and its sex-specific relationship with personality traits, resilience factors and depressive symptoms in the general population. Mol Psychiatry 18(5):607–613, 2013 22665259

Taber KH, Redden M, Hurley RA: Functional anatomy of humor: positive affect and chronic mental illness. J Neuropsychiatry Clin Neurosci 19(4):358–362, 2007 18070837

Waring JD, Etkin A, Hallmayer JF, et al: Connectivity underlying emotion conflict regulation in older adults with 5-HTTLPR short allele: a preliminary investigation. October 8, 2013. Available at: http://www.sciencedirect.com/science/article/pii/S1064748113003357. Accessed August 27, 2014.

Wu N, Li Z, Su Y: The association between oxytocin receptor gene polymorphism (OXTR) and trait empathy. J Affect Disord 138(3):468–472, 2012 22357335

Suggested Cross-References

Well-being is discussed in Chapter 6 ("What Is Well-Being?"), Chapter 7 ("Clinical Assessments of Positive Mental Health"), and Chapter 15 ("Positive Geriatric and Cultural Psychiatry"). Gratitude is discussed in Chapter 9 ("Positivity in Supportive and Psychodynamic Therapy") and Chapter 12 ("Integrating Positive Psychiatry Into Clinical Practice"). Resilience is discussed in Chapter 3 ("Resilience and Posttraumatic Growth") and Chapter 12. Spirituality is discussed in Chapter 2 ("Positive Psychological Traits") and Chapter 10 ("Complementary, Alternative, and Integrative Medicine Interventions"). Optimism is discussed in Chapter 2.

Suggested Readings

The Human Connectome Project. Available at: http://www.humanconnectomeproject.org/. Accessed August 27, 2014.

Jeste DV: Positive psychiatry. Psychiatric News. 2012. Available at: http://psychnews. psychiatryonline.org/newsArticle.aspx?articleid=1182477. Accessed August 27, 2014.

Meeks TW, Jeste DV: Neurobiology of wisdom: a literature review. Arch Gen Psychiatry 66:355–365, 2009

Singh I, Rose N: Biomarkers in psychiatry. Nature 460:202–207, 2009
Zhivotovskaya E: The Biology of Happiness. Positive Psychology News Daily. 2008. Available at: http://positivepsychologynews.com/news/emiliya-zhivotovskaya/200810281108. Accessed August 27, 2014.

14

Positive Child Psychiatry

DAVID C. RETTEW, M.D.

According to the American Academy of Child and Adolescent Psychiatry, a *child psychiatrist* is "a physician who specializes in the diagnosis and the treatment of disorders of thinking, feeling, and/or behavior affecting children, adolescents, and their families" (American Academy of Child and Adolescent Psychiatry 2014). Although it is difficult to argue that these functions are not what most child psychiatrists spend the vast majority of their time doing, there is increasing momentum to broaden this definition and extend the influence and expertise of child psychiatrists into positive aspects of mental functioning. Clinically trained child psychiatrists, psychologists, and other types of counselors speak of themselves as mental *health* professionals, but the truth is that most have been trained as mental *illness* professionals. Most experts in depression, for example, spend little time trying to understand and study happiness, and most authorities on the effects of child abuse and maltreatment get little training on what parents can do to help their children thrive.

The rich and varied chapters of this book illustrate that the slow progress to incorporate aspects of wellness, health promotion, and other areas of positive psychiatry into both the identity of psychiatry as a field and the behaviors of psychiatrists in clinical practice is not due to the lack of a research base for these principles. On the contrary, ample evidence shows that the groundwork has been more than adequately laid. The time has now come for psychiatrists to embrace the notion that a fully competent mental health professional is an expert not only in repairing the processes that make one "not ill" but also in encouraging the processes that make one well.

285

In the 1990s, a movement in psychiatry advocated changing the goal of treatment from *response,* defined as a significant drop in the severity of symptoms, to *remission,* defined as an absence of symptoms and the patient no longer meeting criteria for the target diagnosis. This effort was promoted in part by the pharmaceutical industry and was often described in the course of pharmacological treatment. Psychiatrists are now faced with raising the bar once again from remission to wellness, and medications are clearly inadequate to help patients achieve this level.

Perhaps nowhere is this imperative toward wellness greater than in child psychiatry. Given that child psychiatry is steeped in the developmental perspective with full awareness about the impact on child behavior of parents, schools, peers, and culture, incorporating positive psychiatry elements into child psychiatry would seem like an easy sell. Surprisingly, however, a lot of ground remains to be covered before child psychiatry can be viewed as a field that fully embraces a wellness model in its standard approach. In this chapter, I outline some specific domains of positive psychiatry that can readily be assessed and managed within a child psychiatry framework. Table 14–1 summarizes these areas. Readers are also referred to an excellent review by Hudziak (2008). Following the overview, I offer specific suggestions for incorporating elements of positive psychiatry and health promotion strategies into practice, as well as some recommendations to improve the training of positive psychiatry for the next generation of clinicians and scientists.

Continuum of Mental Functioning

One of the findings that has illuminated the need for psychiatrists to integrate elements of positive psychiatry more fully into their approach has been the accumulating research demonstrating that most aspects of behavior exist along a broad continuum with no clear boundary between what can be considered normal and what can be considered abnormal (Rettew 2013). These findings have countered more traditional disease model perspectives that tend to view those who meet criteria for psychiatric disorders as "having" something that is qualitatively distinct from those who do not meet criteria for a mental illness. When measured quantitatively using instruments that are sensitive to the full range of possibilities, core behaviors related to the majority of child psychiatric disorders, from attention-deficit/hyperactivity disorder (ADHD) (Polderman et al. 2007) to autism (Constantino and Todd 2003), are found to lie along relatively normally distributed curves that do not readily yield consensus as to where the natural line should be between a trait and a disorder. These distributions suggest, but certainly do not prove, that shared elements related to genetics, brain anatomy, physiology, and environmental factors may underlie this full spectrum. A

Table 14–1. Selected domains of wellness in positive child psychiatry

Positive attributes and traits

Nutrition

Physical activity and exercise

Involvement in structured activity

Music and the arts

Reading and limiting screen time

Parenting behavior

Parental mental health

Spirituality and religious involvement

Compassion and giving back to others

Mindfulness

Sleep

limited amount of direct research has confirmed that the forces that may be important in one child who displays a moderate amount of a certain behavior may be similarly important—but perhaps amplified or diminished—in another child who has a much more extreme level of that same behavior (Hettema et al. 2006). Such findings, of course, do not preclude the possibility that more discrete pathological processes may also be in play in some individuals at the tail ends of a distribution.

Elements of Positive Child Psychiatry

True mental health is much more than the absence of mental illness, and wellness is not simply a hedonistic state of doing things that make one feel good all the time. Although scholars and the general public continue to debate the definition of *well-being*, Seligman divides the term into five components: 1) positive emotion, 2) engagement, 3) relationships, 4) meaning and purpose, and 5) accomplishment (Seligman 2011). Obviously, good physical health can also be an important component to mental well-being. The definition of behavioral wellness will, of course, vary among different children and families, and particular families will find some elements of wellness more important than others. The job of psychiatrists is not to impose some rigid definition of wellness on their patients but, rather, to help them identify and reach their own stated goals.

The ingredients that can promote optimal mental health in a child's life are diverse. Here, I very briefly cover some of the areas that have been shown to be important through empirical research and that are the most conducive to the collaborative work among a child, his or her parents, and a child mental health professional. Although they are considered separately, many of these domains feed into one another, inducing a positive "virtuous cycle" that can increase the momentum toward overall health.

Positive Skills and Attributes

Children who are able to achieve a high level of wellness are often found to possess particular traits that help them to be resilient during times of adversity and challenge. Among these attributes are problem-solving skills, the ability to delay gratification, perseverance, emotion regulation capacities, assertiveness, flexibility, and the ability to relax. Some of my own research and that of many others have demonstrated that the temperament trait related to an ability to self-regulate is a component of nearly all types of psychopathology (Rettew 2009). Although many of these characteristics are under a certain amount of genetic influence, ample evidence shows that these skills can be enhanced by intervention targeted directly at the child or by teaching parents to help their children develop these abilities to their full potential (Beck 2011).

Nutrition

Although exaggerated and unproven claims about the effects of specific dietary elements on behavior certainly exist, compelling evidence shows that a healthy diet is an important aspect of optimal mental functioning for children with regard to current functioning and future behavior. In addition to problems stemming from specific nutrient deficiency states, studies have shown links between generally healthier diets (see the U.S. Department of Agriculture's MyPlate initiative at www.choosemyplate.gov/) and lower levels of problem behaviors in nonreferred samples (Jacka et al. 2013). Breakfast can be a particularly important meal for children that is often skipped or quickly consumed with little regard to its nutritional content. Family meals can also be an important time for discussion because mealtimes can often be the only moments during a day that parents and children all congregate in the same place. In addition to addressing the clear problem of child obesity, wide-ranging benefits come from families being able to sit down and enjoy a nutritious meal together.

Physical Activity and Sports Participation

Physical activity is known to have positive effects on mood and depression and can improve symptoms of ADHD (Brown et al. 2013). Playing on a team may also have benefits that go beyond the positive effects of exercise. Participation on a sports team has been found to be linked to less adolescent smoking among teenagers at heightened genetic risk (Audrain-McGovern et al. 2006).

Unfortunately, certain aspects of U.S. culture often conspire to make organized sports more and more challenging to those who may benefit from them the most. As pointed out by Hudziak (2008), twin studies have shown that sports participation is increasingly influenced by genetic factors as one ages. Earlier in childhood, sports participation is explained largely by shared environmental effects, meaning that the family is making a choice about their children's participation. In adolescence, however, genetic effects begin to exert stronger roles. How this phenomenon translates practically is that as children get older, organized sports become more and more the domain of elite athletes, whereas the children who most need to exercise find fewer avenues to do so. Another practical obstacle to regular physical activity is the increasingly popular practice of reducing or eliminating physical activity in the form of recess or physical education during the school day (Barros et al. 2009).

Encouraging more structured sports in addition to regular physical activity can build important skills and attributes such as perseverance, commitment, working as a team, coping with success and defeat, and sacrifice. Structured sports can also provide access to positive role models in the form of coaches. For some children, these experiences become lifelong pursuits that provide scaffolding for socialization and a target for self-fulfillment. Although negative components can also be associated with sports participation, the encouragement of regular physical activity and team sports can help promote what many consider to be a critical element of wellness.

Screen Time and Reading

Children and adolescents spend an astounding amount of time watching television and playing video games. A recent report from the group Common Sense Media documents that present-day American youths spend significantly less time reading compared with youths in previous decades (Common Sense Media 2014). Current recommendations from the American Academy of Pediatrics are that total screen time should be limited to 2 hours per day, on average (American Academy of Pediatrics 2013). Substantial literature shows the link between screen time and negative outcomes, including antisocial behavior, attention problems, and other types of externalizing problems (Strasburger et al. 2010). Concern over screen time generally focuses on the amount of *time* being spent and the opportunities for other pursuits being lost as well as the *content* of what is being viewed or played as inducing anxiety and hypersexual behavior or reinforcing aggressive tendencies. With the advent of smartphones and tablets, children and adolescents now frequently have unfettered access to the Internet in the palms of their hands. These devices present new challenges for parents trying to do their best to limit both the quantity and the type of media being consumed.

One of the frequent victims of increased screen time is reading. A recent report from the group Common Sense Media documents that present-day American youths display a marked reduction in reading time compared with youths in previous decades, with approximately one-third of fourth graders reading at a "below basic" level (Common Sense Media 2014). Regular reading has been linked to a wide range of health outcomes, including improved language development, academic achievement, memory, problem-solving skills, and brain connectivity and reduced stress (Berns et al. 2013). Although some children gravitate toward reading naturally, many others require the encouragement, modeling, and support of parents. One strategy that can work for families is to have children earn their screen time by spending time doing other activities such as reading.

Parenting and Parental Mental Health

Positive parenting involves much more than simply a lack of negative behaviors. Not being negligent or abusive is certainly necessary but hardly sufficient for a child's optimal growth. Rather, positive development involves many other critical elements such as warmth, focused attention, active engagement in a child's life, effective limit setting, and good communication. These factors have been shown to be important in helping typically developing children thrive and are also essential ingredients of family-based approaches for children with emotional-behavioral problems. Maternal warmth, for example, was shown to be a critical factor in reducing relapse in children with bipolar disorder (Geller et al. 2002). Similarly, coaching parents in how to pay active attention to children and how to reinforce positive behaviors is often the founding principle on which parental guidance programs are based, with responses to negative behaviors, such as time-outs, coming later (Forehand and Long 2010). Although it is certainly important to keep in mind that there is no "one size fits all" approach to optimal parenting, a combination of high warmth and effective supervision and limit setting is often a critical combination for many children. This profile has been called the "authoritative style" by Baumrind and Maccoby and Martin (1983).

Being maximally effective as a parent also means that a parent's own mental health is of utmost importance. Substance abuse, depression, ADHD, anxiety, and many other types of psychopathology can affect one's ability to parent maximally, particularly with more challenging children who, partly because of shared genes, may harbor many of the same behavioral challenges. An important study by Weissman and coworkers showed that child behavior can improve when a mother's depression is successfully treated, even without any direct intervention with the child (Weissman et al. 2006).

Unfortunately, the abundance of evidence supporting the need to involve the entire family when working with children with emotional-behavioral problems is in contrast to the very typical practice within child psychotherapy of isolating the child and excluding the parents in treatment (Reiss 2011). Such a technique is often practiced in the name of preserving confidentiality yet has the effect of allowing less optimal parenting practices to persist and to undo gains made in the one-on-one sessions between the child and the therapist. Certainly, the field of psychiatry had its unfortunate era when it seemed like all child behavioral problems were blamed on parents. Now in the age of more "medicalized" treatment, however, the pendulum seems to have swung to the other extreme, with parents often being viewed as almost irrelevant: their behavior an epiphenomenon or a simple reaction to a child's genetically driven tendencies. As psychiatrists increasingly appreciate the bidirectional influences that parents and children have on each other, the ability to engage parents as a critical part of the solution for child psychopathology, whether or not they played a direct role in the problem, will be a vital skill for all clinicians working with youths and families.

Community and Religious Involvements

Children need a sense of belonging and connectedness. Many children are able to get some of these elements from their family. However, many extended families are scattered across wide geographic regions, and children with and without a close-knit family can benefit from being part of larger community groups. The current generation of parents and their children appears to be less oriented toward civic duties and community service than previous generations, and a perhaps related phenomenon is the detectable decline in the current generation's ability to empathize with others (Konrath et al. 2011).

One source of community and feelings of compassion for others is religious groups. Many studies have demonstrated links between improved mental health and being in a religious household, although most of these studies have examined levels of problem behavior rather than wellness per se. Links with reduced aggression, abstaining from substance use, and fewer externalizing problems, among other benefits, have been found (Nonnemaker et al. 2003).

It should be noted that religiosity is not a single construct. Much of the research that links religiosity with positive mental health outcomes relates more to formal attendance and affiliation to organized groups. More private religiosity or a general orientation to spirituality is somewhat distinct and may have different associations with psychopathology (Kendler et al. 2003). Overall, however, the bulk of evidence supports the view that religious affiliation can contribute positively to children's positive mental health.

Obviously, "recommending" religion to families in a clinical appointment can be difficult, although families who are already connected to a positive religious group can be encouraged to get involved and have the children be a part of various activities that are offered. Children and families who are not interested in being part of any organized religious group can also seek out other types of communities and can get involved with many other groups that are devoted to helping others. Beyond the clear benefit to the people they serve, these activities can provide children and adolescents with, at times, some much-needed perspective while also building a sense of compassion and duty.

Mindfulness-Related Practices

The term *mindfulness* refers to a broad group of activities that involves consciously attending to present thoughts and sensations in a nonjudgmental and nonreactive manner. The term encompasses practices anchored in some religions as well as more secular traditions. It includes specific meditation exercises as well as a general state of mind applied in moment-to-moment interactions.

Accumulating research with different models of mindfulness, including mindfulness-based cognitive therapy, has demonstrated the utility of mindfulness in enhancing mental functioning and improving a range of behavioral problems. There is less research on the use of mindfulness in children and adolescents than in adults, but the research that does exist indicates that mindfulness techniques can be very useful for youths, albeit with a smaller effect size (Black et al. 2009).

Music and the Arts

A recent study by Hudziak and colleagues (2014) showed that children who were involved in musical training showed increased cortical thickness in brain areas that have also been implicated in children with attention problems. For many children, artistic pursuits offer an important arena for individual effort, persistence, and creativity, as well as experience with functioning in performance situations. A study looking at the link between singing and well-being demonstrated that similar to the benefits of sports, the positive benefits of singing may be most enjoyed by the "amateurs" rather than those endowed with the most talent and professional potential (Grape et al. 2003). Similarly, other types of artistic expression, such as creative writing, journaling, and visual arts, can provide an important avenue for expression while enhancing qualities of perseverance and teaching children the importance of practice.

Sleep

Although a precise consensus about sleep requirement is lacking, the general thought is that preschool children need between 11 and 12 hours of sleep per night, school-age children need at least 10 hours, and adolescents need between 9 and 10 hours (National Heart, Lung, and Blood Institute 2012). Persistent sleep problems are extremely common, and inadequate sleep has been linked to a number of conditions, including obesity, poor school performance, and behavioral problems in children. Some studies have used designs and analyses that bolster the contention that sleep problems are a true cause, rather than simply an effect, of difficulties such as externalizing problems, particularly for children with certain temperamental predispositions (Goodnight et al. 2007). Research has also shown that many households enact practices that do not enhance sleep, such as having a television or Internet access in the bedroom (American Academy of Pediatrics 2013; Common Sense Media 2014). Thus, it is crucial that clinicians view sleep not only as a symptom of known psychiatric disorders but also as a potential and modifiable cause of overall mental functioning.

In summary, many aspects of wellness have been shown to have implications for helping youths with higher levels of emotional-behavioral problems become less symptomatic and enabling those with less severe difficulties to function at an even higher level. These areas not only contribute to overall well-being but can interact with other dimensions of wellness to create momentum that can flow in both positive and negative directions. The mental health clinician who is able to survey these multiple aspects of wellness and respond in a manner that integrates them with other therapeutic tools at his or her disposal has the best chance of not only helping families overcome the impairment associated with full-fledged psychiatric disorders but also taking them further, from response to remission to wellness. The challenge, then, is having a strategy that allows one to assess these features of positive psychiatry and wellness and bring them into one's scope of everyday practice.

Clinical Application of Positive Child Psychiatry

Incorporating key components of positive psychiatry into one's day-to-day routine can readily be accomplished and does not necessarily require a complete overhaul of standard procedures or entail the abandonment of a careful review of psychiatric symptoms or criteria for specific disorders. For example, our child psychiatry clinic at the Vermont Center for Children, Youth, and Families has adopted many aspects of positive child psychiatry within a model called the Vermont Family Based Approach (VFBA) that was developed by the child psychiatry director, Jim Hudziak. At its core, the VFBA expands the focus of child psychiatry assessment and treatment from illness to wellness and from the individual child to the entire family environment. We try to make an initial assessment of the degree to which a family is able to integrate wellness and health promotion elements into the child's life and, from there, offer monitoring and guidance in these areas as treatment continues. The program can be flexibly applied

by each clinician to suit his or her individual style and emphasis and is implemented by both the patient's child psychiatrist and specific family coaches who
have received additional training in this model. A manual for the approach is
currently in progress, and specific aspects of the model are described in this chapter. In the rest of this section, I discuss the key aspects of the VFBA that may de-
part somewhat from more typical child psychiatry practice.

Assessment of Key Indicators of Child Wellness

An accurate view of many of the previously covered domains of child wellness
requires specific input from both the parents and the child. We have found that
the most effective and comprehensive method to obtain this information is the
use of both informal and more established questionnaires that are sent to families for completion prior to an initial outpatient child psychiatry evaluation.
These questions and other components of a typical psychiatric evaluation are
combined into an instrument called the Vermont Health and Behavior Questionnaire (Hudziak 2008). Areas of investigation include child involvement with
sports and other structured activities, amount of various types of screen time,
degree of family structure and stability, sleep, eating habits, child self-esteem,
level of family conflict and cohesion, parenting practices, and life satisfaction.
This questionnaire is combined with behavioral rating scales such as the Child
Behavior Checklist, Teacher Report Form, and Youth Self-Report (Achenbach
2001), which provide us with a multi-informant view of the child's behavior that
is quantitative and standardized according to age, sex, and culture along multiple
empirically defined dimensions. These questionnaires are returned and scored
before the visit so that they are available to the assessing clinician at the evaluation
and can be reviewed with the family.

A more unique component of the VFBA that is consistent with our emphasis
on overall wellness is the provision to have self- and partner-reported behavioral
assessment questionnaires that pertain to the *parents*. The primary reason for this
additional step is not to provide a more accurate diagnosis of the child (which is
often the main rationale for obtaining a family history of mental health problems)
but to identify emotional-behavioral problems in the parents that may be affecting the entire family environment and might respond to focused interventions,
to the benefit of all family members.

Talking to Families About Wellness and Health Promotion

The wealth of questionnaire information is reviewed by the family coach or
child psychiatrist performing the assessment and is incorporated into an evaluation that lasts at least two sessions and contains all the standard elements of

a typical assessment. Like most evaluations, the evaluation typically concludes with the clinician providing feedback about the findings and a synthesis of his or her impressions, as well as a discussion of possible treatment strategies, if appropriate. In addition to a diagnostic formulation, the clinician conveys the findings obtained with regard to aspects related to the child's strengths, family functioning, and the degree of incorporation of health promotion activities.

An essential but often overlooked aspect of standard child psychiatry treatment relates to an exploration of and discussion among the clinician, child, and parents about what true optimal mental health in the identified patient might look like. All too often, this critical question has been buried as families work hard to overcome crises and seek relief from the pain of various types of symptoms. Although the focus on crises is understandable, discussions about wellness can be invaluable in helping both children and families reframe their goals in more positive terms. They can also reveal areas where the child and the parent have significantly different points of view as a result of temperamental mismatch or other factors. For example, a child might sincerely be content with having a strong connection with a few close friends, whereas a parent might express concern that the child is not generally more popular.

The specifics of how the major findings of an evaluation are conveyed to families is somewhat individualized according to each clinician, although efforts are being made to develop a more structured discussion with the family called the Family Assessment and Feedback Intervention (Ivanova 2013). The goal of this feedback component is not only to provide the important clinical information sought by the family but also to deliver it within a perspective of overall family wellness and to try and motivate the family to take some of the difficult steps that may be required by multiple family members to change a child's more troubled trajectory.

When it comes to discussions about parenting, we have certainly observed that the subject needs to be approached with skill and sensitivity. Many parents bringing their children to treatment already harbor significant guilt that they are responsible for their child's negative behavior but at the same time can become quite defensive at any implication that their parenting skills need some enhancements. Sensing this tension, clinicians can be tempted to fall back on more biological theories and approaches that do not directly target parental behavior. Time and scheduling constraints can also conspire to minimize sessions with parents and push discussions toward less uncomfortable areas such as medication side effects or school performance.

In our clinic's work with parents and parenting, we have found that certain tips and techniques can be helpful in promoting an alliance with families and moving conversations forward in a productive fashion. These tips are summarized in Table 14–2 and involve specific ways to phrase parenting questions, how causes of child behavior are articulated, and how the clinician positions himself or herself as the "expert." For example, one perspective that has proven to be very useful clinically is to reframe the notion that a "bad" parent causes negative child behavior or, conversely, that a "bad" child simply pushes other people's buttons by instead talking about the importance of the parental *override* (Rettew 2013). In this model, a child's behavior can be thought to "create its own weather" and evoke particular responses from parents and other aspects of the environment. However, the parent's response is vital to whether or not the behavior escalates. Although particular responses may be quite natural and understandable (such as reacting with hostility to an irritable child), the ability of a parent to override that response and react in a different way can mean the difference between a minor outburst and a complete behavioral meltdown.

A similarly sensitive topic relates to the parent's own emotional-behavioral wellness. As mentioned, direct assessment of parental psychopathology using standardized instruments is now a part of all of our child psychiatry evaluations. Initial analyses indicate that these instruments reveal quite a bit of parental psychopathology that otherwise would have been missed (Basoglu et al. 2014). The results of these instruments are then shared with the parents, usually without the child being present. Parents frequently seem unsurprised to learn that they themselves struggle with their own mental health disorders, especially if these problems are discussed in a supportive and nonjudgmental manner. Many parents are motivated to work toward improvement not only for their own sake but, primarily, to improve the lives of their children. A frequent challenge is then to find a setting where further evaluation and treatment can take place, given the national shortage of adult mental health professionals. One recent innovation in our clinic has been to offer a parent clinic within the child psychiatry division as a place where the parents of our child patients can been seen and treated according to principles of the family-based approach.

Positive Psychiatry in Ongoing Care

Once the assessment and initial treatment recommendations have been accomplished, it is important to maintain the inclusion of positive psychiatry elements within the overall treatment plan. This goal can be achieved through a variety of means. In our clinic, many of our patients and their parents work with a family coach in addition to seeing a child psychiatrist. For other patients, the child psychiatrist assumes a larger role in ensuring that health promotion activities remain an important focus of intervention. Some clinicians use a more formal approach, with patients and families completing and bringing in monitoring forms related to the amount time being spent on an encouraged activity (e.g., music practice, exercise, reading), with specific "prescriptions" in these areas being written as homework. For others, these factors are addressed more informally, although they remain in the forefront of a comprehensive strategy. Social

Table 14–2. Techniques for improving alliance in discussions of parenting

Evaluation questions

1. As a standard part of the interview, query parents about which parenting practices seem to be going well and which areas may need some improvement. Phrasing the question this way assumes that all parents are doing some things well but are struggling in other areas and conveys that the clinician is not singling them out for this line of questioning.

2. Use questionnaires regarding parenting and family environment that allow the clinician to respond to the parent's own words and ratings.

Framing child behavior

1. Explicitly articulate the belief that parenting is difficult and is even more so when a child has behavioral challenges.

2. Acknowledge that parental behavior is frequently evoked by a child and that the parental response, although perhaps not optimal, is certainly natural and understandable.

3. Invoke genetics as a way to help parents understand that both parent and child may possess similar behavioral dispositions that can serve to amplify both negative and positive interactions.

Parental guidance and coaching

1. Consider teaching principles such as helping a parent override suboptimal responses that can be triggered by children.

2. Remember to honor the parent's status as the person who knows the child the best and what may be in his or her best interests.

3. Convey a certain amount of humility in your role as the parental authority and acknowledge your own imperfections and struggles.

work and case management help can be invaluable to help mobilize resources for families with financial hardship.

Our clinic is also piloting innovative programs that emphasize and promote wellness, such as matching patients with sports mentors and creating parallel groups for children and parents during which a child receives musical training while parents attend a parent behavioral management group. Some of these projects are part of research studies, whereas others represent partnerships with community organizations.

Clearly, many paths can be taken to operationalize a model that embraces positive psychiatry and wellness within the context of child psychiatry. What seems most critical at this point is a perspective that looks beyond traditional psychotherapy and medication treatment as the only routes to recovery and tries to inspire families to prioritize health promotion as part of an overall clinical plan. At the same time, psychiatrists need to be cognizant of their duty as scientists to think critically about their interventions and to look for evidence that supports the added value of these components.

To illustrate how the addition of positive psychiatry can be incorporated within a child psychiatry evaluation, consider the following (composite) vignette.

Clinical Vignette

Ethan is a 10-year-old boy who presents to a child psychiatry clinic because his parents are concerned about a possible diagnosis of ADHD. His mother reports that Ethan does not follow directions at home and that he only seems to "listen" when they yell. He is constantly losing things and cannot keep track of time. There are multiple arguments a day over reasonable limit setting. The school has also noticed difficulty with focus, finishing tasks, and distractibility, although they do not see the degree of oppositionality noted at home. His teacher further notes that Ethan's reading ability seems to be dropping compared with that of his peers.

A standard evaluation focuses on symptoms and, specifically, the criteria for ADHD. Other required elements such as past psychiatric and medical history are also investigated. From this perspective, Ethan does not meet enough ADHD criteria to merit a formal diagnosis, and his family is informed of this outcome and reassured, only to return years later after Ethan's situation has drastically deteriorated.

A broader focus at the initial evaluation that incorporates a positive psychiatry perspective includes queries into many other areas that are important for wellness and health promotion. In this scenario, the clinician learns that Ethan spends about 4 hours per day playing video games and has pulled out of nearly all structured activities. Ethan is rarely physically active. Often, he stays up late into the night playing games on a video console in his room. Because the morning is often so disorganized and rushed, he often skips breakfast. A quantitative assessment of Ethan's level of emotional-behavioral problems reveals that his level of attention problems is around the ninetieth percentile for boys his age. A similar assessment of the parents reveals that Ethan's father may have clinical levels of attention problems and his mother struggles with depression and anxiety.

With such a broad scope of information about so many aspects of Ethan's life and family environment combined with knowledge about where Ethan is on the dimension of attention problems compared with his peers, the clinician now has a number of places to intervene in an effort not only to provide a relief of symptoms but also to help improve the family environment and reengage Ethan into his life. Knowing that Ethan's symptoms are not particularly extreme, the psychiatrist could well decide to hold off on medications, at least in the short term, while concentrating on many areas of Ethan's life that may be contributing to his overall downward trajectory. In Ethan's case, a regular bedtime routine and the removal of the video game system in his room, a policy of earning screen time by reading, a good daily breakfast, regular exercise, and participation in structured activities such as music training, as well as parenting guidance techniques for more effective limit setting, could well be expected to go a long way in improving Ethan's and his family's life together. Referral for the parents for their own possible psychopathology may also significantly reduce tension and provide for more opportunities for positive interactions.

Six months later, Ethan remains somewhat more hyperactive and distractible than most of his peers but is doing much better after some initial resistance to the "new rules." He is not taking medication, although his father now is and notices that his patience with Ethan is much improved. After being told that he had a choice as to what he activity he wanted to do but was required to do something, Ethan now plays basketball and does Tae Kwon Do. The family finds time to sit down together for a quick breakfast each day.

This example illustrates that attention to domains of positive psychiatry and wellness can provide a clinician with many more places to intervene and ways to encourage a family. Through these efforts, energy can be generated that not only stops more problematic trajectories but, in many cases, also reverses a patient's direction and builds positive momentum that enables patients to lead happier and more fulfilling lives.

Education and Training in Positive Psychiatry

It is difficult to imagine how psychiatrists will successfully redefine themselves as leaders in true mental health and wellness without a concerted effort to incorporate positive psychiatry within formal psychiatry residency and fellowship training programs. To date, the vast majority of psychiatric training is devoted to the assessment and treatment of mental disorders, with little time allocated to promoting optimal mental health.

Education of psychiatric trainees occurs through many venues; the most prominent of those include didactic sessions, reading, observation, and supervised clinical experiences. For there to be a substantial shift in perspective of the field, I submit that all of these methodologies need to contain some elements of positive psychiatry. At a recent conference of the American Association of Directors in Psychiatric Residency Training, my colleagues and I unveiled a new didactic seminar in positive child psychiatry that will be given to our incoming class of child psychiatrists (Rettew et al. 2014). Proposed topics for the course are shown in Table 14–3 and reflect many of the chapters contained in this volume. The areas covered include happiness, love, positive parenting, and the neurobiology of wellness. Most of these topics, as well as many others, are also applicable to general residency training programs. The Positive Psychology Center at the University of Pennsylvania (www.ppc.sas.upenn.edu) posts teaching resources online, including full syllabi for educators looking to create and adapt content for their own institution.

Outside of didactic teaching, trainees need to absorb an emphasis on wellness and health promotion that is present among faculty. More formally, these principles need to be discussed in psychotherapy supervision and reinforced

Table 14–3.   Potential topics for a psychiatry residency or fellowship
                 course on positive psychiatry

Topic	Subtopics
Mental wellness	Definitions Components of wellness
Continuum of behavior	Defining boundary of illness Overlap with temperament or personality traits
History of positive psychiatry	Parallels to positive psychology Major thought leaders over time
Happiness	"Pursuit" of happiness Happiness versus fulfillment
Positive traits	Empathy Regulatory skills Executive function
Neurobiology of wellness	Brain imaging studies Genetic influences Common links between psychiatric and nonpsychiatric illness
Resilience	Characteristics associated with resilience Teaching resilience
Religions and spirituality	Differences between religiosity and spirituality Associations with suicide and depression
Mindfulness in psychiatry	Mindfulness-based cognitive therapy Evidence for mindfulness Practice and mindfulness workshop
Positive parenting	Types of parenting styles Secure attachment Parenting controversies and evidence
Prevention of psychiatric disorders	Previous prevention trials for at-risk populations Mental health "checkups"
Love	Why topic is often not discussed Definition Relevance in psychiatry
Applying positive psychiatry to practice	Assessment within evaluations Discussing wellness with families Applications for ongoing care

when trainees present case formulations and treatment plans. Written notes and evaluations need to contain plans that demonstrate that trainees are thinking about wellness in their patients and are communicating the principles of health promotion effectively. Furthermore, medical students, residents, and fellows also need to be taught how to use the various tools available to them to assess wellness as well as how to interact with many non–medically trained professionals (social workers, coaches, teachers) who are skilled at enriching the lives of children and their families.

Specific evaluation components that measure how well students are mastering positive psychiatry in their learning could be developed. Unfortunately, proponents of positive psychiatry missed an opportunity to incorporate these principles into the new psychiatry milestones, a set of specified knowledge, skills, and attitudes in different areas that are now the new standards that will be used to assess all psychiatric residents (Accreditation Council for Graduate Medical Education 2013). The new child psychiatry milestones do contain some wellness items, and regardless, many of the milestones are sufficiently broad that they could be interpreted to include positive psychiatry elements. Further, there is nothing to prevent training programs from requiring competency in positive psychiatry and assessing it directly.

Summary

Child psychiatrists are frequently touted as exerts in mental health, yet in reality their training and practice is much more narrowly focused on mental illness. Such an orientation needs to change if child psychiatrists are going to be able to utilize the increasing compelling literature that demonstrates that 1) most symptoms of child psychopathology exist dimensionally and on a continuum with wellness and 2) various domains of wellness and health promotion, including positive parenting, sleep, nutrition, exercise, and mindfulness practices, can have important benefits for children who struggle with or who are at risk for emotional-behavioral problems. These aspects of positive psychiatry need to be systematically incorporated into child psychiatry evaluations and ongoing care. By doing so, clinicians can identify many more avenues for intervention and improvement beyond the traditional methods of individual psychotherapy and psychopharmacology. The training of the next generation of child psychiatrists needs to reflect these advances in positive psychiatry in order for this field to evolve and be most beneficial to patients.

Clinical Key Points

- Despite the ubiquitous use of the term "mental health," child psychiatrists spend the vast majority of their training focusing on mental illness.

- Research increasingly indicates that most types of clinical symptoms and disorders exist on a broad continuum that spans wellness and illness.

- Many elements of wellness, including exercise, nutrition, the arts, and mindfulness, have been shown to improve mental functioning and improve psychiatric symptoms.

- Incorporating wellness and health promotion more fully into child psychiatric care can be readily accomplished in day-to-day practice.

- The training of new child psychiatrists must include additional education on the domains of positive psychiatry and wellness.

References

Accreditation Council for Graduate Medical Education: The Psychiatry Milestone Project. November 2013. Available at: http://www.acgme.org/acgmeweb/Portals/0/PDFs/Milestones/PsychiatryMilestones.pdf. Accessed August 27, 2014.

Achenbach TMRLA: Manual for the ASEBA School-Age Forms and Profiles. Burlington, University of Vermont Research Center for Children, Youth, and Families, 2001

American Academy of Child and Adolescent Psychiatry: American Academy of Child and Adolescent Psychiatry Web site. 2014. Available at: http://www.aacap.org/. Accessed August 27, 2014.

American Academy of Pediatrics: Children, adolescents, and the media. Pediatrics 132:958–961, 2013

Audrain-McGovern J, Rodriguez D, Wileyto EP, et al: Effect of team sport participation on genetic predisposition to adolescent smoking progression. Arch Gen Psychiatry 63(4):433–441, 2006 16585473

Barros RM, Silver EJ, Stein RE: School recess and group classroom behavior. Pediatrics 123(2):431–436, 2009 19171606

Basoglu F, Rettew DC, Hudziak JJ: How much parental psychopathology is missed during standard child psychiatry evaluations? Poster presented at the 61st annual meeting of the American Academy of Child and Adolescent Psychiatry, San Diego CA, October 2014

Beck JS: Cognitive Behavior Therapy: Basics and Beyond. New York, Guilford, 2011

Berns GS, Blaine K, Prietula MJ, et al: Short- and long-term effects of a novel on connectivity in the brain. Brain Connect 3(6):590–600, 2013 23988110

Black DS, Milam J, Sussman S: Sitting-meditation interventions among youth: a review of treatment efficacy. Pediatrics 124(3):e532–e541, 2009 19706568

Brown HE, Pearson N, Braithwaite RE, et al: Physical activity interventions and depression in children and adolescents: a systematic review and meta-analysis. Sports Med 43(3):195–206, 2013 23329611

Common Sense Media: Children, teens, and reading: a common sense media brief. 2014. Available at: https://www.commonsensemedia.org/research/children-teens-and-reading. Accessed August 27, 2014.

Constantino JN, Todd RD: Autistic traits in the general population: a twin study. Arch Gen Psychiatry 60(5):524–530, 2003 12742874

Forehand RL, Long N: Parenting the Strong Willed Child. New York, McGraw-Hill, 2010

Geller B, Craney JL, Bolhofner K, et al: Two-year prospective follow-up of children with a prepubertal and early adolescent bipolar disorder phenotype. Am J Psychiatry 159(6):927–933, 2002 12042179

Goodnight JA, Bates JE, Staples AD, et al: Temperamental resistance to control increases the association between sleep problems and externalizing behavior development. J Fam Psychol 21(1):39–48, 2007 17371108

Grape C, Sandgren M, Hansson LO, et al: Does singing promote well-being? An empirical study of professional and amateur singers during a singing lesson. Integr Physiol Behav Sci 38(1):65–74, 2003 12814197

Hettema JM, Neale MC, Myers JM, et al: A population-based twin study of the relationship between neuroticism and internalizing disorders. Am J Psychiatry 163(5):857–864, 2006 16648327

Hudziak JJ: Genetic and environmental influences on wellness, resilience, and psychopathology: a family based approach for promotion, prevention, and intervention, in Developmental Psychopathology and Wellness: Genetic and Environmental Influences. Edited by Hudziak JJ. Washington, DC, American Psychiatric Publishing, 2008, pp 267–286

Hudziak JJ, Albaugh MD, Ducharme S, et al: Cortical thickness maturation and duration of music training: health-promoting activities shape brain development. J Am Acad Child Adolesc Psychiatry 53(11):1153–1161, 2014 25440305

Ivanova M: Family Assessment and Feedback Intervention (FAFI): A Training Manual. Burlington, University of Vermont, Department of Psychiatry, 2013

Jacka FN, Ystrom E, Brantsaeter AL, et al: Maternal and early postnatal nutrition and mental health of offspring by age 5 years: a prospective cohort study. J Am Acad Child Adolesc Psychiatry 52(10):1038–1047, 2013 24074470

Kendler KS, Liu XQ, Gardner CO, et al: Dimensions of religiosity and their relationship to lifetime psychiatric and substance use disorders. Am J Psychiatry 160(3):496–503, 2003 12611831

Konrath SH, O'Brien EH, Hsing C: Changes in dispositional empathy in American college students over time: a meta-analysis. Pers Soc Psychol Rev 15(2):180–198, 2011 20688954

Maccoby EE, Martin JA: Socialization in the context of the family: parent-child interaction, in Handbook of Child Psychology, 4th Edition, Vol 4. Edited by Mussen PH. New York, Wiley, 1983, pp 1–101

National Heart, Lung, and Blood Institute: How much sleep is enough? February 2012. Available at: http://www.nhlbi.nih.gov/health/health-topics/topics/sdd/howmuch.html. Accessed July 2, 2014

Nonnemaker JM, McNeely CA, Blum RW; National Longitudinal Study of Adolescent Health: Public and private domains of religiosity and adolescent health risk behaviors: evidence from the National Longitudinal Study of Adolescent Health. Soc Sci Med 57(11):2049–2054, 2003 14512236

Polderman TJ, Derks EM, Hudziak JJ, et al: Across the continuum of attention skills: a twin study of the SWAN ADHD rating scale. J Child Psychol Psychiatry 48(11):1080–1087, 2007 17995483

Reiss D: Parents and children: linked by psychopathology but not by clinical care. J Am Acad Child Adolesc Psychiatry 50(5):431–434, 2011 21515190

Rettew DC: Temperament: risk and protective factors for child psychiatric disorders, in Comprehensive Textbook of Psychiatry, 9th Edition, Vol 2. Edited by Sadock BJ, Sadock VA, Ruiz P. Philadelphia, PA, Lippincott, Williams & Wilkins, 2009, pp 3432–3443

Rettew DC: Child Temperament: New Thinking About the Boundary Between Traits and Illness. New York, WW Norton, 2013

Rettew DC, Althoff RR, Hudziak JJ: Happy kids: teaching trainees about emotional-behavioral wellness, not just illness. Poster presented at the 43rd Annual Conference of the American Association of Directors in Psychiatric Residency Training, Tucson, AZ, March 12–15, 2014

Seligman MEP: Flourish: A Visionary New Understanding of Happiness and Well-Being. New York, Free Press, 2011

Strasburger VC, Jordan AB, Donnerstein E: Health effects of media on children and adolescents. Pediatrics 125(4):756–767, 2010 20194281

Weissman MM, Pilowsky DJ, Wickramaratne PJ, et al; STAR*D-Child Team: Remissions in maternal depression and child psychopathology: a STAR*D-child report. JAMA 295(12):1389–1398, 2006 16551710

Suggested Cross-References

Sleep is discussed in Chapter 11 ("Preventive Interventions") and Chapter 12 ("Integrating Positive Psychiatry Into Clinical Practice"). Nutrition is discussed in Chapter 12.

15

Positive Geriatric and Cultural Psychiatry

MARÍA J. MARQUINE, PH.D.

ZVINKA Z. ZLATAR, PH.D.

DANIEL D. SEWELL, M.D.

The U.S. population is becoming increasingly older and more diverse. Aging is usually accompanied by declines in physical and mental abilities, and ethnic and racial minorities tend to be disadvantaged in terms of income, education, and access to care. Thus, both older adults and ethnic and racial minorities represent vulnerable segments of the population. Identifying ways to foster positive mental health among these groups is increasingly important in efforts to improve the nation's mental health.

In the first part of this chapter, we discuss well-being in older age and the associated concept of *successful aging,* as well as positive psychological traits and their role in promoting successful aging. Ongoing scientific research suggests that these positive traits and the development of interventions that bolster them have the potential to reduce the current and future burden of mental and physical health problems in older persons in the United States and the world. In the second portion of this chapter, we summarize what is currently known about achieving

This work was supported, in part, by National Institutes of Health grant T32 MH019934 and by the University of California, San Diego Center for Healthy Aging and Sam and Rose Stein Institute for Research on Aging.

successful mental health outcomes in the two largest racial and ethnic minorities in the United States while keeping in mind that the key factors that lead to positive mental health may vary among and within ethnic and racial groups. Two clinical vignettes have been included to highlight how increasing understanding of successful aging may have immediate and practical clinical benefits.

Older Adults

Older Adults in the United States

Data from the 2010 U.S. census show that there were 40 million adults 65 years and older in 2010, representing 13% of the overall U.S. population. It is estimated that by 2030, one in every five Americans will be older than 65. Furthermore, the number of older adults living in the United States will more than double by 2050, reaching approximately 89 million and composing 20% of the population (Figure 15–1). This exponential growth in the number and proportion of older adults in the United States is unprecedented in the history of this country and reflects a broader worldwide phenomenon that will spawn many health care–related challenges. Aging is usually accompanied by declines in physical and mental abilities that affect various domains of function and quality of life; thus, as the world ages, it will be imperative for health care professionals to identify factors that foster well-being and quality of life in older adults and to develop interventions that take into account these important concepts.

Positive Psychiatry of Aging

Health care–related challenges associated with unparalleled growth in older population brackets include increasing numbers of older adults with mental illness. The number of older individuals living with serious mental illness is expected to triple over the next 25 years. Although much of the research in old age psychiatry has focused on mental illness, recently, a call has been made for the development of a new positive psychiatry of aging that focuses "not simply on symptom relief, but on recovery and promotion of successful ageing" (Jeste and Palmer 2013, p. 81). This movement is part of a large and growing idea that health care professionals should not only recognize and treat symptoms but also promote well-being. For old age psychiatry, this idea translates into a focus on successful aging. To date, no clear consensus on a single definition of successful aging exists. Health care professionals, however, are increasingly aware that subjective (self-report) assessments of successful aging or well-being in older age provide meaningful and valuable information above and beyond the perspective obtained from objective evaluation instruments that quantify physical, cognitive, and social disability.

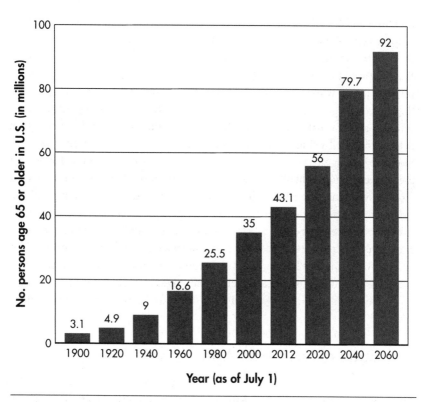

FIGURE 15–1. Number of persons age 65 or older in the United States from 1900 to 2060 (in millions).

Source. Reprinted from Administration on Aging: Future Growth, December 2012. Available at: http://www.aoa.gov/Aging_Statistics/Profile/2013/4.aspx. Original source is U.S. Census Bureau, Population Estimates and Projections.

If *successful aging* is defined as the lack of physical and cognitive disability, older adults, as a group, tend to fare worse than their younger counterparts. It is well known that as people age, they are more likely to experience a number of medical conditions, such as heart disease, stroke, arthritis, and chronic pain. Similarly, although certain cognitive abilities (e.g., vocabulary and world knowledge) tend to improve with age, most cognitive functions (e.g., processing speed, attention, learning, and memory) tend to decline. When they become pronounced, these declines in physical and cognitive abilities cause clinically significant functional losses and result in dementia. Despite this inverse association between increasing age and decreasing physical and cognitive functioning, older adults tend to report higher levels of well-being than do younger adults, suggesting that life satisfaction and general well-being do not necessarily decease with age and might even increase. For example, a study examining change in life satisfaction over a period of 8 years in 899 older adults between ages 62 and 95 found increases in life satisfaction, even after taking into account important demo-graphic factors and self-perceived health (Gana et al. 2013). Similarly, another study of community-dwelling older adults showed that most older adults believe that they are aging successfully (Jeste et al. 2013). Even older adults with chronic physical illness who would not meet objective disability-based criteria perceive themselves as aging successfully (Strawbridge et al. 2002). Taken together, these findings suggest that factors other than physical functioning play a key role in determining well-being in older age and in an individual's perception of whether he or she is aging successfully. Importantly, evidence also indicates that factors that predict well-being might differ by age group. For example, Hamarat and colleagues (2001) investigated the relationship between perceived stress and coping ability in relation to life satisfaction across different age groups. Perceived stress was found to be a better predictor of life satisfaction for younger adults, and coping resource effectiveness was a better predictor of life satisfaction for middle-age and older adults. These findings highlight the importance of studying well-being and sat-isfaction with life separately at different life stages to avoid erroneous assump-tions that might occur from applying findings from younger groups to older adults.

Predictors of Successful Aging

Are there any identified predictors of successful aging or well-being in older adults? Although research in this area remains scarce, using empirical methods to derive a dimensional model of successful aging, Vahia and colleagues (2012) identified various domains of aging that appeared to influence successful aging. These do-mains included physical, emotional and mental, and psychosocial protective fac-tors. Resilience, a personality characteristic that moderates the negative effects of stress and negative experiences and promotes adaptation to new challenges, is emerging as one of the key psychosocial protective factors. At least some aspects of resilience have been found to be higher in older adults compared with younger persons. For example, older adults have been found to be more resilient with re-spect to emotional regulation ability and problem solving but less resilient with respect to resilience based on social support (Gooding et al. 2012). Resilience in older adults has been associated with better physical and mental health, and it may also play a role in the recovery from physical injury, counteracting the nega-tive effects of illness, and reducing mortality. Furthermore, the effects of resilience on successful aging seem to be comparable to the effects of physical health on suc-cessful aging (Jeste and Palmer 2013), highlighting the importance of resilience in promoting successful aging. It is important to note that the association between resilience and indicators of successful aging appears to be present even in the more vulnerable segments of the older adult population, such as those with lower income and living in rural communities.

Contributors to resilience in older persons are likely to be multifactorial and have not yet been fully elucidated. Importantly, age might affect not only levels of resilience but also which factors might be most important in promoting it. Some factors, such as perceptions of poor health, low energy, and increased hopelessness, have been associated with low levels of resilience regardless of age, whereas mental illness and physical dysfunction are particularly predictive in older adults (Gooding et al. 2012). The potential for age to be associated with differences in resilience factors was confirmed by a study of 1,395 community-dwelling women older than 60 that found that the factors underlying a resilience scale were somewhat different from those previously reported among younger adults (Lamond et al. 2008). Findings such as these highlight that different psychological processes may underlie resilience at different ages.

Although much work still needs to be done to identify key correlates of resilience among older adults, social (Lamond et al. 2008) and spiritual support are two such factors that have consistently been associated with increased resilience. For example, characteristics that have been labeled "social connectedness," "a head-on approach to challenge," and "spiritual grounding" are salient to resilience in older women. The study by Lamond and colleagues (2008) also found various correlates of resilience, including social engagement, emotional well-being, fewer cognitive complaints, optimism, and self-rated successful aging. A longitudinal study of 3,581 British participants older than 50 showed that participants with high social support preadversity and during adversity had a 40%–60% increased likelihood of resilience compared with those with low social support (Netuveli et al. 2008).

Although *spirituality* is emerging as a *tool* by which persons promote and maintain resilience in later life, which leads to increased well-being, it has also been posited as an important *predictor* of well-being in older age, independent of the effect of other factors. For example, Lawler-Row and Elliott (2009) found that spiritual well-being and prayer contributed to the prediction of psychological well-being, subjective well-being, physical symptoms, and depression, even when the contributions of age, gender, healthy behaviors, and social support were taken into account (Lawler-Row and Elliott 2009).

Another important predictor of successful aging and well-being in older adults is *optimism*. In a population-based study conducted in Britain, optimism predicted quality of life over a period of 7–8 years above the effect of biomedical factors (Bowling and Iliffe 2011). Interestingly, optimism appears to affect objective physical functioning as well as subjective well-being. For example, Brenes et al. (2002) found that optimism was associated with walking performance after controlling for demographic and health variables in a group of 488 community-dwelling older adults with knee pain. Perhaps more importantly, optimism predicts subjective physical functioning better than objective physical functioning does in older adults. A longitudinal study over 6 months that included 309 older adults (ages 65–85) with multiple medical problems found that health-specific optimism partially explained the relationship between fitness and perceived physical functioning and that health-specific optimism predicted perceived physical functioning better than did objective physical functioning. Some of the mechanisms by which optimism may affect well-being in older age include increased meaning in life, social support, and self-efficacy.

Another important predictor of successful aging and well-being in older age is engagement in *leisure-time activities*. Leisure activities include physical activity and exercise and cognitive, artistic, and social engagement. Participation in regular physical activities that decrease sedentary time has emerged as an important preventive strategy against cognitive decline as well as a method to reduce symptoms of depression and improve cardiovascular health in older adults. Simple walking interventions have shown that physical activity leads to brain changes that support more efficient cognitive functioning (Colcombe et al. 2006). Moreover, cognitive engagement that challenges the brain to learn something new is also important in maintaining brain health and well-being in late life (Park et al. 2014). Similarly, participating in social events such as attending church, choir singing, and interacting with others through art has been associated with successful aging and well-being. For example, women who participate in the Red Hat Society, a leisure organization for elderly women, have reported multiple psychosocial health benefits from their involvement in that organization, including creating happy moments, responding to transitions and negative events, and enhancing the self, all of which lead to increased well-being (Son et al. 2007).

For the purpose of clarity, we have attempted to present findings investigating predictors of successful aging or well-being in older age in a simple and systematic fashion. It is important, however, to bear in mind that other factors may play a role and the associations among these elements are likely to be quite complex. For example, a number of studies posit that perception of control or self-efficacy might have an important role in explaining the association between optimism and well-being; however, the nature of these associations is not clear. Some studies find that optimism affects well-being independently of and in addition to the effect of self-efficacy, and some indicate that self-efficacy plays a mediating role, whereas others find that self-efficacy modifies the association between optimism and well-being, such that optimism affects well-being only in those with low self-efficacy. Although clinical researchers in the field of successful aging and health care professionals are still far from understanding these complex associations and how they affect well-being and life satisfaction in older age, the current state of knowledge indicates that scientists must continue to investigate the complexity and multidirectionality of the associations among these factors. With a better understanding of these concepts and their associations, health care professionals can begin to develop appropriate interventions that bolster resilience, optimism, social support, spirituality, and leisure time activities to ultimately improve the quality of life of older adults and potentially prevent mental and physical problems that accompany the aging process.

Clinical Vignette

Leila, a 73-year-old woman from a rural town in the southern region of the United States, presents to her mental health professional with complaints of depression and debilitating diabetic neuropathy. Leila is a full-time caregiver for her husband of 45 years, who now has moderate Alzheimer's disease. She reports that she is unable to find respite and feels it is hard for her to get out of bed in the morning because she feels hopeless about her future and the health of her husband. Her social circle is very limited, and she has no family members nearby to help her care for her husband. From a successful aging perspective, treatment of Leila would consist of not only prescribing medication for her depression and neuropathic pain but also bolstering her quality of life by increasing her social support. Her treatment includes increasing social support to have an alternative caregiver for her husband a couple of times per week, so that she can attend bingo night at her local community center (which she reported is an activity she really enjoys). Attending bingo night serves not only as respite from caregiving duties but also as an opportunity to socialize and make new friends. Leila also loves to paint, so part of her treatment plan is to schedule a biweekly afternoon for painting while her husband takes a nap. To aid in decreasing her depression and chronic pain, daily 20-minute walks with her husband are scheduled, which will have beneficial effects not only for Leila but also for her husband, because structured activities have been found to be helpful for individuals living with moderate Alzheimer's disease. After 4 months of treatment, during which the goals were gradually achieved, Leila reports that she has found a "new purpose in life" and has made new friends who are supportive and have helped her feel as though she is "not alone anymore." "My life has changed drastically. Even though the pain is still there and my caregiving duties remain a major part of my life, my quality of life has improved thanks to the support I am receiving from my friends. Doing fun activities makes me feel good about myself and gives me a sense of purpose."

Racial and Ethnic Minorities

Although there are a number of racial and ethnic minorities in the United States, each facing unique challenges, in this chapter we focus on achieving successful mental health outcomes, which is a central part of successful aging, in the two largest racial and ethnic minority groups in the United States, namely, Hispanics/Latinos and blacks/African Americans. "Hispanic or Latino origin," as ascertained by the 2010 U.S. Census Bureau, refers to persons of Cuban, Mexican, Puerto Rican, South or Central American, or other Spanish culture regardless of race. Thus, Hispanics can be of any race. "Black" or "African American" refers to a person who has origins in any of the black racial groups of Africa. (In this chapter the terms "black" or "African American" are used interchangeably to describe a person with origins in any of the black racial groups of Africa.)

Although these ethnic and racial groups have important differences, which might affect the nature and predictors of positive mental health outcomes, both Hispanics and African Americans tend to have lower incomes, higher poverty rates, and lower rates of health insurance compared with non-Hispanic whites. Thus, they represent segments of the U.S. population that are vulnerable to poor mental health outcomes. The key factors that enhance well-being and lead to positive mental health might vary among ethnic and racial groups given the differing life experiences and vulnerabilities among minority groups. Identifying ways to foster positive mental health is particularly important among these groups and may also yield information that could benefit older individuals who are not members of these ethnic and racial groups.

Hispanics

Hispanics in the United States

Hispanics are the largest minority group in the United States. In 2012, there were 53 million Hispanics living in the United States, representing 17% of the general population, and it is expected that by 2060 Hispanics will make up a third of the U.S. population (U.S. Census Bureau 2012) (Figure 15–2). When studying Hispanics in the United States, researchers should bear in mind that there is significant diversity among Hispanics because they vary in a number of characteristics, including country of origin or descent, language use, race, and immigration history. These variations between and within Hispanic subgroups might affect both positive mental health outcomes and their predictors. Nevertheless, it is also important to recognize that most Hispanics share certain cultural values, such as familism (key role of the family) and collectivism (importance placed on the group rather than the individual). The Spanish language and the immigrant experience are also other common bonds. To understand mental health outcomes and predictors, it is important to keep in mind both the shared and the unique experiences of different subgroups of Hispanics.

Hispanic Paradox

Compared with other ethnic and racial groups, Hispanics, as a group, tend to have lower socioeconomic status and other adverse social circumstances and thus, not surprisingly, tend to have higher rates of some chronic medical conditions, such as diabetes and obesity. However, Hispanics also tend to fare better with regard to other health outcomes, such as birth and mortality rates, a trend that has been referred to as the *Hispanic paradox*. In fact, in the United States, Hispanics are the group with the longest approximate life expectancy at birth (81 years) when they are compared with non-Hispanic whites (79 years) and non-

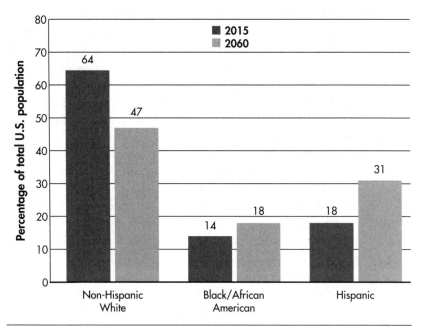

FIGURE 15–2. Population by race and Hispanic origin: 2015 and 2060 (percent of total population).

Source. Based on U.S. Census Bureau data: "Percent Distribution of the Projected Population by Race and Hispanic Origin for the United States: 2015 to 2060." Available at: http://www.census.gov/population/projections/data/national/2012/summarytables.html.

Hispanic blacks (75 years). Although mixed evidence exists with regard to the prevalence of psychiatric morbidity among Hispanics and important differences might occur among subgroups of Hispanics, most reports indicate that Hispanics, particularly those who are immigrants, experience lower rates of mental health disorders than their non-Hispanic white counterparts (for a review, see U.S. Department of Health and Human Services 2001). Less is known about positive mental health outcomes and their predictors in Hispanics. Identification of possible strengths in Hispanics leading to this paradoxical effect on mental health could provide key insights for Hispanic mental health. Furthermore, understanding what Hispanics do to reduce the likelihood of mental disorders could be of value for all Americans.

Well-Being in Hispanics

Research findings regarding well-being in Hispanics living in the United States have been mixed. Most population-based studies suggest that Hispanics might have lower life satisfaction than other ethnic and racial groups and that level of life satisfaction might be similar across Hispanic subgroups based on country of origin (e.g., Barger et al. 2009; Coverdill et al. 2011). However, there are conflicting findings regarding whether these ethnic disparities in life satisfaction might be accounted for or "explained" by differences in socioeconomic status and other potential determinants of life satisfaction that vary across ethnic groups. In an analysis of General Social Survey data (Coverdill et al. 2011), Latinos showed lower quality of life than non-Latinos, and this difference persisted *even after* the role of years of education, employment, marital status, age, gender, and frequency of attendance at religious events was taken into account. In a study of two cross-sectional, representative samples of U.S. adults (National Health Interview Survey [Centers for Disease Control and Prevention 2004] and Behavioral Risk Factor Surveillance System [Centers for Disease Control and Prevention 2013], together representing more than 350,000 individuals), Hispanics were also less likely to be very satisfied with their lives than non-Hispanic whites. Interestingly, however, these disparities in life satisfaction were eliminated after adjustments for socioeconomic status and were reversed when socioeconomic status, health, and social relationships were taken into account (Barger et al. 2009). Recent findings involving English-speaking older Hispanics and a demographically matched group of non-Hispanic whites were consistent with the earlier findings and suggest that older Hispanics might, in fact, be more satisfied with their lives (Marquine et al. 2014).

Key Predictors of Well-Being Among Hispanics

Hispanics have an array of cultural tools that equip them to cope with stress and life challenges. Various studies show that family, community, faith, and feelings of belongingness or self-identification with the group may all play important roles in bolstering resilience and well-being among Hispanics. *Acculturation* is a key concept in understanding mental health outcomes among Hispanics. It refers to the process by which members of one cultural group adopt the beliefs and behaviors of another, usually the more dominant group. The protective cultural factors listed above are particularly strong in newly arrived immigrants and less strong in acculturated Hispanics. Although the association between acculturation and these factors is quite complex and may vary by aspects of these constructs and by Hispanic subgroup, their effectiveness appears to wear off in subsequent generations as Hispanics acculturate more fully into the dominant society (usually the non-Hispanic white culture).

Spirituality and religiosity play a salient role in the Hispanic culture. A high proportion of Hispanics report affiliation with a religious group, and Hispanics tend to use religion and spirituality as coping mechanisms more readily than do non-Hispanic whites (Pew Research Center's Religion and Public Life Project 2014). Furthermore, religiosity also seems to have a positive impact on Hispanic health, particularly mental health. Among Mexican Americans, weekly church attendance was found to reduce the risk of mortality over and above a host of other factors (i.e., sociodemographic characteristics, cardiovascular health, activities of daily living, cognitive functioning, physical mobility and functioning, social support, health behaviors, mental health, and subjective health) (Hill et al. 2005). Interestingly, in a study of Mexican American families caring for older relatives with disability, religiosity and religious coping were related to the mental health and burden of caregivers but were not associated with caregivers' subjective physical health (Herrera et al. 2009).

When attempting to understand the association of religiosity and spirituality to mental health outcomes in Latinos, researchers should keep in mind that the nature of these links might differ by distinct dimensions of this construct. Organizational religiosity (i.e., public practice of religious rituals) appears to have a positive impact on mental health (Herrera et al. 2009) and to reduce the risk of mortality (Hill et al. 2005) among Mexican Americans. Similarly, individual experiences of religiosity and spirituality also appear to have a positive effect on mental health among Hispanics (Herrera et al. 2009; Marquine et al. 2014). For example, research has found that increased daily experiences of spirituality among older Hispanics play a key role in explaining why Hispanics also show increased life satisfaction compared with older non-Hispanic whites (Marquine et al. 2014). Consistently, in a study of Mexican American families caring for older relatives with disability, caregivers who reported higher levels of intrinsic religiosity (i.e., internalized religion) were less likely to perceive their caregiving role as burdensome (Herrera et al. 2009). In contrast, nonorganizational religiosity (i.e., private practice of religious rites) was associated with worse mental health. Although the reasons for these differential associations have yet to be elucidated, they highlight the need for a better understanding of these complex relationships. Overall, it appears that among Hispanics, religious and spiritual beliefs tend to have a positive impact on mental health, yet some aspects of these beliefs may have an unintended negative impact.

Familism, or family orientation, is one of the most widely shared cultural values among Hispanics, and it refers to feelings of mutual obligation, reciprocity, and solidarity toward one's family. Its positive effect on mental health has been established widely. For instance, familism has been linked to psychological well-being among Mexican American adults and Puerto Rican mothers of children with mental retardation and to reduced burden in Hispanic dementia caregivers (Losada et al. 2006). In addition, parental warmth significantly reduced alcohol use among Latino adolescents, and family warmth was protective against relapse for Mexican Americans with schizophrenia (López et al. 2004). Despite these positive associations between familism and well-being among Hispanics, it is important to keep in mind that not all aspects of familism are necessarily advantageous. For example, negative interactions among family members can have detrimental effects on well-being.

More broadly, *perception of social support* is also beneficial to mental health among Latinos. It has been shown to play an important role in academic well-being among Latino youths and to buffer the effects of perceived discrimination and other risk factors for poor outcomes in this context (Perez et al. 2009). *Hispanic neighborhood composition* has been consistently linked to better health outcomes, including mental health outcomes (Shell et al. 2013). The protective effect of high neighborhood Hispanic composition on mental health appears to be mediated by higher levels of social support and lower levels of discrimination and stress. Living in a neighborhood with high Hispanic composition may buffer against stress by reinforcing a sense of identity and ethnic pride and fostering social support through increased neighborhood solidarity and trust.

Among Hispanics, those who are immigrants have a lower prevalence rate of mental disorders than those born in the United States. One of the potential factors that might contribute to the resilience of Hispanic immigrants is what has been called *dual frame of reference*. This term refers to the tendency for Hispanic immigrants to use their families back home as reference points for assessing their lives in the United States. The fact that social and economic conditions are usually worse in their homelands might lead immigrants to feel less distressed about the stressors of their daily lives in the United States. Another factor that could foster resilience and well-being among Hispanic immigrants might relate to having *collective achievement goals*. In other words, Hispanics often have a high aspiration to succeed not only for their own personal benefit but also to help their families back home (U.S. Department of Health and Human Services 2001).

African Americans

African Americans and Mental Health

According to the U.S. Census Bureau, in July 2012 there were 44 million African Americans in the United States, which is approximately 14% of the overall population, making this group the second largest ethnic or racial minority group in the United States. It is estimated that by 2060 there will be 77 million African Americans, constituting 18% of the general U.S. population (U.S. Census Bureau 2012) (Figure 15–2). Similar to Hispanics, African Americans are diverse and are becoming even more so each year. Most African Americans are of west and central African descent and are descendants of enslaved blacks in the United States, but this group also includes an increasing number of immigrants from African nations who have immigrated since the abolition of slavery as well as immigrants from Caribbean, Central American, and South American nations.

Although the heterogeneity within the African American population should be kept in mind, as a group, African Americans typically show mental health outcomes that are similar to or better than those of whites, an unexpected pattern given the disproportionate exposure of African Americans to psychosocial stressors (see U.S. Department of Health and Human Services [2001] for a review). This trend has been termed the *race paradox in mental health*. However, it is worth noting that when certain mental health disorders, such as major depressive disorder, affect African Americans, these disorders are usually untreated and are more severe and disabling compared with those in non-Hispanic whites. Evidence also shows that some disorders, such as schizophrenia and depressive disorders and bipolar disorders, have a high likelihood of misdiagnosis among African Americans. This misdiagnosis appears to be due to a number of reasons, including differences in how African Americans express symptoms of emotional distress, distrust in the health care system, and symptom underreporting due to the stigma surrounding mental illness in this community.

Findings contrasting well-being among African Americans and whites have been mixed. Some evidence indicates that well-being and life satisfaction might be increased in African Americans compared with whites. For example, among family caregivers of persons with dementia, African Americans reported increased life satisfaction compared with whites (Clay et al. 2008). However, other studies indicate that there might be differences among subgroups of blacks, such that happiness may be comparable among older whites and African Americans with no ancestral ties to the Caribbean but decreased in Caribbean blacks (Lincoln et al. 2010).

Key Predictors of Well-Being Among African Americans

The race paradox in mental health has been attributed to presumed stronger *social ties* among African Americans. Consistent with this notion, increased life satisfaction among African American family caregivers of persons with dementia was partially explained by increased satisfaction with social support in this group compared with whites (Clay et al. 2008). However, a population-based study of 4,086 individuals found few race differences in the quantity and quality of friendships and fictive kinships (persons who are unrelated by either blood or marriage but regard one another in kinship terms) between racial groups, and these small differences did not explain the race paradox in mental health (Mouzon 2014). Regardless of whether social ties explain racial differences in well-being, social support has been consistently associated with well-being among African Americans (Taylor et al. 2001). Interestingly, a study examining a wide variety of social support networks and their relationship to well-being among African Americans found that subjective family closeness was the strongest and most consistent predictor of life satisfaction among a host of other variables assessing size of family, friend, and neighbor networks; frequency of contact with family, friends, and neighbors; interaction patterns; and presence of fictive kin and a nonkin confidant. Consistently, contact with neighbors and community engagement have been found to be associated positively with well-being among African Americans (Taylor et al. 2001).

To cope with difficult life situations, African Americans often turn not only to family members and their community but also to religion and spirituality. Of all the major racial and ethnic groups in the United States, African Americans are the most likely to report a formal religious affiliation (87%). Even more than two-thirds of those who report no formal affiliation say that religion is somewhat or very important in their lives (Pew Research Center's Religion and Public Life Project 2014). Several studies have indicated that religion may be an important source of resilience and a key predictor of mental health outcomes, including well-being and life satisfaction, for African American adults (e.g., Taylor et al. 2001). For example, a study on a national sample of African Americans showed that frequency of attending religious services is positively associated with life satisfaction (Taylor et al. 2001). Similar findings have been reported across studies despite differences in designs, methodologies, measures of religious involvement, and outcomes. The pathways by which religiosity might affect well-being are likely to be multifactorial. Both the ability to find meaning in life based on religion and the expansion of an individual's social connectedness appear to be some of the major ways in which religion benefits mental health, particularly among African Americans.

Clinical Vignette

Edgar, a 40-year-old man of Mexican origin, presents to his primary care physician for treatment of diabetes. In the context of reviewing his diabetes treatment history, Edgar reports recent difficulty adhering to his medical regimen because of feelings of "not caring anymore," apathy, and irritability. The physician recommends mental health treatment to treat these symptoms of depression. Although Edgar is initially reluctant to start mental health treatment, he agrees to do so after encouragement from his wife and children. The mental health professional follows a positive mental health perspective and focuses his treatment on identifying factors that will not only treat the symptoms of depression but also foster mental wellness. Over the course of treatment, the clinician learns that although the patient holds a high-level administrative position at a company, his family of origin had a low socioeconomic status, and Edgar immigrated to the United States illegally at a young age with his family. His father passed away after a hit-and-run accident soon after the family came to the United States, and his mother was left to care for the family. As the older child, Edgar left school prematurely to help his family financially; however, he was able to graduate from college at age 30 with support from his church and a neighbor. His symptoms of depression started 6 months ago, after his younger son was born, and were related to his fears of being unable to provide financially for his growing family. In addition to prescribing an antidepressant, the clinician focuses treatment on identifying and building on the resources that have been helpful to Edgar in fostering his resilience. The clinician helps Edgar to structure time to spend with his children to foster his emotional connection and his sense of contributing to his family in more ways than just financially. The clinician also encourages Ed-

gar to engage more actively with his church, from which he had distanced himself over that past few years. After 5 months of treatment, Edgar's symptoms improve. The patient gradually discontinued use of the antidepressant after both he
and his mental health professional agreed that pharmacotherapy was no longer warranted. Edgar returns to see the mental health professional 3 months later for a
scheduled follow-up. He denies any symptoms of depression and reports an enhanced sense of well-being, which he attributes to the support from his family
and church.

Summary

Even though older adults tend to experience more physical and mental disabilities than younger adults, research has found that successful aging is not only
possible but also more common than ageist beliefs have previously suggested.
For years, it has commonly been believed that older adults are not very resilient
or amenable to change (Perkins 2014). Research results regarding the positive
effects of leisure time activities and the personality traits that enhance resilience
in aging, some of which have been presented in this chapter, highlight the important fact that older adults can change and continue to benefit from learning
and experience even into very old age. Focusing on and bolstering positive personality traits and behavioral activities that improve well-being and successful
aging, such as resilience, optimism, social support, and leisure activities, continue
to be a promising avenue to possibly delay or prevent disability and to maintain
well-being in old age. Future community-level and individualized interventions
to promote successful aging in older adults should take into account these factors
and should also explore their complex associations. Achieving the goal of promoting successful aging has the potential to greatly reduce the global burden
of physical and mental illness associated with the rapidly growing older adult
population.

Hispanics and African Americans constitute a large proportion of the U.S.
population. Despite having a number of sociodemographic characteristics that
place them at risk for poor mental health outcomes and despite the considerable
heterogeneity within these ethnic and racial minorities, as a group, they tend to
fare as well as or better than non-Hispanic whites in some mental health outcomes. Both Hispanics and African Americans have an array of cultural tools
that equip them to cope with stress and life challenges, including increased religiosity and spirituality and social connectedness. Recognizing and fostering
these elements might prove to be crucial for increasing well-being and enhancing mental health in these vulnerable segments of the U.S. population. In addition, introducing and fostering elements such as familism or spirituality in older
individuals who are not members of these racial and ethnic minorities could
also prove clinically beneficial.

Clinical Key Points

- Despite the increase in physical and mental disability that usually accompanies the aging process, successful aging is not only possible but also more common than previously thought.

- Fostering positive personality traits (e.g., optimism and resilience) and behavioral activities, such as engagement in physical, cognitive, and social activity, can play a key role in aging successfully.

- Although Hispanics and African Americans are disadvantaged in terms of a number of sociodemographic characteristics, they have an array of cultural tools that equip them to cope with stress.

- Although the considerable heterogeneity between and within Hispanics and African Americans should be kept in mind, spirituality and social connectedness have a particularly important role in enhancing positive mental health among these groups.

- Introducing and fostering spirituality and social connectedness in individuals who are not members of these ethnic and racial minority groups can also have important clinical benefits with regard to successful aging.

References

Administration on Aging: Future growth. December 2012. Available at: http://www.aoa.gov/Aging_Statistics/Profile/2013/4.aspx. Accessed August 27, 2014.

Barger SD, Donoho CJ, Wayment HA: The relative contributions of race/ethnicity, socioeconomic status, health, and social relationships to life satisfaction in the United States. Qual Life Res 18(2):179–189, 2009 19082871

Bowling A, Iliffe S: Psychological approach to successful ageing predicts future quality of life in older adults. Health Qual Life Outcomes 9:13, 2011 21388546

Brenes GA, Rapp SR, Rejeski WJ, et al: Do optimism and pessimism predict physical functioning? J Behav Med 25(3):219–231, 2002 12055774

Centers for Disease Control and Prevention: National Health Interview Survey. January, 2004. Available at: http://www.cdc.gov/nchs/data/series/sr_10/sr10_218.pdf. Accessed August 27, 2014.

Centers for Disease Control and Prevention: Behavioral Risk Factor Surveillance System. March 19, 2013. Available at: http://www.cdc.gov/brfss/about/about_brfss.htm. Accessed August 27, 2014.

Clay OJ, Roth DL, Wadley VG, et al: Changes in social support and their impact on psychosocial outcome over a 5-year period for African American and White dementia caregivers. Int J Geriatr Psychiatry 23(8):857–862, 2008 18338341

Colcombe SJ, Erickson KI, Scalf PE, et al: Aerobic exercise training increases brain volume in aging humans. J Gerontol A Biol Sci Med Sci 61(11):1166–1170, 2006 17167157

Coverdill JE, Lopez CA, Petrie MA: Race, ethnicity and the quality of life in America, 1972–2008. Soc Forces 89:783–806, 2011

Gana K, Bailly N, Saada Y, et al: Does life satisfaction change in old age: results from an 8-year longitudinal study. J Gerontol B Psychol Sci Soc Sci 68(4):540–552, 2013 23103381

Gooding PA, Hurst A, Johnson J, et al: Psychological resilience in young and older adults. Int J Geriatr Psychiatry 27(3):262–270, 2012 21472780

Hamarat E, Thompson D, Zabrucky KM, et al: Perceived stress and coping resource availability as predictors of life satisfaction in young, middle-aged, and older adults. Exp Aging Res 27(2):181–196, 2001 11330213

Herrera AP, Lee JW, Nanyonjo RD, et al: Religious coping and caregiver well-being in Mexican-American families. Aging Ment Health 13(1):84–91, 2009 19197693

Hill TD, Angel JL, Ellison CG, et al: Religious attendance and mortality: an 8-year follow-up of older Mexican Americans. J Gerontol B Psychol Sci Soc Sci 60(2):S102–S109, 2005 15746025

Jeste DV, Palmer BW: A call for a new positive psychiatry of ageing. Br J Psychiatry 202:81–83, 2013 23377203

Jeste DV, Savla GN, Thompson WK, et al: Association between older age and more successful aging: critical role of resilience and depression. Am J Psychiatry 170(2):188–196, 2013 23223917

Lamond AJ, Depp CA, Allison M, et al: Measurement and predictors of resilience among community-dwelling older women. J Psychiatr Res 43(2):148–154, 2008 18455190

Lawler-Row KA, Elliott J: The role of religious activity and spirituality in the health and well-being of older adults. J Health Psychol 14(1):43–52, 2009 19129336

Lincoln KD, Taylor RJ, Chae DH, et al: Demographic correlates of psychological well-being and distress among older African Americans and Caribbean black adults. Best Practices Ment Health 6(1):103–126, 2010 21765812

López SR, Nelson Hipke K, Polo AJ, et al: Ethnicity, expressed emotion, attributions, and course of schizophrenia: family warmth matters. J Abnorm Psychol 113(3):428–439, 2004 15311988

Losada A, Robinson Shurgot G, Knight BG, et al: Cross-cultural study comparing the association of familism with burden and depressive symptoms in two samples of Hispanic dementia caregivers. Aging Ment Health 10(1):69–76, 2006 16338817

Marquine MJ, Maldonado Y, Zlatar Z, et al: Differences in life satisfaction among older community-dwelling Hispanics and non-Hispanic Whites. Aging Ment Health Nov 17, 2014 [Epub ahead of print] 25402813

Mouzon DM: Relationships of choice: can friendships or fictive kinships explain the race paradox in mental health? Soc Sci Res 44:32–43, 2014 24468432

Netuveli G, Wiggins RD, Montgomery SM, et al: Mental health and resilience at older ages: bouncing back after adversity in the British Household Panel Survey. J Epidemiol Community Health 62(11):987–991, 2008 18854503

Park DC, Lodi-Smith J, Drew L, et al: The impact of sustained engagement on cognitive function in older adults: the Synapse Project. Psychol Sci 25(1):103–112, 2014 24214244

Perez W, Espinoza R, Ramos K, et al: Academic resilience among undocumented Latino students. Hisp J Behav Sci 31:149–181, 2009

Perkins MM: Resilience in later life: emerging trends and future directions. Gerontologist January 15, 2014 [Epub ahead of print] 24429377

Pew Research Center's Religion and Public Life Project: U.S. Religious Landscape Survey. 2014. Available at: http://religions.pewforum.org/. Accessed August 27, 2014.

Shell AM, Peek MK, Eschbach K: Neighborhood Hispanic composition and depressive symptoms among Mexican-descent residents of Texas City, Texas. Soc Sci Med 99:56–63, 2013 24355471

Son JS, Kerstetter DL, Yarnal C, et al: Promoting older women's health and well-being through social leisure environments: what we have learned from the Red Hat Society. J Women Aging 19(3–4):89–104, 2007 18032255

Strawbridge WJ, Wallhagen MI, Cohen RD: Successful aging and well-being: self-rated compared with Rowe and Kahn. Gerontologist 42(6):727–733, 2002 12451153

Taylor RJ, Chatters LM, Hardison CB, et al: Informal social support networks and subjective well-being among African Americans. J Black Psychol 27:439–463, 2001

U.S. Census Bureau: Percent distribution of the projected population by race and Hispanic origin for the United States: 2015 to 2060. Available at: http://www.census.gov/population/projections/data/national/2012/summarytables.html. Accessed January 8, 2015.

U.S. Department of Health and Human Services: Mental health: culture, race, and ethnicity: a supplement to mental health: a report of the Surgeon General. Rockville, MD, U.S. Department of Health and Human Services, Substance Abuse and Mental Health Services Administration, Center for Mental Health Services. 2001. Available at: http://www.ncbi.nlm.nih.gov/books/NBK44243/pdf/TOC.pdf. Accessed August 27, 2014.

Vahia IV, Thompson WK, Depp CA, et al: Developing a dimensional model for successful cognitive and emotional aging. Int Psychogeriatr 24(4):515–523, 2012 22050770

Suggested Cross-References

Well-being is discussed in Chapter 6 ("What Is Well-Being?"), Chapter 7 ("Clinical Assessments of Positive Mental Health"), and Chapter 13 ("Biology of Positive Psychiatry"). Culture is discussed in Chapter 16 ("Bioethics of Positive Psychiatry").

Suggested Readings

Administration on Aging—United States Department of Health and Human Services. Available at: http://www.aoa.gov/. Accessed August 27, 2014.

Centers for Disease Control and Prevention—Black or African American Populations. Available at: http://www.cdc.gov/minorityhealth/populations/remp/black.html. Accessed August 27, 2014.

Centers for Disease Control and Prevention—Healthy Aging. Available at: http://www.cdc.gov/aging/aginginfo/index.htm. Accessed August 27, 2014.

Centers for Disease Control and Prevention—Hispanic or Latino Populations. Available at: http://www.cdc.gov/minorityhealth/populations/REMP/hispanic.html. Accessed August 27, 2014.

Depp CA, Jeste DV: Successful Cognitive and Emotional Aging. Washington, DC, American Psychiatric Publishing, 2010

Gambert SR: Be Fit for Life: A Guide to Successful Aging: A Wellness, Weight Management, and Fitness Program You Can Live With. Singapore, World Scientific Publishing Company, 2010

Landry R: Live Long, Die Short: A Guide to Authentic Health and Aging. Austin, TX, Greenleaf Book Group Press, 2014

National Institute on Aging-Health Topics. Available at: http://nia.nih.gov/health/topics. Accessed August 27, 2014.

O'Brien M: Successful Aging. Concord, CA, Biomed General, 2005

The Red Hat Society. Available at: http://redhatsociety.com/. Accessed July 14, 2014.

Small G, Vorgan G: The Alzheimer's Prevention Program: Keep Your Brain Healthy for the Rest of Your Life, 2012

U.S. Department of Health and Human Services: Mental health: culture, race, and ethnicity: a supplement to mental health: a report of the surgeon general. Rockville, MD, U.S. Department of Health and Human Services, Substance Abuse and Mental Health Services Administration, Center for Mental Health Services. 2001. Available at: http://www.ncbi.nlm.nih.gov/books/NBK44243/pdf/TOC.pdf. Accessed August 27, 2014.

16

Bioethics of Positive Psychiatry

AJAI R. SINGH, M.D.

Two fundamental ethical questions must be briefly addressed right at the beginning. First, why should ethical considerations even be a concern, given that science is essentially value neutral? Second, why should psychiatrists be concerned with the bioethics of a nascent branch of psychiatry when other considerations are more pressing and bioethical considerations right at the inception may impede, rather than accelerate, progress?

The answer to the first question is that although *pure* science is essentially value neutral, *applied* science and the related procedures and interventions are not. Since applied sciences are directly concerned with human beings and society, they cannot remain value neutral. Like general psychiatry, positive psychiatry is fundamentally an applied science; hence, its procedures and treatments have ethical implications.

The answer to the second question is that the problems facing this nascent field will be shaped by the emergence of dilemmas that are created by science and technology but cannot be solved by them. Many of these problems will be related to health care issues and preferences, and the skill sets that bioethics can provide will help resolve these issues. Rather than impede progress, bioethics

I wish to express my grateful thanks to Barton W. Palmer, Ph.D., for constructive inputs and helpful assistance with this chapter and to Dilip V. Jeste, M.D., for inviting me to contribute to this volume.

will set limits and safeguards right from the beginning, which will only help to accelerate sound progress. Also, biomedical fields, which neglect bioethical considerations early on in their course, inevitably face and have to undergo objections and consequent course corrections later. This also will be preempted.

Some Important Definitions

Positive Psychiatry

Positive psychiatry means promoting well-being by adopting scientific interventions that result from identifying positive psychosocial attributes and processes that positively affect the prevention, treatment, rehabilitation, and relapse of patients with psychiatric disorders in particular and medical diseases in general.

In Chapter 1, "Introduction: What Is Positive Psychiatry?," *positive psychiatry* is defined as "the science and practice of psychiatry that seeks to understand and promote well-being through assessment and interventions" involving positive psychosocial attributes in "people who have or are at high risk of developing mental or physical illnesses." In his 2013 presidential address to the American Psychiatric Association, Jeste noted, "I expect that the future role of psychiatry will be much broader than treating psychiatric symptoms. It will seek to enhance well-being of people with mental or physical illnesses. That is positive psychiatry. We will learn more about brain processes responsible for these traits, and we will seek new ways to promote resilience, optimism, and wisdom through psychotherapeutic interventions" (Jeste 2013, p. 1105).

Positive Psychology

In contrast to positive psychiatry, positive psychology is primarily concerned with using psychological theory, research, and intervention techniques to understand the positive, adaptive, creative, and emotionally fulfilling aspects of human behavior (Seligman 2006). Its aim is a psychology of positive human functioning that achieves scientific understanding of and effective interventions to build thriving individuals, families, and communities (Seligman and Csikszentmihalyi 2000). The intent of positive psychology is to "catalyze a change in the focus of psychology from preoccupation only with repairing the worst things in life to also building positive qualities" (Seligman and Csikszentmihalyi 2000, p. 6). Rather than merely treating psychiatric disorders, positive psychologists seek to make normal life more fulfilling and to find and nurture genius and talent (Compton 2014).

Larger Mandate and Paradigm Shift

Whereas the goal of positive psychology is to incorporate the larger mandate of psychology, which is to make life better for all people, not just the mentally ill (Seligman 1999), the goal of positive psychiatry is to incorporate the larger mandate of psychiatry, which is not only to treat psychiatric symptoms but also to enhance the well-being of those with mental or physical illnesses (Jeste 2012). The paradigm shifts that both positive psychology and positive psychiatry champion are 1) going beyond psychopathology to well-being in the normally functioning population (positive psychology) and 2) going beyond psychopathology to well-being in the patient population (positive psychiatry). Between them, these two fields cover the entire gamut of the population to be served, with the final result being going beyond psychopathology to well-being in the general population, both normal and sick (positive mental health).

Positive Mental Health

Positive mental health is a superordinate category that includes both positive psychiatry (which predominantly studies behaviors of people with mental health disorders and also some behaviors of people without mental health disorders) and positive psychology (which predominantly studies behaviors of people without mental health disorders and also some behaviors of people with mental health disorders). It involves work and research in the fields of psychology and psychiatry and interdisciplinary studies. In other words, if positive mental health is the parent, positive psychology is the elder sister and positive psychiatry the younger.

Why should there be such a distinction at all? It is necessary to demarcate areas of connect and disconnect so that no unnecessary blurring of boundaries occurs. Practitioners in all fields know what their legitimate domains are, what areas they should avoid transgressing into, and where they need to positively interact with and affect the other branches while staying within their own boundaries.

Core Concepts in the Bioethics of Positive Psychiatry

To study the bioethics of positive psychiatry, a brief working knowledge of the following concepts is required: bioethics, principlism (including the four principles of beneficence, nonmaleficence, autonomy, and justice), double effect, common and specific morality, specification, and balancing. These concepts are central to the discussion that follows.

Bioethics

Bioethics is a branch of practical ethics in the philosophy of biology and medicine that deals with the propriety and impropriety of procedures and issues connected with them. By procedures I mean interventions—for example, abortion, euthanasia, surrogacy, organ transplantation, cloning, gene therapy, and human genetic engineering. By issues I mean concepts such as suicide, patients' rights, advocacy, health care rationing, life extension arguments, and so forth.

Principlism

Beauchamp and Childress' (2009) seminal work in biomedical ethics, *Principles of Biomedical Ethics,* details an approach that is often simply called *principlism,* which contains four biomedical ethical principles:

1. *Beneficence* (i.e., patient welfare, or, in Latin, *salus aegroti suprema lex*). A practitioner should act in the best interest of the patient. Patient welfare comes first; everything else depends on it. This principle is the cornerstone of medicine, and it cannot be abandoned at any stage.
2. *Nonmaleficence* (i.e., "first, do no harm," or, in Latin, *primum non nocere*). Even if a practitioner cannot do good, he or she should never cause his or her patient harm. Some *hurt* is understandable as part of a procedure, but *harm* is never permissible (Singh and Singh 2006). For example, a surgeon's incision hurts but is sanctioned under the principle of beneficence because it is meant to carry out a much needed surgery. However, the same incision harms when it is meant to carry out an organ removal without the patient's knowledge and consent (Singh and Singh 2006).
3. *Autonomy* (i.e., consent, or, in Latin, *voluntas aegroti suprema lex*). A patient has the right to refuse or choose treatment. Coercion, forced or subtle, is unethical.
4. *Justice* (i.e., fair treatment for all). Justice concerns equity, the distribution of scarce health resources, and the decision of who gets what treatment (fairness and equality). It also requires that every patient gets fair treatment irrespective of ethnicity, creed, religion, nationality, and so forth.

In other words, a medical practitioner works primarily for the welfare of his or her patient (beneficence); should never cause harm, even if he or she cannot provide care and comfort (nonmaleficence); should respect the patient's right to choose and refuse treatment (autonomy); and should give fair treatment irrespective of geographic, cultural, and ideological considerations (justice).

Double Effect

In addition to the four fundamental principles, we also consider what is known as the *double effect*. Originating in Thomas Aquinas's ideas on homicidal self-defense, double effect is a bioethical concept that states that a single action may produce two types of consequences. In medical ethics, it is usually regarded as the combined effect of beneficence and nonmaleficence. An often-cited example of double effect is using morphine or its analogues in a terminal patient. Morphine can have the beneficial effect of easing pain and suffering. Simultaneously, because it is a respiratory depressant, it can also have the maleficent effect of shortening the patient's life (Randall 2008).

Common Morality, Particular Morality, Specification, and Balancing

Common morality is the set of norms shared by all persons committed to morality. It is not merely *a* morality, in contrast to other moralities. It is applicable to all persons in all places, and we rightly judge all human conduct by its standards (Beauchamp and Childress 2009, p. 3). An example of common morality is the moral principle that all physicians, irrespective of their geography, should work for the welfare of patients (beneficence).

Different from common morality, which contains universal moral norms, "particular moralities" contain nonuniversal moral norms that arise from different cultural, religious, and institutional sources. Whereas common morality provides general rules of morality, particular morality indicates how these general rules are applied in particular cases. For example, when an American Christian physician treats a Chinese Confucian patient, he or she should expect the patient's opinion on death, rebirth, and immortality to be different from his or her own and respect the patient's right to make end-of-life decisions on the basis of his or her own beliefs.

Specification provides the content relevant to a specific context. For example, the ethical code adopted by surgeons is different from that of psychiatrists, and the specific ethical code dictates which ethical and clinical guidelines are put into practice. Specification also indicates which cultural norms should be considered inviolate in treatment.

Balancing entails what to do and what to avoid and also the act of balancing and adjudicating between two goods. It also involves developing sound judgment and acting according to justice. It is important for reaching sound judgments in individual cases. For example, what should a physician do with regard to life support systems for a patient in a permanent vegetative state? Both removing life support and continuing it can be justified from different standpoints, so they appear to be equally good. Balancing primacy of life (absolutist stance) and a dignified exit to a life no longer worth living (utilitarian stance) will depend on the belief system of the patient, relatives, and physician and the law of the land.

The Case for Positive Psychiatry: Salient Research Findings

The progress of positive mental health in the last two decades has been dotted with numerous studies showing the beneficial effects of a number of positive psychosocial characteristics and attributes that have been identified and validated by quantitative studies and meta-analytic reviews. Prominent qualities include resilience (Stewart and Yuen 2011), optimism (Rasmussen et al. 2009), personal mastery (Mausbach et al. 2007), wisdom (Jeste and Harris 2010), religion and spirituality (Vahia et al. 2011), social relationships and support (Holt-Lunstad et al. 2010), and engagement in pleasant events (Uchino 2006). As reviewed in Chapter 13, "Biology of Positive Psychiatry," a growing number of studies suggest that such positive attributes are tightly linked to human biology. Also, these positive attributes are associated with significant positive health outcomes exemplified by longevity, better functioning, and reduced susceptibility to psychiatric disorders such as depression, as well as to cardiovascular, metabolic, and other physical diseases (Jeste 2012).

The Case for Beneficence: Application to Positive Psychiatry

The bioethical principle of beneficence, which is the cornerstone of medicine and its major, if not only, justification, is of interest here. All studies, interventions, and research are justified only if this fundamental principle is upheld. Which raises the question: does positive psychiatry stand the test of beneficence? In identifying positive psychosocial characteristics that affect health outcomes and recovery, positive psychiatry is attempting to pinpoint precisely those aspects that help recovery and are in the best interest of the patient. Therefore, it passes the test of beneficence very well. The following clinical vignette encapsulates the positive psychosocial factors and highlights the beneficent role the psychiatrist may have in relation to them.

Clinical Vignette

Barbara, a 55-year-old businesswoman, lost her husband in a car accident 15 years ago. She was an educated homemaker before that. Following her husband's sudden demise, she was devastated. She experienced prolonged grief and slipped into depression. She underwent psychiatric treatment in which, along with being prescribed medication, she was encouraged to look into strengthening her existent positive traits (resilience, self-mastery, and spirituality), to learn new ones such as optimism and wisdom, and to develop strong social relationships and social support.

Barbara took over the reins of the family business, established herself as an alternative to her husband with the partners and clients, and brought up her two children (resilience). She took charge of her emotions and grief (personal mastery) and became part of a musical group that had strong bonds among members (social relationships and social support). She was devoted to a certain spiritual group whose weekly meetings she attended regularly (religious and spiritual practices). Whenever in doubt, Barbara sought guidance from her "guru," whose wisdom had always helped her sail through major obstacles (wisdom). Diagnosed with type 2 diabetes 4 years prior to her husband's death, she controlled it with exercise, diet, yoga, and a single morning dose of a metformin and glimeperide combination (personal mastery). Barbara's zest for life and looking on the brighter side of things never diminished through all this (optimism). Not wanting to take any risk with her mental health, she continued to visit her psychiatrist twice a year just to confirm all was well with her (controlled optimism).

Barbara managed her depression following strengthening of positive psychosocial factors by her psychiatrist (beneficence). She managed her business, the education of her children, and her own diabetes through her optimism, resilience, engagement in pleasant events, personal mastery, strong social relationships and social support, religious and spiritual practices, and wisdom (positive psychosocial factors).

Encouraging these and other positive factors, finding their additional nuances through scientific studies, and incorporating them in interventions that stand the test of beneficence is the next step forward for the field of positive psychiatry.

The Case for Caution: Nonmaleficence, Autonomy, and Justice

Optimism

Even though positive psychosocial attributes are useful for the individual and society, there are several potential ethical issues of concern in the practice of positive psychiatry. Even if data support the principle of beneficence, the principles of nonmaleficence, autonomy, and justice and resolving potential double effects also must be fulfilled.

Let us consider the case of optimism for which there is extensive support. Every positive characteristic has a potential downside; for example, people who are too optimistic may indulge in risky behaviors because of a belief that they would survive (double effect). This belief may result in the neglect of risk factors and warning signs, even if the patient is properly informed. "Controlled" optimism, even "controlled" pessimism, may be more advisable in certain situations.

Clinical Vignette

Daniel was informed of the warning signs of a heart attack after an anginal attack and angioplasty. When he developed retrosternal pain a year later, he shrugged it off, saying it was just "gas" and it often happened to him (*pseudo-optimism*). He held the opinion that doctors alarmed patients unduly so they could make more money.

His wife was more realistic. However, Daniel often labeled her as unduly alarmist (*pseudo-optimistic labeling*) because he thought she took medical advice rather too seriously, thinking of the worst-case scenario immediately. Not trusting her husband's bravado, she called their daughter, a physician, who also lived in the area. She immediately rushed her father to the intensive cardiac care unit, and Daniel was found to have developed extensive myocardial infarcts. He was immediately put on emergency measures and survived.

Daniel's pseudo-optimism would have cost him his life. His wife's controlled pessimism, which made her aware of a perilous situation, was better in this situation. Daniel's medically trained daughter had controlled optimism: she heeded the warning signs but was optimistic that prompt treatment would help her dad, which was the outcome. Psychiatric counseling for depressive symptoms that Daniel developed later could convince him to move from pseudo-optimism to controlled optimism.

As the clinical vignette about Daniel illustrates, it is necessary to promote only "due" optimism in the sick—that is, optimism that helps patients see the brighter side of things and believe in their recovery and helps them face difficult situations with humor and courage but prevents false bravado and treatment noncompliance through pseudo-optimism and pseudo-optimistic labeling. Promoting blanket optimism without clarifying its nuances can amount to maleficence. In other words, to ensure that the principle of nonmaleficence is not violated, psychiatrists and other health care professionals must exercise abundant caution with the espousal of optimism by noting that it also can have a downside (double effect).

Resilience

Let us examine nonmaleficence with regard to another positive attribute: resilience. Numerous studies show its positive side, but future studies may show downsides to positive attributes; for example, excessive pain tolerance and resilience may lead to delayed diagnosis of cancer until it becomes inoperable (double effect). This amounts to *pseudoresilience*, the result of pseudo-optimism often born out of denial.

Clinical Vignette

Grant, a physician, had been experiencing extensive weight loss for the last year. Acquaintances who met him infrequently were alarmed at his weight loss and his look of premature aging. However, most of his family members had not noticed the changes because they saw him daily. Although his wife did notice his weight loss and told him to see a doctor, he brushed her suggestions aside, saying that he himself was a doctor (pseudoresilience).

Grant still managed to enjoy his work and workouts, saying with good humor that he could now eat anything and not put on weight. He also felt excessive thirst but laughed it off, saying it was good he had to follow the advice he gave his patients—drink more water. Lately, he had developed difficulty sleeping, which he brushed off, attributing it to a defective mattress. Having always been resilient in life, he felt all would be well with a good exercise and diet schedule (pseudoresilience due to pseudo-optimism, which led to denial). Fearing the worst, malignancy or AIDS, Grant chose to adopt the strategy of denial.

More recently, however, Grant developed sexual dysfunction. His wife insisted they both undergo whole-body checkups. Grant's blood sugar was found to be 630 mg/L, and retinal damage had already set in.

His physician counseled him on the perils of such pseudoresilience. Grant immediately took charge of the situation. Although he had never taken medications in his life, he promptly began an efficient regimen of medication, diet control, exercise, and yoga (proper resilience). Grant's blood sugar was well under control in 3 months and remained so over the next 2 years. His retinal damage was arrested, as determined at 1- and 2-year follow-up appointments.

As this vignette illustrates, it is necessary to tease out proper resilience from pseudoresilience. The former is beneficent; the latter is maleficent. Hence, promoting blanket resilience without clarifying its potential downside can be a form of maleficence.

It is also necessary to avoid *forced* resilience and pseudoresilience. The promotion of pseudoresilience may give rise to a blame game. For example, the implication that resilience is associated with faster recovery from a disorder could result in blaming patients who do not recover quickly for not trying to be more resilient (double effect). The physician must beware that in his or her misplaced benevolent paternalism, he or she does not harm the patient's self-esteem and damage the very cause the physician espouses.

Clinical Vignette

Karl is a gastroenterologist who greets his patients cheerfully and is aware of the psychosomatics of gastrointestinal tract disorders. Recently, he read about the role of optimism and resilience in getting well. He enthusiastically advises his patients to change for the better, giving examples of how emotions control the gastrointestinal tract (e.g., when anxious before an exam or test, some people experience intestinal hurry).

Patients who get well are great ego boosters for Karl. However, those who do not get well become a challenge he finds difficult to explain. He makes a blanket judgment, blaming them for not being resilient and optimistic enough. He warns them that they had better change and become more optimistic and resilient in life if they want to get well, without offering patients ways to do so (resilience promotion by pseudo means). He will not refer his patients to a psychotherapist, claiming psychotherapy is a waste of time and that he is a competent enough psychotherapist himself because he keeps abreast of psychosomatics.

Karl does not realize that having knowledge and having the expertise to implement it are two different things. His tendency to blame his patients who do not recover for not being resilient or optimistic enough is one form of resilience promotion by pseudo means and amounts to harm, albeit unintentional. Although his espousal of resilience is well intentioned, not implementing it correctly amounts to maleficence and is an example of double effect.

Autonomy

Intrinsic to autonomy is the patient's right to refuse or choose his or her treatment. The evidence for positive psychosocial interventions should be presented to the patient before he or she is expected to comply with procedures that enhance them or to modify his or her habitual responses. Moreover, the patient has the right to give or refuse consent to one or more of the procedures the physician or psychiatrist may consider better suited for the patient, except if the patient is legally incompetent, in which case a competent legal health care proxy must take over. Even if the chances of a legally incompetent person adopting positive measures such as optimism, resilience, and wisdom are remote, such safeguards (consent, intervention of a health care proxy) are necessary. The safeguard of health care proxy is also needed for special populations such as children, older people with mild or major cognitive impairment, and people who are otherwise not fully competent to provide consent for treatments.

Justice

As described in the earlier subsection "Principlism," in the field of bioethics, the term *justice* essentially means fairness in the procedures that are adopted and involves all of the other three principles (beneficence, nonmaleficence, and autonomy). It is involved at various levels in bioethics. Beneficence should be adopted, but in a fair manner. Nonmaleficence should be exercised, but in an equally fair manner. Patient autonomy should be respected, but in a fair manner. Justice also means that decisions should be made and treatments should be offered irrespective of sexual orientation or preference, color, creed, nationality, or religion (justice).

Clinical Vignette

Anne is a physician who always keeps herself abreast of the latest developments in her branch of medicine and adopts only those procedures she knows will benefit her patients (beneficence). She would never carry out any procedure that she knows would harm her patients (nonmaleficence). She is careful to explain the procedure to be carried out to her patients without unduly alarming them, informs them fully about the benefits and risks involved, and performs the procedure only after obtaining a valid patient consent (autonomy). Anne behaves in this manner with all of her patients, irrespective of their sexual orientation or preference, color, creed, nationality, or religion.

Anne not only is a good physician but also follows the laws of justice. In fact, she is a good physician only because she carries out sound procedures in a fair manner.

Justice has further nuances that need to be elaborated. It essentially means not crossing the line from beneficence to condescending paternalism (e.g., a doctor making decisions for a patient, brushing aside his or her objections), not becoming so obsessed with nonmaleficence that due beneficence is ignored (e.g., advocating against and/or not giving legally permitted involuntary treatment), not adopting maleficence in the garb of beneficence (e.g., adopting nonscientific or obsolete procedures in the name of treatment), and not giving absolute value to patient autonomy and forgetting that such autonomy is relative (e.g., not treating a patient who is incompetent to give consent). Justice also means offering all facilities equally to all patients, irrespective of their ethnicity, culture, sexual orientation, or religion or creed. Discrimination on any count amounts to maleficence and nonbeneficence.

How can justice be of concern in positive psychiatry? A health care professional who is not just may not provide the best care for his or her patients, as illustrated by the following examples. A positive psychiatrist who emphasizes greater social connectivity as an important positive psychosocial method may brush aside a patient's basic introversion and the stress induced in the patient when he or she is forced to become social. A patient who has successfully adopted controlled pessimism as a coping mechanism may be forced into optimism, which previously has not worked for him or her. A patient may be offered homegrown advice or folk remedies as scientifically validated advice in psychotherapy. A patient may be deprived of the benefits of becoming optimistic, becoming resilient, having greater social connectivity, and concentrating on pleasant events because the psychiatrist believes that patient has a poor-prognosis psychiatric disorder such as schizophrenia with negative symptoms or early cognitive decline likely to lead to Alzheimer's disease. A positive psychiatrist may similarly lay undue emphasis on resilience to prevent normal grieving, which takes its own time to resolve. The psychiatrist may encourage the patient to move past grief prematurely. This may encourage the patient to pursue reckless behaviors such as attending all-night parties and entering into one-night stands, which carry their own risks of sexually transmitted diseases in addition to rebound grief.

Clinical Vignette

Helen allows her patients to decide between the methods of positive psychiatry after offering them information and counsel. She takes care that she never presents her "hunches" as scientifically proven, but nevertheless does present them as "hunches," for the patient to adopt or reject. Moreover, she keeps abreast of developments in the field and offers the latest information on positive psychiatry to her patients, irrespective of their race, creed, religion, sexual orientation, or socioeconomic status. She never forces her personal preferences on her patients and helps them develop their own strategies based on their basic strengths, preferences, and shortcomings. She never rushes her patients into choosing this or that process, but she does gently prod them forward to make a purposeful decision about which process to adopt. Helen is not only a good positive psychiatrist but also a just one.

Justice demands that in a nondiscriminatory manner, health care professionals respect patients' autonomy to decide which method to adopt, give only scientifically validated advice, exercise due discretion in factors with scarce but emerging evidence, and avoid rushing patients into procedures. Clearly, a just person is one who embodies a judicious mix of benevolence and nonmaleficence in his or her actions, with respect for others' autonomy. In other words, justice embodies the other three biomedical principles. A just person is also one who distributes his or her expertise equally.

Conflicts Among Values

An understanding based on common morality, specific morality, specification, and balancing will help if conflicts among the values occur. Useful rules of thumb are as follows (Singh and Singh 2009): beneficence is the bedrock of medicine, nonmaleficence is its conscience, justice is its sentinel, and autonomy is its crowning glory (common morality).

Each principle is dynamically linked to the other. However, in case of conflict, autonomy and then justice may need to be compromised and temporarily suspended, although most reluctantly, in special circumstances, such as involuntary treatment (specific morality).

That leaves beneficence and nonmaleficence. Which of the two is more essential? The answer is beneficence (balancing). Beneficence can never be forsaken. Can nonmaleficence be forsaken then (balancing)? It need not be. If properly implemented, nonmaleficence is built into beneficence (specification) (Singh and Singh 2009).

In psychiatric therapy, beneficence and nonmaleficence are paramount and may occasionally need to override autonomy and justice when they conflict (e.g., involuntary treatment). In psychiatric research, however, autonomy and justice are paramount and must override beneficence and nonmaleficence when they conflict (specification and balancing).

From this discussion of conflicts, two important principles emerge:

1. Beneficence can never be forsaken (common morality) (Singh and Singh 2009). Beauchamp and Childress (2009) identify beneficence as one of the core values of health care ethics, and Pellegrino and Thomasma (1988) argue that beneficence is the sole fundamental principle of medical ethics.
2. Autonomy and justice may occasionally need to be overridden by beneficence and nonmaleficence in therapy. However, beneficence and nonmaleficence always need to be overridden by autonomy and justice in research (Singh and Singh 2009).[1]

Let us see how these considerations apply to the bioethics of positive psychiatry.

Clinical Vignette

Sanjay, an Indian emigrant to the United States who teaches Indian philosophy, develops cardiovascular disease with depressive symptoms and insists on maintaining a pessimistic outlook on life. The positive psychiatrist advises that a change in attitude toward optimism would help. He presents data that optimism has been studied in the context of a number of serious medical conditions, including cardiovascular disease, and has been shown to be associated with less illness-related distress, higher quality of life and satisfaction, and lower incidence of depression (Carver et al. 2010). The psychiatrist also presents the results from a meta-analysis of 83 studies of optimism that found a significant relationship between optimism and physical health outcomes, including cardiovascular outcomes, physiological markers (including immune function), cancer outcomes, and outcomes related to pregnancy, physical symptoms, pain, and mortality (Rasmussen et al. 2009).

Sanjay still insists on maintaining his pessimistic outlook toward life, presenting metaphysical arguments that life is essentially full of suffering (the Buddhist position) and that the world is an illusion (the Advaita Vedanta position on maya).

---

[1]It should be noted that there are objections to this position. Tassano (1999), for example, has questioned the notion of beneficence having priority over autonomy at times. He argues that autonomy violations more often only prioritize the state's or the "supplier group's" interest over that of the patient. Although this statement may be true when maleficent intentions are cloaked as beneficence, it may also lead to such an obsession with nonmaleficence that due beneficence is ignored (e.g., when one may need to "dare to care" as in the case of involuntary treatment).

The psychiatrist has to decide between his duty of beneficence based on scientific findings and Sanjay's autonomy to continue to hold on to cultural and religious beliefs that hamper his recovery. Also, the psychiatrist must consider the need to be just by not imposing his views on Sanjay.

What does the psychiatrist do? In ordinary circumstances, the psychiatrist would present the scientific findings and respect the patient's autonomy and allow Sanjay to decide whether he accepts the findings. The psychiatrist would wait for Sanjay to integrate the findings with his metaphysical beliefs. However, what if Sanjay resists, and his pessimism, according to the psychiatrist, is mainly responsible for the lack of recovery? Does the psychiatrist say this directly to Sanjay? Beneficence prompts him to do so. Should the psychiatrist decline to continue to treat Sanjay, given that by allowing Sanjay to stick to his beliefs, the psychiatrist is causing harm to the patient (nonmaleficence)? What about justice? Being fair to the patient gives Sanjay the right to decide what advice he follows and therefore to continue to stick with his pessimism. However, being fair to the patient's interests enjoins the psychiatrist to persevere to change the patient's belief on the basis of scientific evidence, especially because the patient's belief directly affects his recovery and sense of well-being.

In this case, should the psychiatrist be just to Sanjay's autonomy or to his or her own notion of beneficence? How does the psychiatrist adjudicate? Here the psychiatrist seems well within his duties of beneficence and nonmaleficence to help Sanjay to modify his beliefs, and the psychiatrist needs to judiciously use his intuitive sense of justice by ascending in his thinking to a critical moral level wherein he adjudicates between two or more goods and maximizes utility (Hare 1984). Although the psychiatrist accepts that Sanjay has the right to hold on to his pessimism as a general metaphysical position and as a general rule to make sense of life and living, the psychiatrist would be right to noncoercively persevere with helping Sanjay modify his pessimistic outlook to become more optimistic in his attitude toward his ailment, life, and living so that Sanjay can recover from his cardiovascular condition. In fact, leaving Sanjay to his pessimistic outlook would amount to maleficence and injustice. In other words, the psychiatrist should help Sanjay adopt optimistic means to aid his recovery even though he may continue to retain a generally pessimistic philosophy of life (both specification and balancing are involved here).

Therefore, in psychiatric therapy, beneficence and nonmaleficence are paramount and may, in certain circumstances, need to be given precedence over autonomy and justice, as they are ordinarily understood, when they conflict. This preference is only to maximize utility and promote due beneficence and should never be used as a means to practice overt or covert maleficence. Moreover, it must be noted that the final right to decide to accept a psychiatrist's advice, even if it is in the patient's best interest, lies solely with the patient unless he or she is legally incompetent.

Next, let us consider the case of research and imagine Sanjay is a participant in a research study on the role of optimism in cardiovascular cases. The same arguments are presented on both sides. The patient decides to stick to his pessimism and demands that his autonomy be respected. The researcher will present data but will stop short of trying to modify the patient's attitudes if he resists.

Here, the patient's autonomy and justice trump the psychiatrist's notions of beneficence and nonmaleficence because as a research subject, Sanjay has the *absolute* right to accept or reject a certain therapy. In the case of therapy, however, the psychiatrist is well guided to continue to encourage attitude modification, even though he accepts the patient's *final* right to persist with or modify his attitude. Such bioethical balancing gives the much-needed specifications that correctly guide a morally sound positive psychiatrist.

Other Unforeseen Negative Consequences of Positive Attributes

Other unforeseen negative consequences of positive attributes could arise. For instance, some people may be more comfortable being asocial rather than having a large social network. An example of the potential harm that could arise in this situation is provided in the following hypothetical vignette.

Clinical Vignette

Caleb, age 56, is a shy, reserved person by temperament who has enjoyed good health all through life. He has a small circle of friends with whom he is happy, and he enjoys a quiet, contented life. Six months ago, Caleb heard about recent findings that greater social connectivity was a positive psychosocial factor and that brain plasticity meant newer neuronal connections could be established at any age. He started socializing with great vigor, stimulating his brain with vigorous cerebral activities such as prolonged animated discussions, giving speeches at various functions, continuously interacting via e-mail in social groups, and spending hours on Facebook and Twitter accounts. He started keeping his cell phone on 24/7 so that he did not miss any opportunity to interact with new and old acquaintances.

After a few months, the excitement got the better of Caleb, and he started losing sleep. He developed spells of severe headaches with giddiness. He started feeling exhausted most of the time, with bouts of irritability over small matters, something that had never happened to him before. He was subsequently diagnosed with moderate hypertension. Thus, a man who had led an otherwise disease-free life until this change he forced on himself developed a chronic ailment.

Caleb's physician started him on medication, which led to only mild improvement. Noting Caleb's irritability and lack of sleep, his physician felt depression might be a contributing factor and referred Caleb to a psychiatrist. In treatment, Caleb revealed his changed lifestyle and the reasons. Psychotherapy helped him realize he should lead a more relaxed lifestyle suited to his basic temperament. Along with medication, Caleb reduced his excessive social connectivity and returned to his previous way of living. As a result, his symptoms are under control.

Social stimulation has its positive effects. However, as the above vignette illustrates, excessive and unregulated social connectivity and stimulation unsuited to basic temperament could potentially have negative consequences (double effect). When suggesting the positive effects of positive psychiatric interventions, psychiatrists should equally emphasize the potential harm due to excess and sudden introduction, especially to patients who may get carried away.

Cross-Cultural Differences

The need to consider cross-cultural differences in positive psychiatry is discussed in detail in Chapter 15, "Positive Geriatric and Cultural Psychiatry," so here I only briefly consider the unique ethical dilemmas that may arise in a cross-cultural context. In particular, while emphasizing positive psychosocial factors, positive psychiatrists may neglect important cultural differences and unwittingly coerce homogenization (double effect). Eastern cultures seem to stress the role of spirituality more than that of humor, whereas the reverse may be true for Western cultures. Such differences should not be seen as problematic. The need to understand and judiciously combine such differences in different patients without adopting a straitjacket rule should prevent the informed positive psychiatrist from committing unintended harm.

Furthermore, another risk is creating a homogeneous society in which everyone is apparently optimistic, social, resilient, and so on, but people are actually struggling to cope with sudden changes that overenthusiastic physicians or psychiatrists forced on them or they forced on themselves, which frequently occurs because of information bombardment from the Internet and other media. This homogenization may be akin to eugenics (double effect). The widely varying tapestry of human beings adds color and variety to human living. Society needs optimistic, irreligious, socializing people as much as it needs religious, asocial, wise beings. Also, human beings have myriad means of coping, and different psychosocial factors can be equally good. There is no need to unduly promote one over the other.

Seeking Answers to Hitherto Unresolved Issues

Positive psychiatry still has a vast area to cover. Just identifying positive factors such as optimism, resilience, personal mastery, social cooperativeness, and wisdom is not enough. This identification is necessary but not sufficient. In calculating the balance among the bioethical principles described earlier, it is necessary to tease out the individual, synergistic, and even antagonistic roles of these various components. In other words, we must proceed from common morality to particular morality with specification and balancing.

For example, is it possible that mutually antagonistic psychosocial factors could exist? That wisdom may correlate more with an asocial attitude than with greater social connectivity? That social connectivity may correlate well with engagement with pleasant activities but may correlate poorly with self-transcendence? What about synergistic psychosocial factors? Does wisdom synergize with self-transcendence? Does resilience synergize with optimism? Does social connectivity synergize with engagement with pleasant events?

Processes that may be enthusiastically applied in the general populace may require more restrained application in an ailing populace. How much resilience, optimism, wisdom, and social connectivity should psychiatrists consider appropriate in people with psychoses, and at which stage of their recovery should patients exhibit these traits? To what degree will individuals with different neuroses and personality disorders exhibit these same traits? Often, well-wishers have already given these individuals the common-sense advice to "be optimistic," "take adversity in stride," "go on a vacation," or "be in jovial company," and that advice has not worked. Often, individuals come to psychiatric treatment only after trying to take such advice fails. If the psychiatrist also starts giving out such common-sense advice, how does the patient benefit?

Another question that must be answered is related to efficacy. Are these positive psychosocial factors predominantly important in treating psychosomatic conditions and helping the geriatric population prolong longevity and lead a more meaningful life in spite of physical and cognitive decline? Should these factors be studied and applied more in those areas than in the treatment of general psychiatric and medical disorders? Currently, the clinical cases and research evidence are mainly related to psychosomatic disorders and the geriatric population. Further study will be needed to answer these questions.

Further study will also be needed to clarify which psychosocial factors are genuine and which are "pseudo" psychosocial factors. Research will be necessary to discriminate resilience from pseudoresilience, optimism from pseudo-optimism, wisdom from pseudowisdom, and spirituality from pseudospirituality. This determination will be based on what effect the psychosocial factor has on a patient's well-being, not on psychiatrists' notions and value judgments. For example, proper resilience will lead to a patient's well-being; pseudoresilience will lead to ill health.

Another issue to be resolved is related to the allocation of resources and basic expertise. Would it not be appropriate for psychiatrists to concentrate scarce resources on remedies they know best? They are experts in handling psychopathology; that is their expertise and training. There is so much psychopathology that needs to be treated and understood. A strong case can be made for the argument that the limited resources psychiatrists have need to be judiciously harnessed and directed mainly toward the goal of treating and researching psychiatric disorders, rather than foraying into territories best handled by educationists, social thinkers, and preachers and religious reformers, who have always talked of the value of wisdom, optimism, resilience, spirituality, self-transcendence, social connectivity, and cooperativeness.

A further fundamental problem must also engage our attention here. In their preoccupation to establish scientifically verifiable models, is it possible that psychiatrists are making discrete entities out of factors that are integrally and synergistically related to each other and are best understood in relation to one another? Is it possible that these positive psychosocial factors are being artificially separated to suit the scientific convenience of categorizing and standardizing?

All of the unanswered questions in this section are legitimate ones that positive psychiatry will need to address in the next decade.

Some Other Cautionary Viewpoints

In defining the parameters of positive psychiatry, positive psychiatrists must address cross-cultural differences, keep in mind that average may not mean healthy, and specify whether attributes are considered traits or states and in which contexts these attributes are applicable. Also, if positive psychiatry is beneficial, whom does it benefit: individuals or society or both? And how does it benefit them: for fitting in or for a deviance that sets a new trend? Vaillant (2012) raises these questions about positive mental health, but they are equally applicable to positive psychiatry. Linden (2012) raises the important philosophical issue of first defining what *positive* means and whether *positive* and *healthy* are synonyms. Another question that needs to be clarified is the relation between health and illness. Karlsson (2012) raises the issue of real-life implementation of the core features of positive mental health and indicates that these features must be integrally related to where mental health professionals think society should be headed, whereas Stein (2012) considers it debatable whether interventions to improve positive mental health should necessarily fall within the purview of mental health clinicians.

Task for the Future

Positive psychiatry is in its infancy. A number of studies show that it holds promise. Its background and scope have been well established in that it will consider all psychosocial factors that make living positive and worthwhile for psychiatric patients in particular and all patients in general. Moreover, its methods will be based on quantitative data and biology. Positive psychiatry thus holds the promise of making the patient both an object and an agent of change.

The task of determining the nuances of positive psychosocial factors should occupy researchers for the next decade. Serious researchers should be aware that there could be unanticipated long-term negative consequences of interventions (behavioral or biological) that seek to enhance positive factors (double effect). Hence, any negative reports on positive factors and any suggested modifications should be taken seriously and not brushed aside as being unduly alarmist. Taking negative findings seriously would be the best way to couple beneficence (doing good) with nonmaleficence (do no harm) and prevent avoidable double effects.

Summary

Positive psychiatry seeks to move beyond a narrow definition of psychiatry as a medical subspecialty restricted to the treatment of psychiatric disorders to a psychiatry of the future that will develop into a core component of the overall health care system (Jeste 2012). Its foundation has been well laid by an emphasis on quantitative data and biology. The bioethical implications of the findings from positive psychiatry and its interventions as an applied science need to be carefully studied at each stage of its development so that the four biomedical principles of beneficence, nonmaleficence, autonomy, and justice are never violated and serve as conscience keepers for the future growth of this promising branch.

Because positive psychiatry is an applied science, all further work will be judged on the basis of the following four basic questions: 1) Does it help the patient (beneficence)? 2) Does it cause minimal hurt and no harm (nonmaleficence)? 3) Does it take into account the valid consent of the patient (autonomy)? 4) Ultimately, is it fairly distributed to benefit the target populace in a nondiscriminatory manner, and do stakeholders have recourse to judicial measures to reconcile any conflicts arising between the physician or psychiatrist, the patient, and the patient's relatives (justice)? Those intimately involved in the propagation of positive psychiatry must ensure that interventions and progress pass this litmus test, and positive psychiatry must be subjected to this test within the broader field of positive mental health from time to time so that there is greater consensus over whether its forward progress is being made with the greatest of beneficence and minimal maleficence and few violations of autonomy and justice.

Clinical Key Points

- Positive psychiatry seeks to move beyond, but not neglect, psycho-pathology and to achieve better living and well-being in spite of psychopathology.

- The four biomedical principles of beneficence, nonmaleficence, autonomy, and justice coupled with an understanding of common morality, specific morality, specification, and balancing are important in setting the bioethical agenda of positive psychiatry.

- Beneficence (i.e., patient welfare) is a key test, and positive psychiatry passes it very well because of its emphasis on positive psychosocial factors such as resilience, optimism, social connectivity, wisdom, personal mastery, and religion and spirituality, with interventions based on scientific evidence from quantitative data and biology.

- However, positive psychiatrists must beware of promoting pseudo manifestations of positive psychosocial factors and the potential double effects that could be created as a result (nonmaleficence). Positive psychiatrists must also never override patient autonomy by steamrolling patients into accepting positive psychosocial factors (autonomy) and must be careful to fairly allocate scarce resources irrespective of a patient's color, creed, religion, or ethnicity (justice).

- Positive psychiatry has many connections with positive psychology, its sister discipline, and with positive mental health, its parent discipline. However, professionals in each discipline should know their areas of connect and disconnect so they work in synergy and avoid undue domain conflicts later.

References

Beauchamp TL, Childress JF: Principles of Biomedical Ethics, 6th Edition. New York, Oxford University Press, 2009

Carver CS, Scheier MF, Segerstrom SC: Optimism. Clin Psychol Rev 30(7):879–889, 2010 20170998

Compton WC: An Introduction to Positive Psychology, 5th Edition. Belmont, CA, Wadsworth Publishing, 2014

Hare R: The philosophical basis of psychiatric practice, in Psychiatric Ethics. Edited by Bloch S, Chodoff P. Oxford, UK, Oxford University Press, 1984, pp 30–45

Holt-Lunstad J, Smith TB, Layton JB: Social relationships and mortality risk: a meta-analytic review. PLoS Med 7(7):e1000316, 2010 20668659

Jeste DV: Positive psychiatry. 2012. Available at: http://psychnews.psychiatryonline.org/newsarticle.aspx?articleid=1182477. Accessed August 27, 2014.

Jeste DV: A fulfilling year of APA presidency: from DSM-5 to positive psychiatry. Am J Psychiatry 170(10):1102–1105, 2013 24084815

Jeste DV, Harris JC: Wisdom—a neuroscience perspective. JAMA 304(14):1602–1603, 2010 20940386

Karlsson H: Problems in the definitions of positive mental health. World Psychiatry 11(2):106–107, 2012 22654941

Linden M: What is health and what is positive? The ICF solution. World Psychiatry 11(2):104–105, 2012 22654939

Mausbach BT, Patterson TL, Von Känel R, et al: The attenuating effect of personal mastery on the relations between stress and Alzheimer caregiver health: a five-year longitudinal analysis. Aging Ment Health 11(6):637–644, 2007 18074251

Pellegrino E, Thomasma D: For the Patient's Good: The Restoration of Beneficence in Health Care. New York, Oxford University Press, 1988

Randall F: Ethical issues in cancer pain management, in Clinical Pain Management: Cancer Pain, 2nd Edition. Edited by Sykes N, Bennett MI, Yuan C-S. London, Hodder Arnold, 2008, pp 93–100

Rasmussen HN, Scheier MF, Greenhouse JB: Optimism and physical health: a meta-analytic review. Ann Behav Med 37(3):239–256, 2009 19711142

Seligman MEP: The president's address. Am Psychol 54:559–562, 1999

Seligman MEP: Learned Optimism: How to Change Your Mind and Your Life, 6th Edition. New York, Pocket Books, 2006

Seligman ME, Csikszentmihalyi M: Positive psychology: an introduction. Am Psychol 55(1):5–14, 2000 11392865

Singh A, Singh S: To cure sometimes, to comfort always, to hurt the least, to harm never. Mens Sana Monogr 4(1):8–9, 2006 22013325

Singh AR, Singh SA: Notes on a few issues in the philosophy of psychiatry. Mens Sana Monogr 7(1):128–183, 2009 21836785

Stein DJ: Positive mental health: a note of caution. World Psychiatry 11(2):107–109, 2012 22654942

Stewart DE, Yuen T: A systematic review of resilience in the physically ill. Psychosomatics 52(3):199–209, 2011 21565591

Tassano F: The Power of Life or Death: Medical Coercion and the Euthanasia Debate. Oxford, UK, Oxford Forum, 1999

Uchino BN: Social support and health: a review of physiological processes potentially underlying links to disease outcomes. J Behav Med 29(4):377–387, 2006 16758315

Vahia IV, Depp CA, Palmer BW, et al: Correlates of spirituality in older women. Aging Ment Health 15(1):97–102, 2011 20924814

Vaillant GE: Positive mental health: is there a cross-cultural definition? World Psychiatry 11(2):93–99, 2012 22654934

Suggested Cross-References

Social factors are discussed in Chapter 3 ("Resilience and Posttraumatic Growth"), Chapter 4 ("Positive Social Psychiatry"), Chapter 5 ("Recovery in Mental Illnesses"), Chapter 11 ("Preventive Interventions"), and Chapter 12 ("Integrating Positive Psychiatry Into Clinical Practice"). Culture is discussed in Chapter 15 ("Positive Geriatric and Cultural Psychiatry").

Suggested Readings

Gordon J-S: Bioethics. Internet Encyclopedia of Philosophy: A Peer Reviewed Academic Resource. Available at: http://www.iep.utm.edu/bioethic/. Accessed August 27, 2014.

Jeste DV: APA President Dilip Jeste, MD, explains positive psychiatry—video interview. Available at: http://www.psychcongress.com/video/breaking-news-apa-president-dilip-jeste-md-explains-positive-psychiatry-video-interview-11554. Accessed August 27, 2014.

Marcum JA: Philosophy of Medicine. Internet Encyclopedia of Philosophy: A Peer Reviewed Academic Resource. Available at: http://www.iep.utm.edu/medicine/#H3. Accessed August 27, 2014.

Seligman MEP: APA 1998 Annual Report. The President's Address. Positive Psychology Center. Available at: http://www.ppc.sas.upenn.edu/aparep98.htm. Accessed August 27, 2014.

Wikipedia: Bioethics. Available at: http://en.wikipedia.org/wiki/Bioethics. Accessed August 27, 2014.

Index

*Page numbers printed in **boldface** type refer to tables or figures.*

mHealth. *See* Mobile health
MHRM. *See* Mental Health Recovery
    Measure
Mild cognitive impairment (MCI), 197
Mind-body medicine, **196,** 199–204
Mind-body techniques, 9, **196,** 199
Mindfulness, 229
    biomarkers associated with, 277
    conscientiousness and, 37
    positive child psychiatry and, 292
Mindfulness-based cognitive-behavioral
    therapy (MBCT), 247–248
Mindful physical exercise, 199, 206
Minnesota Multiphasic Personality
    Inventory, 113
Misery, xvii
MMRS. *See* Multidimensional Measure-
    ment of Religiousness/Spirituality
Mobile health (mHealth), 120–121, 122,
    122
Morality, 329–330
Mothers and Babies Internet Project, 231
Mother Theresa, 57
MRI. *See* Functional magnetic resonance
    imaging
MRT. *See* Master Resilience Training
    Course
Multidimensional Measurement of Reli-
    giousness/Spirituality (MMRS), 38
Music, positive child psychiatry and, 292
MyPlate, 288

Narcissism, coping and, 62
Narcotics Anonymous, 105
National Alliance on Mental Illness, 105
National Health Interview Survey, 194
Nature, 247
NDA-PAE. *See* Neurobehavioral disor-
    der associated with prenatal alcohol
    exposure
Negative emotions, adaptive, 55–56
Neurobehavioral disorder associated
    with prenatal alcohol exposure
    (NDA-PAE), 222–223
Neurobiology, positive psychology and, 6

Neurocircuitry
    brain regions in, 267, **268–269,** 271
    positive psychiatry and, 262–273
NFP. *See* Nurse-Family Partnership
Nicomachean Ethics, 83
Nonmaleficence, 328, 344
Norepinephrine, 277
    personal mastery and, 26
Nottingham Health Profile, 113
Nurse-Family Partnership (NFP),
    224–225
Nutrition, 10, 232, 247
    positive child psychiatry and, 288

Omega-3 fatty acids, 195, 197, 214
Opti-Brain Center, 265
Optimism, 2, 6, 19–43, **242, 268,**
    331–332,
    in aging adults, 309
    biomarkers associated with, 276–277
    clinical implications and interven-
        tions, 21–22
    clinical vignette of, 332
    description of, 20
    positive psychiatry and, 265–266
    relationship between health and, 21

Pain, positive psychological interven-
    tions for, 159–161
PANAS. *See* Positive and Negative Affect
    Schedule
Paré, Ambroise, 67
Parenting. *See also* Family-based services
    parental mental health, 290–291
    programs, 225
    techniques for improving alliance in
        discussions of, **297**
Pastoral care, 203–204
Patient-centered outcomes research
    (PCOR), 112
Patient-Centered Outcomes Research
    Institute (PCORI), 112
Patient-Reported Outcome Measure-
    ment Information System
    (PROMIS), 115